Mind, Brain, Body, and Behavior

Biomedical and Health Research

Volume 62

ISSN 0929-6743

Mind, Brain, Body, and Behavior

Foundations of Neuroscience and Behavioral Research
at the National Institutes of Health

Ingrid G. Farreras   EDITOR-IN-CHIEF

Caroline Hannaway   EDITOR

Victoria A. Harden   EDITOR

2004

IOS
Press
Amsterdam • Berlin • Oxford • Tokyo • Washington, D.C.

ISBN 1-58603-471-5
Library of Congress Control Number: 2004113434

Publisher
IOS Press
Nieuwe Hemweg 6B
1013 BG Amsterdam
The Netherlands
fax: +31 20 620 3419
e-mail: order@iospress.nl

Distributor in the UK and Ireland
IOS Press/Lavis Marketing
73 Lime Walk
Headington
Oxford OX3 7AD
England
fax: +44 1865 750079

Distributor in the USA and Canada
IOS Press, Inc.
4502 Rachael Manor Drive
Fairfax, VA 22032
USA
fax: +1 703 323 3668
e-mail: iosbooks@iospress.com

Contents

Part III: Scientists' First-Person Accounts

Directors' Foreword

To appreciate the groundbreaking discoveries we have made in recent years in the field of neuroscience–from the mapping of human disease genes to sophisticated imaging studies of the brain and insightful investigations of cognition and behavior–we must first understand the context of what came before, in the last half century. Fifty years ago we had only just discovered the structure of DNA. Now we can analyze the expression of thousands of genes in an afternoon.

Our forebears laid the vital groundwork needed to make progress against neurological and mental disorders. A large portion of that foundation was built in the intramural laboratories at the National Institutes of Health (NIH)–by the pioneering scientists who founded and staffed the National Institute of Mental Health (NIMH) and the National Institute of Neurological Diseases and Blindness (NINDB, predecessor of the National Institute of Neurological Disorders and Stroke).

We now have powerful tools and methods at our disposal thanks to the efforts of these early neuroscientists, who fueled the engine of discovery and changed the nature of the scientific questions that can be asked today. Without them, we would not have the remarkable breakthroughs in genomics, imaging, and many other areas that help us bring novel treatments to the millions of Americans who so desperately need them.

The two institutes were joined early, almost from the inception of the NIH. Formerly the PHS's Division of Mental Hygiene, the NIMH was established as part of the NIH in 1949. Congress established the NINDB in 1950, but without the funds it needed, at first, to establish its own research program. The first director of the NINDB had to rely on the generosity of the first director of the NIMH, and its scientific director–Seymour S. Kety. Kety hired researchers for both institutes on the basis of their skills and put them to work in laboratories that were set up to study basic mechanisms of brain function, rather than disease-specific investigations. The camaraderie and collegiality of the laboratories was palpable, according to those early researchers. The discoveries and advances that resulted were numerous.

In 1960, when more funding became available, the joint NIMH-NINDS basic research program was separated, and each developed its own intramural research program. With subsequent rapid advancements, the neurosciences have become more and more specialized, which has meant tremendous growth at the NIH. Neuroscience programs have spilled over the borders of its campus in Bethesda, with several satellite offices now scattered throughout the Bethesda/Rockville area.

Along with that growth has come a less connected, more fragmented scientific neuroscience community at the NIH, even though the most exciting discoveries of the last decade tell us that similar, and in some cases, the same biological mechanisms underlie both neurological and psychological disorders. For example, common mechanisms of nerve cell degeneration probably underlie Alzheimer's disease, vascular dementia, and the depression that follows stroke. Similar alterations in the mechanisms of the neurotransmitters serotonin and dopamine can cause thought disorders, such as schizophrenia, or movement disorders, such as Parkinson's disease.

To lead the re-integration of the neurosciences, and recapture the stimulating collaborative nature of the early laboratories, the NIH has created a National Neuroscience Research Center. This Center, located in the newly constructed John E. Porter Neuroscience Building on the Bethesda campus, will house physicians and scientists from the eleven different NIH institutes involved in neuroscience research, grouped according to their research interests rather than their institute affiliation.

This bold initiative will increase the pace of discovery in all areas of neuroscience. Thus, we hope to continue the longstanding tradition of the NIH as the crucible for many of the most exciting discoveries in the neurosciences. Trends in research may come and go, but there has always been unwavering support at the NIH for the intramural programs, and its researchers–who make up the nation's largest and most outstanding concentration of neuroscientists.

Thomas I. Insel, Ph.D.
Director, NIMH

Story C. Landis, Ph.D.
Director, NINDS

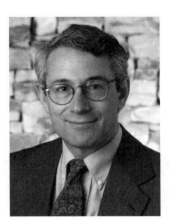
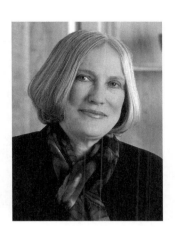

Historical Foreword

Often glorified and sometimes criticized, the National Institutes of Health (NIH) has nevertheless become one of the most important, if not the most important, biomedical research organizations in the world. Its intramural program has included scientists who have made major contributions; its extramural program has enabled universities and medical schools throughout the United States to build major research and training programs.

Although its origins date back to the late nineteenth century, the NIH began to take its modern shape shortly after the end of World War II. To be sure, the National Cancer Institute was created in 1937, but its budget remained relatively insignificant. During World War II, Surgeon General Thomas Parran, one of the most influential figures to occupy that office, undertook a campaign to expand the Public Health Service's authority to award grants to investigate a variety of diseases. Shortly thereafter he succeeded in assuming responsibility for research contracts awarded by the Committee on Medical Research of the Office of Scientific Research and Development. These wartime research contracts became the foundation for the phenomenal expansion of the NIH extramural research program. After 1945 the NIH began to grow rapidly. With each passing year, fiscal appropriations increased at an exponential rate.

Slowly but surely the number of institutes also began to proliferate. The passage of the National Mental Health Act in 1946 was but a beginning. It not only provided for the establishment of the National Mental Health Advisory Council and the National Institute of Mental Health (NIMH), but also contributed to the creation of a biomedical lobby that included Mary Lasker, Florence Mahoney, Representative John Fogarty, and Senator Lister Hill. In succeeding decades these and other figures played significant parts in expanding the role of the NIH. In 1949 the NIMH came into existence, followed by the National Institute of Neurological Diseases and Blindness (NINDB) in the following year.

In the immediate postwar years there was little to suggest that the NIH would replace philanthropic foundations as the primary source of research and training funding. To be sure, the act of 1946 gave the National Mental Health Advisory Council the function of recommending grants and the NIMH to create an intramural research program. Nevertheless, Robert H. Felix, the head of the NIMH from 1949 to 1964, proved to be one of the most adroit federal administrators of his generation. He developed close relationships with key congressional figures, and reinforced the growing belief that medical science had the ability to uncover the etiology of diseases and to develop effective therapies. In this sense he mirrored, or helped to shape, the growing public faith in the ability of science, medicine, and technology to create a better world.

Despite the importance of the NIH, its history has been neglected. Admittedly, policy studies allude to its role. This is particularly true for the NIMH, largely because the voluminous records pertaining to its policy role and extramural program have been retained. Little attention, however, has been given to the intramural research program, if only because relatively few primary sources have survived. This volume seeks to fill the historical void. The first two parts of the book, written by Dr. Ingrid Farreras, provide descriptive accounts of the NIMH and the NINDB intramural programs and their laboratories and branches during the 1950s, including their research activities. The third part of the book includes the recollections of some of the prominent individuals who were associated with these intramural programs in the 1950s. Their recollections help to compensate for the paucity of primary source materials.

The NIMH and the NINDB brought together biomedical and social scientists who played important roles in shaping their disciplines and raising novel questions. By this time the boundary lines between psychiatry and neurology had begun to sharpen. Before World War II, by contrast, these lines were blurred. Both specialties, for example, claimed jurisdiction over many disorders. Indeed, in the 1920s some individuals began to identify themselves as neuropsychiatrists. After World War II, the two specialties began to grow apart. Psychiatry emphasized psychodynamic and psychoanalytic approaches; neurologists were preoccupied with somatic concerns. Nevertheless, the individuals associated with the intramural programs of the NIMH and the NINDB were rarely in conflict, and many worked on common problems.

This volume provides insights not only into their work, but the relationship between institutional and governmental structures and the manner in which they influenced the direction taken by individual scientists. Neither biomedical nor social science research, after all, occurs in a vacuum. The nature of the questions asked and the subjects that are selected to be investigated often reflect broader scientific, intellectual, and political currents. The recollections of the individuals in the intramural program juxtaposed alongside whatever primary sources have survived also provide an equally fascinating contrast. To what extent are individual researchers aware that the choices they make are related to broader social and environmental factors? And what is the relationship between history and memory?

Can the study of history provide us with a narrative that offers policy guidance? The answer to this ostensibly simple question is extraordinarily complex. History, to be sure, does not offer concrete lessons. Nevertheless, it suggests broad themes that are useful to keep in mind when considering policy decisions. In addition, it helps to develop an awareness of the complexities and ambiguities inherent in all scientific research. This volume can serve not only as an important stimulus to further research dealing with the evolution of the NIH intramural programs, but also provides a perspective that can illuminate contemporary policy debates about the nature and direction of biomedical and social science research as well as the relationships between government and science.

Gerald N. Grob, Ph.D.
Henry E. Sigerist Professor of the History of Medicine Emeritus
Rutgers University, New Brunswick, NJ

Preface

The initial idea for this book emerged as the Office of NIH History was organizing a symposium on the research conducted in the 1950s by the National Institute of Mental Health (NIMH) and the National Institute of Neurological Diseases and Blindness (NINDB, today the National Institute of Neurological Disorders and Stroke) during the first decade of their existence. The goal of the symposium was to capture as many first-person accounts of the 1950s as possible from scientists from both institutes and to have these individuals document, first, their personal recollections of the broad scientific ideas and debates of the time; second, the organizational structures at the NIH that supported or hindered research; and third, the factors that caused lines of research to move from one direction to another.

Although the book was originally conceived as a volume of proceedings, the organizers soon realized that the twelve symposium speakers' chapters would benefit from being placed in a broader context. The historical literature on the intramural programs of the NIMH and the NINDB is very limited. What was needed was a detailed description documenting the history of the institutes and situating for readers the individuals, events, and research referred to by the scientists.

This volume will then provide two different but complementary perspectives, i.e., a historical one and a scientific one. The two will offer different kinds of analysis; each approach asking different questions, employing different methods, and relying on different sources of evidence. The historical portion attempts to portray the institutional context in which the scientific research was conducted. The chapters by individual scientists offer their perspectives on the research in which they participated at these two institutes during the 1950s.

It is a pity that, partly because of the large amount of funding devoted to the extramural program as compared to the intramural program, so little is known of the history of the NIH intramural programs in neurology and mental health. The intramural programs have been very influential over the years and are fertile ground for historical research in the biomedical sciences. However, the scant published literature and archival material available have meant that historians and other scholars have not easily been able to devote themselves to a detailed investigation. The history that can be written depends on the records that are kept and the resources at hand. In this book, for instance, the NIMH intramural program can be discussed more fully than that of the NINDB because more records and scientists from that program are available. The hope is that the publication of a volume such as this will spur scientists and administrators from both institutes to collect, preserve, and donate their archival materials to the Office of NIH History and the National Library of Medicine. The book also aims to serve as a catalyst for new areas of descriptive and analytical research by historians and other scholars of biomedical science.

Part I of this volume begins with a history of the establishment of the United States Public Health Service (PHS) and how its Division of Mental Hygiene was the precursor of today's NIMH. An overview of the national mental health program, with a discussion of the National Mental Health Act and the establishment of the National Mental Health Advisory Council, leads to an organizational description of the institute, including both its extramural and intramural programs. A similar history of the establishment of the NINDB is introduced and tied to that of the NIMH. The two institutes shared a joint intramural basic research program throughout the 1950s. This was created by the first director of basic research, Seymour S. Kety. In 1956, Kety stepped down and Robert B. Livingston took his place. Short segments describe the programs that Livingston developed or encouraged. A concluding section discusses the transition between Livingston and his successor, John C. Eberhart. The first part of the book ends with descriptions of the other components of the intramural programs of these institutes; namely, the separate NIMH and NINDB clinical research programs.

Part II of this volume presents succinct reviews of the research conducted by the fifteen laboratories and branches of the NIMH and the NINDB intramural basic and clinical research programs. These reviews include available photographs of 1950s scientists and the names of the laboratory, branch, and section chiefs. A list of all of the laboratory and branch members identified can be found in the appendices.

Following this historical background, Part III provides twelve varied recollections of scientists and administrators who were at the two institutes during the 1950s. The current director and former scientific director of the NINDB also offers her view of how that original 1950s research has changed over the course of time.

The volume has four appendices. Appendix A is an organizational chart of both institutes, highlighting the joint basic research program of the institutes and the individual clinical programs. Appendix B presents lists of all of the members of each laboratory and branch at the NIMH and the NINDB during the 1950s. Appendix C provides citations of landmark papers published by some of the laboratories and branches (whenever they were provided by individual scientists) resulting from the 1950s research (up to a 1965 publication date). Appendix D provides a list of selected primary and secondary sources related to the history of both of these institutes.

The editors would like to acknowledge a number of individuals and organizations whose assistance made this book possible. The initial idea for this book emerged from a symposium on research at the NIMH and the NINDB in the 1950s that was co-sponsored by the NIMH, the NINDS, and the Office of NIH History. The two institutes' generous financial support of the symposium, the production of this volume, and the Editor-in-Chief's DeWitt Stetten, Jr., Memorial Fellowship was indispensable. The symposium's Scientific Advisory Committee, consisting of Drs. Mortimer Mishkin, Roscoe O. Brady, and Allan F. Mirsky, was invaluable in assisting us in locating many of the 1950s scientists and shaping the symposium's program.

Drs. Mishkin, Brady, Robert A. Cohen, Cosimo Ajmone-Marsan, Philip G. Nelson, S. Harvey Mudd, and Richard A. Littman were most generous with their time and expertise in commenting on drafts of the scientific portions of this book. Drs. Cohen, Mishkin, Ajmone-Marsan, Littman, James E. Birren, Melvin L. Kohn, Detlev Ploog, Sid Gilman, and Morris B. Parloff, were most responsive to on-going queries we had throughout the project.

We would like to thank Drs. Gerald N. Grob, Thomas I. Insel, Story C. Landis, Robert Desimone, and the twelve scientists for their contributions. We are also grateful to Jan Lazarus and Belle Waring, History of Medicine Division, National Library of Medicine, Jules Asher at the NIMH, and Pamela Jones at the NINDS for providing us with most of the photographs in this volume. Special thanks go to Brooke Fox, Office of NIH History archivist, for her assistance locating archival materials and scanning, labeling, and organizing the photographs obtained. Pamela Jones at the NINDS and Richard Pine at the NIMH, were very helpful providing us with information on the history of their institutes' budgets. Marilyn Farreras and Vassilios Karapanos combed through 14 volumes of *Annual Reports* of the two institutes in order to compile the names of all of the NIMH and NINDB 1950s scientists appearing in Appendix B. Buhm Soon Park and Sarah Leavitt, Office of NIH History, provided archival and technical assistance.

We would also like to thank the many NIMH and NINDB scientists from the 1950s who, since the symposium in April 2003, have generously donated to the Office of NIH History short memoirs, write-ups, photographs, reprints, curriculum vitae, and correspondence. It is from materials such as these that more detailed and analytical histories can be written. We encourage other scientists to donate as well.

Dr. Robert A. Cohen was the most ardent supporter of this book. As the remaining administrator from that time period, he spent an inordinate amount of time locating information for us, explaining things that were unclear or missing from our materials, and providing us with answers to questions no one else could answer. The Editor-in-Chief would like to dedicate this book to him.

Ingrid G. Farreras, Ph.D., Caroline Hannaway, Ph.D.,
and Victoria A. Harden, Ph.D.
Office of NIH History, Bethesda, MD

Contributors

Cosimo Ajmone-Marsan, M.D., was Professor Emeritus and Director of the Electroencephalography Laboratory in the Department of Neurology at the University of Miami School of Medicine, until his retirement in 1997. He came to the NINDB from the Montreal Neurological Institute in January of 1954 as Chief of the Electroencephalography and Clinical Neurophysiology Branch. He remained with the NINDB until 1979 when he left for the University of Miami.

James E. Birren, Ph.D., has just retired as Associate Director of the UCLA Center on Aging in Los Angeles, California. He joined the Public Health Service in 1947, after serving during World War II at the U. S. Naval Medical Research Institute. He was assigned to the program on aging of the National Heart Institute but in 1950 transferred to the NIMH and in 1953 joined the newly formed Laboratory of Psychology as Chief of the Section on Aging in the basic research program. In 1963, he transferred to the National Institute of Child Health and Human Development to head its program on aging. In 1965, he moved to the University of Southern California to develop the Gerontology Center.

Robert A. Cohen, M.D., Ph.D., retired from the NIH in 1981, where he had served as Deputy Director of NIMH Intramural Research since 1968. He was Director of Clinical Research at the NIMH from 1952-1968 and subsequently Director of the Division of Clinical and Behavioral Research. He was in active duty in the Medical Corps of the U.S. Naval Reserve during World War II, was a consultant in psychiatry at the National Naval Medical Center and a member of the Panel on Human Relations and Morale of the Department of Defense from 1946 to 1952. He was Associate Physician and Clinical Director at Chestnut Lodge Hospital before coming to the NIH in 1952.

Joel Elkes, M.D., is Professor Emeritus at the Johns Hopkins University, the University of Louisville, and McMaster University in Hamilton, Ontario. He came to the NIMH in 1957 to found the Clinical Neuro-pharmacology Research Center at St. Elizabeths Hospital in Washington, D.C., and, in 1963, moved on to the Johns Hopkins University where he served as Henry Phipps Professor and Director of the Department of Psychiatry and Behavioral Sciences until 1975. His work has contributed to the founding of the new science of psychopharmacology, a science dealing with the play of chemical influences on mental life, and the place of drugs in the management and treatment of mental illness.

Ingrid G. Farreras, Ph.D., is Assistant Professor of Psychology at Hood College in Frederick, Maryland. She has also been a DeWitt Stetten, Jr., Memorial Fellow in the History of Biomedical Sciences and Technology at the Office of NIH History since 2001. Her research interests include the efforts to professionalize the field of clinical psychology during the first half of the twentieth century and the history of David Shakow's NIMH Laboratory of Psychology. She has a chapter in the forthcoming book by Wade E. Pickren and Stanley F. Schneider (Eds.): *Psychology and the National Institute of Mental Health: A Historical Analysis of Science, Practice, and Policy* (Washington, D. C.: American Psychological Association Press.)

Sid Gilman, M.D., is the William J. Herdman Professor and Chair of the Department of Neurology at the University of Michigan Medical School, where he has been since 1977. He is also Director of the University of Michigan Alzheimer's Disease Research Center. He is a member of the Institute of Medicine of the National Academy of Sciences and a past President of the American Neurological Association. He has also held faculty and hospital appointments at Harvard Medical School and Columbia Presbyterian Medical Center. His research is in vestibular and cerebellar physiology and in the pathophysiological processes underlying the cerebellar ataxias, Parkinson's disease, the parkinsonian syndromes and Alzheimer's disease. He serves on numerous journal editorial boards and has published over 400 scientific papers, book chapters, and abstracts, including several co-authored or edited books.

Lloyd Guth, M.D., is a Visiting Researcher at the Reeve-Irvine Research Institute at the University of California at Irvine School of Medicine since 2000. He enlisted in the Public Health Service and was appointed to the Section on Development and Regeneration of the Laboratory of Neuroanatomical Sciences at the NINDB in 1954. In 1961, he was promoted to Section Chief of Experimental Neurology and developed a new program in which he investigated trophic functions of the nervous system. In 1975, he accepted an academic appointment at the University of Maryland School of Medicine where he continued research on trophic influences of nerve on muscle and initiated a new program on spinal cord injury. In 1990, he joined the faculty at the Department of Biology at the College of William and Mary.

David A. Hamburg, M.D., is President Emeritus of the Carnegie Corporation of New York, having been President from 1983 to 1997. He came to the NIH as Chief of the Adult Psychiatry Branch in 1958. He left in 1961 and went on to Stanford University where he served as Professor and Chair of the Department of Psychiatry and Behavioral Sciences and Reed-Hodgson Professor of Human Biology. He then served as President of the Institute of Medicine of the National Academy of Sciences, Director of the Division of Health Policy Research and Education and John D. MacArthur Professor of Health Policy at Harvard University. His research interests have included behavioral, endocrine, and genetic factors in response to stressful experience; factors influencing healthy adolescent development; and various aspects of human aggression, conflict resolution, and violence prevention. He is the author or editor of several books and has served on policy advisory boards, including the President's Committee of Advisors on Science and Technology for the White House. He has received several awards and honors, including the Presidential Medal of Freedom.

Caroline Hannaway, Ph.D., is a Historical Consultant. She was a faculty member at the Johns Hopkins Institute of the History of Medicine and edited the *Bulletin of the History of Medicine* for eleven years. She directed the Francis C. Wood Institute for the History of Medicine of the College of Physicians of Philadelphia (1990-1992). Her research interest in eighteenth- and nineteenth-century French medicine is longstanding, and she co-edited with Ann La Berge the volume, *Constructing Paris Medicine* (1998). Her research in twentieth-century American medicine has included analyzing, with Victoria Harden, the National Institutes of Health response to AIDS and the development of cochlear implants. She has co-edited with Victoria Harden and John Parascandola, *AIDS and the Public Debate: Historical and Contemporary Issues* (1995).

Victoria A. Harden, Ph.D., is Director of the Office of NIH History and the Stetten Museum, a post she has held since the office was created in 1986. In 1992, she oversaw the establishment of the DeWitt Stetten, Jr., Fellowship in the History of Biomedical Sciences and Technology, designed to bring scholars in the humanities and social sciences to the NIH to study aspects of its history. Dr. Harden is the author of *Inventing the NIH: Federal Biomedical Research Policy, 1887-1937* and *Rocky Mountain Spotted Fever: History of a Twentieth-Century Disease*. She is the editor, with Harriet R. Greenwald, of *NIAID Intramural Contributions, 1887-1987*; with Guenter Risse, of *AIDS and the Historian*; and with Caroline Hannaway and John Parascandola, of *AIDS and the Public Debate: Historical and Contemporary Perspectives*.

Melvin L. Kohn, Ph.D., did research in the NIMH's Laboratory of Socio-Environmental Studies from 1952 to 1985, serving as Chief of that Laboratory from 1960 until he left the NIMH to become Professor of Sociology at the Johns Hopkins University. His research is in the field of social structure and personality. His work is cross-national, comparing the United States to Poland and Japan. He has published several books and numerous journal articles, including many in languages other than English. He is a past President of the American Sociological Association and a Fellow of the American Academy of Arts and Sciences. His international work has included serving as a member of the Scientific Advisory Board of the Max-Planck Institute für Bildungsforschung in Berlin, the U.S.-U.S.S.R. Commission on the Humanities and Social Services of the American Academy of Learned Societies, and the Soviet Academy of Sciences.

Irwin J. Kopin, M.D., is currently Scientist Emeritus in the Section on Clinical Neurocardiology of the NINDS. He began his NIH career as a Research Associate in the Laboratory of Clinical Science at the NIMH in 1957, went on to head the Section on Medicine in this Laboratory and then became Laboratory Chief. In 1983, he became NINDS Scientific Director, a post he held for more than a decade. He also headed the Clinical Neuroscience Branch for several years. He has served on numerous committees, won several medals and awards, participated in many scientific advisory boards and professional societies, and served as co-editor or editorial board member for more than 20 scientific journals. He has authored or co-authored more than 700 articles, reviews, and book chapters that together constitute a major part of current scientific knowledge about catecholamines.

Guy McKhann, M.D., is Professor of Neurology and Neuroscience and founding Director of the Zanvyl Krieger Mind/Brain Institute at the Johns Hopkins University. Previously, he served as the Associate Director for Clinical Research and Acting Clinical Director at the NINDS. His research has included work on multiple sclerosis, Alzheimer's disease, and, most recently, the neurological and cognitive outcomes in people following coronary bypass surgery. He has authored, edited, or co-authored over 200 publications including a neurology textbook and a book about aging and the brain for the general public. He has served as an advisor in many settings, from the Vatican to the public television station WETA on issues relating to the brain. He is a past President of the American Neurological Association and serves on many other advisory committees and boards.

Richard L. Sidman, M.D., is currently Professor Emeritus of Harvard Medical School and a member of the Department of Neurology of the Beth Israel Deaconess Medical Center in Boston. He came to the NIH in 1956 and spent two years as a Senior Assistant Surgeon in the Laboratory of Neuroanatomical Sciences at the NINDB. He left to go to Harvard Medical School where he was appointed Bullard Professor of Neuropathology in 1968 and reached emeritus status in 1999. A member of the National Academy of Sciences and a Fellow of the American

Academy of Arts and Sciences, he has published four books and more than 200 scientific papers on neuroanatomy, neuropathology, and neurogenetics. His main contributions have been as a pioneer in working out modern concepts on patterns of cell genesis and cell migration in the developing mammalian brain and in using genetic disorders in mice to analyze diseases causing malformations, premature neuronal death, and disorders of myelination. His current work is in the use of neural stem cells.

Donald B. Tower, M.D., Ph.D., came to the NINDB in 1953 as Chief of the Section on Clinical Neurochemistry, and moved on to be Chief of the Laboratory of Neurochemistry. He was Acting Associate Director for Extramural Programs in 1967 and 1968 and became the NINDS Acting Director in 1973 and Director in 1974. During his tenure as Director, until 1981, the institute was renamed the National Institute of Neurological and Communicative Disorders and Stroke. He is a pioneer in brain chemistry and investigated the biochemistry of the epileptic focus in excised brain tissue.

Abbreviations

AHAP
Shakow Papers
Archives of the History of American
Psychology
University of Akron
(Akron, OH)

NARA
National Archives and Records
Administration
(College Park, MD)

NIH Report
National Institutes of Health
Reports for fiscal years, 1950-51,
and 1951-52
(Bethesda, MD)

NIMH Annual Report
National Institute of Mental Health
Annual Report
(Bethesda, MD)

NINDB Annual Report
National Institute of Neurological
Diseases and Blindness Annual Report
(Bethesda, MD)

NLM
Modern Manuscripts Collection
History of Medicine Division
National Library of Medicine
(Bethesda, MD)

ONH
Office of NIH History
National Institutes of Health
(Bethesda, MD)

I

Historical Background

Ingrid G. Farreras

Mind, Brain, Body and Behavior
I. G. Farreras, C. Hannaway, and V. A. Harden (Eds.)
IOS Press, 2004

Establishment of the National Institute of Mental Health

Historical Background to the National Mental Health Program

The United States Marine Hospital Service (forerunner of the United States Public Health Service [PHS]) was established on July 16, 1798, when Congress passed an act that would allow for the creation and payment of hospitals that would care for sick and injured or disabled Merchant Marines in exchange for a 20-cent monthly deduction from each sailor's or marine's pay.[1] The Service was reorganized in 1870 with a Surgeon General based in Washington, D.C., overseeing its administration. During the late 1800s, the PHS's services were expanded to include the medical inspection of immigrants to the United States.[2] This included screening for mental illness, drug addiction, and alcoholism to avoid admitting immigrants who might become a "public charge."[3] In order to be free from any political pressure, however, the Commissioned Corps–consisting of physicians, dentists, engineers, and pharmacists–was established in 1889 to administer the national health program.[4]

On January 19, 1929, Congress enacted Public Law 70-672,[5] which authorized establishing two federal "narcotic farms for the confinement and treatment of persons addicted to the use of habit-forming narcotic drugs."[6] The first narcotic farm was not opened until May 29, 1935, in Lexington, Kentucky,[7] and the second on November 8, 1939, near Fort Worth, Texas. Both were intended exclusively for the treatment of addicted patients–mostly inmates transferred from Federal prisons–who had committed offenses, as well as a few who voluntarily sought treatment. By 1942, however, the farms began admitting mentally ill patients so as to alleviate the patient load of St. Elizabeths Hospital in Washington, D.C.[8]

The 1929 Act also established the Narcotics Division within the PHS. It was to serve four purposes: 1) administering the two narcotic farms; 2) studying drug addiction and its best treatment and rehabilitation; 3) disseminating information on this research and treatment; and 4) providing states with advice on the care, treatment and rehabilitation of addicts.[9] The following year, on June 14, 1930, Public Law 71-357[10] moved the Narcotics Division to the Division of Mental Hygiene and the functions of the new division, headed by physician Walter L. Treadway, were enlarged to include: 1) providing medical and psychiatric care in federal penal and correctional institutions; and 2) studying the "etiology, prevalence, and means for the prevention and treatment of mental and nervous diseases."[11]

Apart from the two narcotic farms, the PHS's Division of Mental Hygiene was quite small, but it nonetheless followed a set of principles that would lead to a national mental health program: the recognition and treatment of the mentally ill; the investigation of the nature and etiology of mental disorders; the training of personnel to work in the field of mental hygiene; the development of measures to reduce mental illness; the search for solutions to the economic problems resulting from mental illness; and the uncovering of the community sources of mental illness.[12]

World War II (WWII), however, interrupted the development of such a national mental health program. The PHS ceased to advise the states, the Fort Worth narcotic farm began accepting mentally ill patients from the armed services, and the large number of war discharges and casualties demonstrated "the tremendous toll mental illness took on the national welfare."[13] Mental illness filled more hospital beds than any other cause: treatment was lengthy; prognoses were pessimistic; and relapse rates were high.[14] By August 1945, 1.8 million men had been rejected for service for neuropsychiatric reasons, by far the largest cause for rejection. Combined with mental and educational deficiencies, this meant that 4.8 million, or 32 percent of the 15 million American men who had been examined for duty by December 1944, were found to be unfit for service.[15] Of those who had been inducted but subsequently discharged, 40 percent were for neuropsychiatric reasons. Following the war, 25 percent of general hospital beds and 10 percent of psychiatric hospital beds were filled by neurologically disabled veterans, and by

April 1946, 44,000 of 74,000 (60 percent) Veterans Administration (VA) hospital beds were filled with neuropsychiatric patients alone, costing at least $40,000 per bed.[16]

Eight million Americans–or 6 percent of the American population at the time–were also found to be suffering from some mental disorder and the economic consequences of this were profound. Professional personnel to treat these patients, however, was seriously lacking. There were only 3,500 psychiatrists nationwide at the beginning of the war and the shortages of trained personnel in two other related mental health fields–psychologists and psychiatric social workers–were very large.[17] Knowledge of and research on the etiology, treatment, and prevention of mental illness were also significantly lacking.[18] Toward the end of the war, this lack of personnel, knowledge, understanding, and treatments led to a new national awareness of mental illness, of its problems, its costs, and the need for effective intervention.[19]

The National Mental Health Act

The Superintendent of the Division of Mental Hygiene, physician Lawrence Kolb, had pursued the idea of establishing a research center–similar to the existing National Cancer Institute (NCI)–that would focus on mental illness.[20] When he retired in 1944, he was followed by physician Robert Hanna Felix, who combined his background in epidemiology, community-based mental health training, and public health to draft a bill for a National Neuropsychiatric Institute.

Felix expanded Kolb's ideas to include a training and service component.[21] By February 1945, Mary Switzer, special assistant to Watson Miller, the administrator of the Federal Security Agency, and Felix had visited Gladys Harrison and Sidney Saperstein in the General Counsel's Office. The two worked with them in drafting the bill in very broad language. Felix and Switzer were then introduced to Congressman J. Percy Priest (R) of Tennessee, Chairman of the Labor and Public Welfare Committee, who introduced Felix's bill into Congress in March 1945.[22]

The bill was to focus on three things: research, training, and community services. Toward these three goals, the bill sought an appropriation of $10 million as well as an additional $4.5 million for the creation of a National Neuropsychiatric Institute and a National Mental Health

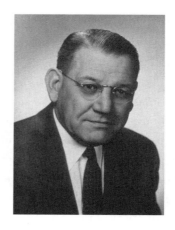

Robert H. Felix, M.D.
*Courtesy of the National Library
of Medicine*

Advisory Council. The Neuropsychiatric Institute would conduct, as well as help fund, research on the etiology, prevention, diagnosis, and treatment of mental illness. The program would also fund the training of mental health professionals through individual fellowships, institutional grants, and state aid. Finally, the bill would help expand existing community mental health services and establish additional clinics and treatment centers.[23] These goals raised a number of concerns, ranging from criticisms and fears of legislating socialized medicine to those of overburdening the federal budget and of federal interference with state social welfare programs.[24]

President Harry S. Truman signed the bill, Public Law 79-487,[25] on July 3, 1946, but the bill's name was changed from the National Neuropsychiatric Institute Act to the National Mental Health Act.[26] The new name had been a matter of contention. Following World War II, mental, rather than neurological, problems were at the forefront of the nation's attention. The psychiatric establishment, because of its prevalent psychoanalytic emphasis, leaned toward mental health rather than neurology. Thomas Parran, the Surgeon General, leaned strongly toward the label of neuropsychiatry due to its scientific connotations. The powerful American Medical Association, however, opposed what it saw as a first step toward socialized medicine.[27] Winfred Overholser, the Superintendent of St. Elizabeths Hospital, who unsuccessfully pushed for the institute to be a part of St. Elizabeths, believed the proposed term, neuropsychiatric, was too narrow. Karl Bowman, president of the

American Psychiatric Association, believed it was not appropriate and suggested the new agency be named the National Psychiatric Institute. John C. Whithorne, the first representative of the American Psychiatric Association on the National Research Council, urged the use of the term "mental health" "to emphasize the aim toward which many different disciplines might contribute."[28]

The proposed institute's name was changed to the National Institute of Mental Health (NIMH), to reflect a broad and optimistic mission of promoting mental health and combating mental illness.[29] This contrasted with the missions of the other NIH institutes, the NCI or the National Heart Institute (NHI), for example, which focused on disease conditions.

The National Mental Health Advisory Council

The NIMH's authorization for construction and equipment of hospitals and laboratory facilities was increased to $7.5 million but because the Act's programs did not require that they be conducted at the NIMH, no money was appropriated by Congress for the operation of the NIMH.[30] Only the Greentree Foundation, a small organization from New York, provided Felix with $15,000. Felix used this money to finance the first two National Mental Health Advisory Council (NMHAC) meetings on August 15-16, 1946, and January 1947. The NMHAC was charged with implementing the Act's goals and looking out for the public's interest, from reviewing research and training grant applications to advising the Surgeon General on all PHS programs involving mental health.[31] It originally consisted solely of six experts whom Felix himself recommended to the Surgeon General.[32] Felix described the first selection as follows:

> I proposed a list to [Surgeon General Dr. Thomas] Parran....Some of those people were picked for political or pay-off reasons....the law said that 2 could be chosen for 3 years, 2 for 2 years, and 2 for 1 year, so we were to draw the names out of a hat. So we put a name in a hat and drew it out and that way we got what we wanted....Frank [F.] Tallman and George [S.] Stevenson....were chosen for 1 year. George Stevenson...was a pay-off to the National Committee for Mental Hygiene....Frank Tallman...was a pay-off to the

Congressman of Ohio, Brown [who had helped get the bill through]....[David M.] Levy,...[Edward A.] Strecker,... [William C.] Menninger,...and [John] Romano...were not chosen for any pay-off purposes. These were all strong men.[33]

By December 1950, the Council would come to consist of twelve members–six experts on mental illness and six lay members–who review-ed research and training proposals and then made recommendations to the Surgeon General.

Organization of the National Institute of Mental Health

The PHS's Division of Mental Hygiene administered the Act's program until it was formally established as one of the National Institutes of Health (NIH).[34] The Act's first appropriation was passed in 1947 for the 1948 fiscal year and when the NIMH became an official institute of the NIH on April 15, 1949, it took over the division's functions as ad-ministrator of the National Mental Health Act program, marking the beginning of the federal government's large-scale support of research in mental health.[35]

This did not come about easily. In the beginning, the research appropriations were minimal–the first appropriation consisted of about $400,000–and the National Institute of "Head Feelers" was small and non-threatening.[36] Increasingly larger appropriations, however, translated into the PHS appointing a First Reorganization Committee that planned to reorganize and dismember the new NIMH in order to partake of the newly acquired riches.[37] These parties wanted to place the research component within the NIH, the training component partly within the NIH as well as within the Office of Education (in the Bureau of State Services), the community services component within the Bureau of State Services, and the two narcotic hospitals within the Division of Hospitals of the Bureau of Medical Services.[38]

Felix, however, believed that the national mental health program would be destroyed if the Act's three components were torn apart; its strength lay in its being a solid, integrated program under one person's direction. As a result, he approached the director of the NIH, Rolla Eugene Dyer, and asked for the NIMH to become one of the NIH

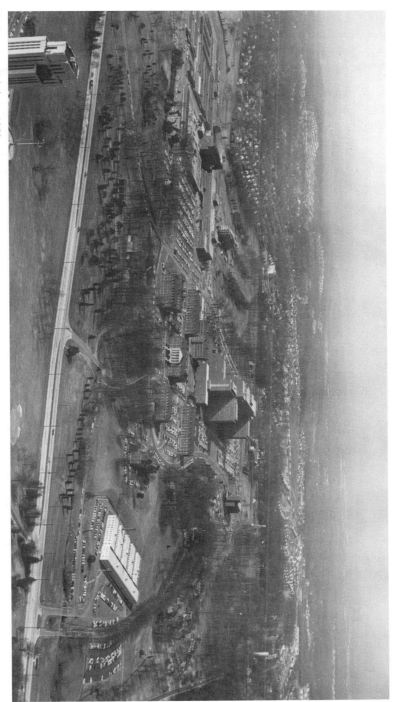

NIH Campus aerial photo, 1960
Courtesy of the Office of NIH History

institutes. Dyer objected to the training and community services components which Felix wanted to bring on board but he finally agreed, in exchange for the transfer of the Lexington and Fort Worth narcotic farms to the Division of Hospitals within the Bureau of Medical Services.[39]

When the NIMH became one of the institutes of the NIH, the PHS Division of Mental Hygiene was abolished. Given the lack of knowledge at the time about the etiology, prevention, and treatment of mental illness, the NIMH readily decided that it would support and fund research in any field related to mental illness. Such a broad mission was important; the NIMH did not share the prestige of the other NIH institutes at the time. In Felix's words:

> This wasn't the most friendly climate....I got nothing but misunderstanding....We weren't respectable. Clinical research in psychiatry wasn't even research. There wasn't any basic research going on. We weren't doing any physiology, or chemistry and so forth. All we did was listen to people talk and then draw hypotheses and say that they were facts. We were sloppy in the way we did things. You could see the hostility, and you could see the fear of us. These guys were a little nervous about these psychiatrists. As one guy told me one time..."I don't like to sit in a Directors' staff meeting with you because I think all the time you're trying to psych me [out], and I'm on my guard from the minute I walk in the room, until you walk out. I don't like you around."[40]

Felix and the NMHAC thus decided that mental health research would never be targeted research. As Felix said, "[W]e would never say, 'We want to do research in so and so,' but rather this would be free research in order that we could sift and mine the largest amount of dirt, to see where there was pay."[41]

In addition to research focusing on mental illness, the NIMH was unique in that it incorporated a social mission—including training and services in addition to research. It also went beyond basic and clinical biomedical research to include and support behavioral and social science research.[42] The NIMH's operating programs consisted of four principal branches: a Community Services Branch (consultant services to states);

a Training and Standards Branch (training grants and stipends); a Research Grants and Fellowships Branch (non-federal research); and an Office of the Scientific Director (intramural research).[43] The first three branches comprised the extramural program of the institute. Tables 1 and 2 indicate the funding allocated to each program and the distribution of funding within the intramural research program:

Table 1. NIMH Funding History–Appropriations
(in thousands of dollars)

	Research			Training			Community Mental Health Program	Research Management and Support	NIMH Total
	Extramural	Intramural	Total	Clinical	Research	Total			
1948	$473	$102	$575	$1,107	$277	$1,384	$4,025	$267	$6,251
1949	716	137	853	1,336	334	1,670	5,806	152	8,481
1950	1,203	265	1,468	3,182	796	3,978	5,698	193	11,337
1951	794	524	1,318	1,605	401	2,006	5,787	252	9,363
1952	1,629	757	2,386	3,018	755	3,773	3,403	251	9,813
1953	1,828	1,016	2,844	3,206	801	4,007	3,396	227	10,474
1954	2,834	1,599	4,433	3,572	893	4,465	2,657	186	11,741
1955	3,869	2,715	6,584	3,664	916	4,580	2,648	218	14,030
1956	4,364	3,489	7,853	5,289	1,322	6,611	3,219	275	17,958
1957	8,123	4,826	12,949	9,811	2,453	12,264	4,653	140	30,006
1958	13,367	5,692	19,059	11,386	2,846	14,232	4,993	173	38,457
1959	18,092	6,386	24,478	15,898	3,974	19,872	5,167	336	49,853
1960	24,916	7,024	31,940	23,095	5,774	28,869	6,300	361	67,470

Source: Compiled from NIMH data

Table 2. NIMH Intramural Funding History–By Priority
(in thousands of dollars)

	Basic Brain	Schizophrenia	Depression	Aging	Child	Anxiety	Behavioral Medicine	Other	Total
1948	$ 35	$ 0	$ 0	$ 0	$ 0	$ 0	$ 0	$ 67	$ 102
1949	37	0	0	0	0	0	0	100	137
1950	100	0	0	0	0	0	0	165	265
1951	367	0	0	0	0	0	0	157	524
1952	592	0	0	0	0	0	0	165	757
1953	298	110	153	66	110	33	66	180	1,016
1954	565	170	238	102	170	51	102	201	1,599
1955	1,113	281	394	169	281	84	169	224	2,715
1956	1,439	367	514	220	367	110	220	252	3,489
1957	2,039	505	707	303	505	152	303	312	4,826
1958	2,300	595	832	357	595	178	357	478	5,692
1959	2,559	699	978	419	699	210	419	403	6,386
1960	3,011	721	1,009	432	721	216	432	482	7,024

Source: Compiled from NIMH data

NIMH Extramural Program

The Community Services Branch, headed by James V. Lowry, surveyed regional mental health resources, needs, and problems and provided grants-in-aid and other assistance to help states develop and strengthen their mental health programs. The Training and Standards Branch, headed by Seymour D. Vestermark, provided grants to individuals and institutions for training in mental health and to "increase the supply of psychiatrists, psychologists, psychiatric nurses, and psychiatric social workers."[44] The Research Grants and Fellowships Branch was headed by Lawrence Coleman Kolb, son of Lawrence Kolb, until 1949. Psychologist John C. Eberhart succeeded him and the branch provided fellowships and grants to individuals and institutions throughout the country conducting research on mental and neurological disorders.

The four key disciplines in mental health, psychiatry, psychology, social work, and psychiatric nursing, were represented and developed at the new institute. A 1952 analysis of the first five years of the NIMH research grant program reveals that over $5 million were spent on 165 projects focusing on "the etiology of mental illness, development or evaluation of treatment methods, normal child development, studies of the nervous system, and the relation of environmental stress to mental health and illness."[45] Sixty-four percent of all of the applications were submitted by psychiatrists and psychologists, who received 70 percent of all of the funds. Although medical schools carried out most of the nation's health and medical research at that time, they only received 11 percent of the funds directed toward mental health research. Forty-three percent of all of the applications were submitted by colleges and universities, receiving 52 percent of the funds.[46]

Psychiatry, however, clearly took the lion's share of the funding available from the NIMH extramural program. Although the Training and Standards Branch tried to bring in all four disciplines, the NMHAC and the Training and Standards Branch committee needed a mechanism that would decide how to distribute the funds. Because the psychiatrist was seen as "a very key person in the mental health program [without whom there] probably couldn't be much of a program" and because of psychiatrists' higher salaries vis-à-vis those of the other disciplines, a

"40-20-20-20" formula was developed whereby psychiatry would obtain 40 percent of the funds and psychology, social work, and psychiatric nursing 20 percent each.[47] One of Felix's oral histories pointedly describes this mechanism:

> I am so ashamed of this that I hoped to forget it. This is part of the old power struggle....[The Training and Standards Branch was] having a lot of good applications coming in and some of the very best applications coming in were from psycholog[ists], who are natural born grant writers, grantsmen and also statisticians....Some of the prettiest applications we ever got....Well, some of the people began to get nervous ...because...one year, for instance, they took them right as they came down the line. Sixty or seventy percent of the money would have gone to psychology. Because they were ready and the rest weren't and so this was bitterly protested that you couldn't do anything without psychiatrists. They were captain[s] of the team, everybody else followed them and here are these others getting out of line and there would be rebellion in the ranks. So the council passed a resolution that...under the law you can't make a grant unless approved by council....Therefore, council set as its policy that they would not approve grants other than in the proportion of 40 for psychiatry, 20 for each of the other three and there was nothing left for anybody else. There was a lot of screaming...In those days there was one psychologist on the council and some laymen, who were mostly psychiatry oriented....I was opposed to it but it was obvious that it was not going to get anywhere. And that 40-20-20-20 stayed in for several years.[48]

NIMH Intramural Program

The Office of the Scientific Director was involved in the intramural research conducted at the institute's own laboratories, the NIH Clinical Center, and in the field (at the Addiction Research Center at the Lexington narcotic farm and in Hagerstown, Maryland).[49] The intramural research program's mission was broad and multidisciplinary:

> ...lacking definite clues to the etiology or best methods of treatment of mental illness, it is wisest to support the best research in any and all fields related to mental illness, whether clinical or non-clinical, basic or applied, empirical, methodological, or theoretical, in the medical, biological, social, or behavioral sciences.[50]

Three smaller staff branches that reported to the Office of the Director also existed: a Biometrics Branch, a Publications and Reports Branch, and a Professional Services Branch. The Biometrics Branch, headed by Morton Kramer, compiled, analyzed, and evaluated statistical data on the national incidence and prevalence of mental illness, acted as a consultant to outside agencies, and obtained a census of patients in mental institutions. The Publications and Reports Branch, under Albert S. Altman, produced and disseminated scientific and technical information in pamphlets, articles, films, posters, and other materials for professional and lay education. The Professional Services Branch, headed by Dale Cameron until 1950, when Joseph Bobbitt succeeded him, consisted of advisors to the institute director on the long-range planning of the national mental health program, formulating objectives and assessing program progress and effectiveness.[51]

The NIMH's philosophy in the 1950s, whether in the extramural or intramural programs, was that the government should provide individuals and institutes with the maximum amount of freedom and not hamper their progress by directing or regimenting their activities.[52] In Felix's words:

> I never, ever would tolerate controlling research or education. I felt that if we compromised the freedom of intellectual thought, the freedom of research, if we compromised academic freedom, we [would have] compromised more than we would ever gain back if we found the answer to schizophrenia tomorrow. The minds have to be free.[53]

Notes

1. Federal Security Agency, "PHS-SG History of the Public Health Service, Ch. 1, p. 1," Folder: Organization of the PHS (History), Box 4: 1939-1973, WW Entry 2: Organizational Management 1937-1973, RG 90, NARA; Ralph Chester Williams, *The United States Public Health Service, 1798-1950* (Washington, D.C.: Commissioned Officers Association of the United States Public Health Service, 1951); Bess Furman, *A Profile of the United States Public Health Service, 1798-1948* (Washington, D.C.: U.S. Department of Health, Education, and Welfare, 1973); Fitzhugh Mullan, *Plagues and Politics: The Story of the United States Public Health Service* (New York: Basic Books, 1989).

2. See Alan Kraut, *The Huddled Masses: The Immigrant in American Society, 1880-1921* (Arlington Heights, IL: Harlan Davison, 2001) and Alan Kraut, *Silent Travelers: Germs, Genes, and the "Immigrant Menace"* (New York: Basic Books, 1994).

3. John Parascandola, "Background Report on the Organizational History of Mental Health and Substance Abuse Programs in the PHS," (Public Health Service, September 1993), unpublished manuscript, 2; Mullan, *Plagues and Politics.*

4. Federal Security Agency, "PHS, What is the PHS? October 1945," Folder: Historical Chronology in the Origin of the PHS and HSMHA, Box 5: 1955-1973, WW Entry 2: Organizational Management 1937-1973, RG 90, NARA. A Public Health Service Act signed by President Franklin D. Roosevelt on July 3, 1944, allowed scientists and nurses also to be commissioned. For a history of the Commissioned Corps, see Williams, *USPHS*, Mullan, *Plagues and Politics*, and Furman, *Profile of the PHS.*

5. 45 Stat. L. 1085.

6. Jeanne L. Brand, "Antecedents of the NIMH in the Public Health Service," in *An Historical Perspective on the National Institute of Mental Health (Prepared as sec. 1 of the NIMH Report to the Wooldridge Committee of the President's Scientific Advisory Committee) Mimeograph*, eds. Jeanne L. Brand and Philip Sapir (February 1964), 5; Parascandola, "Background Report," 6. These farms were planned and designed largely by Lawrence Kolb, Superintendent of the Division of Mental Hygiene from 1938 to 1944. *Mental Health Challenges: Past and Future. Proceedings of a Conference on the Twenty-Fifth Anniversary of the National Mental Health Act. June 28 and 29, 1971* (Washington, D.C., 1971); Caroline J. Acker, *Creating the American Junkie: Addiction Research in the Classic Era of Narcotic Control* (Baltimore, MD: Johns Hopkins University Press, 2002); Furman, *Profile of the PHS*; Williams, *USPHS*, 51-52, 335.

7. This later became the Addiction Research Center within the NIMH's intramural basic research program.

8. For a history of St. Elizabeths Hospital, see Frank Rives Millikan, *Wards of the Nation: The Making of St. Elizabeths Hospital, 1852-1920* (Washington, D.C., 1989) and Frank Clark, *St. Elizabeths Hospital for the Insane* (Washington, D.C., 1906). See also: St. Elizabeths Hospital Medical Society, *Proceedings of the Annual Meetings* (Washington, D.C.); St. Elizabeths Hospital, *Clinics and Collected Papers of St. Elizabeths Hospital* (St. Louis); and Arcangelo R. T. D'Amore and A. Louise Eckburg, *Symposium on William Alanson White: The Washington Years 1903-1937* (St. Elizabeths Hospital, Washington, D.C.: U.S. Dept. of Health, Education and Welfare, Publication No. (ADM) 76-298, 1976).

9. Federal Security Agency, Public Health Service, National Institutes of Health, National Institute of Mental Health, The Organization and Functions of the National Institute of Mental Health, August 15, 1950, Organization 1950, Box 1, "1935," Historical Development of NIMH, RG 511, NARA, hereafter cited as NIMH Organization-1950, Box 1); Parascandola, "Background Report."

10. 46 Stat. L. 585.

11. *Mental Health Challenges*, 4.

12. Brand "Antecedents of the NIMH;" Williams, *USPHS*.

13. Brand "Antecedents of the NIMH," 7.

14. Edward D. Berkowitz and Susan LaMountain, "Organizational Change at the National Institutes of Health: Historical Case Studies, National Institute of Mental Health," (Prepared at the request of the Institute of Medicine, National Academy of Sciences, January 13, 1984), unpublished paper, 2.

15. Brand "Antecedents of the NIMH;" Robert A. Cohen, "Studies on the Etiology of Schizophrenia," in *NIH: An Account of Research in its Laboratories and Clinics*, eds. DeWitt Stetten, Jr., and W. T. Carrigan (New York: Academic Press, 1984), 13-34; Lewis P. Rowland, *NINDS at 50: An Incomplete History Celebrating the Fiftieth Anniversary of the National Institute of Neurological Disorders and Stroke* (Bethesda, MD: National Institutes of Health, Publication No. 01-4161, 2001).

16. James G. Miller, "Clinical Psychology in the Veterans Administration," *American Psychologist* 1 (1946): 181-9.

17. Berkowitz and LaMountain, "Organizational Change at the NIH."

18. Brand "Antecedents of the NIMH."

19. Meredith P. Crawford, "Rapid Growth and Change at the American Psychological Association: 1945-1970," in *The American Psychological Association: A Historical Perspective*, eds. Rand B. Evans, Virginia Staudt Sexton, and Thomas C. Cadwallader (Washington, D.C.: American Psychological Association, 1992).

20. Kolb had succeeded Treadway in 1938.

21. Dale Cameron, oral history interview by Eli Rubinstein, 1978, transcript, NIMH Oral History Collection, 1975-1978, OH 144, NLM.

22. Robert Felix, oral history interview by Eli Rubinstein, May 27-28, 1975, transcript, NIMH Oral History Collection, 1975-1978, OH 144, NLM; Robert Felix, oral history interview by George Rosen, February 8, 1963, transcript, Folder Felix, Box 1, MSC 203, NLM. Mary Lasker, a wealthy New York entrepreneur married to millionaire Albert Lasker, and Senator Claude Pepper, who "had sponsored bills that created five of the first six disease-oriented institutes," were also influential in pushing for NIH legislation (Rowland, *NINDS at 50*, 6).

23. Jeanne L. Brand, "The National Mental Health Act of 1946: A Retrospect," *Bulletin of the History of Medicine* 39, no. 3 (1965): 231-45; NIMH Organization-1950, Box 1.

24. Berkowitz and LaMountain, "Organizational Change at the NIH."

25. 60 Stat. L. 421.

26. Felix, oral history by Rubinstein; Gerald N. Grob, *From Asylum to Community: Mental Health Policy in Modern America* (Princeton, NJ: Princeton University Press, 1991).

27. Robert Felix, oral history interview by Milton J. E. Senn, March 8, 1979, transcript, Folder Felix, Box 2, OH 76, NLM.

28. *Mental Health Challenges*, 27. Robert Felix, oral history interview by Jeanne Brand, March 18, 1964, transcript, Folder Felix, Box 3, OH 149, NLM.

29. Felix, oral history by Rosen.

30. Brand, "National Mental Health Act."

31. *Mental Health Challenges.*

32. Felix, oral history by Rubinstein.

33. Ibid., 50-51. Consultants to the National Mental Health Advisory Council included S. Allen Challman, Frank Fremont-Smith (Josiah Macy, Jr., Foundation), Nolan D. C. Lewis, and William Malamud, as well as guests such as Daniel Blain (Veterans Administration), Joseph Bobbitt (PHS), Dale Cameron (PHS), Rolla E. Dyer, Sam Hamilton, Mary Lasker, Winfred Overholser, Mary Switzer, Dael Wolfle (American Psychological Association), and Ralph C. Williams.

34. In the late 1940s, the PHS consisted of three branches: the NIH, the Bureau of Medical Services, and the Bureau of State Services. The NIH was the research arm of the PHS.

35. *NIH Report, 1950-1951;* National Institute of Mental Health, *Research in the Service of Mental Health: Report of the Research Task Force of the National Institute of Mental Health* (Bethesda, MD: National Institutes of Health, Publication No. (ADM) 75-236, 1975).

36. Felix, oral history by Rosen.

37. Ibid.

38. Ibid.; Felix, oral history by Senn; Felix, oral history by Brand.

39. Felix, oral history by Senn; Felix, oral history by Rosen; Felix, oral history by Brand.

40. Felix, oral history by Rosen, 44-45.

41. Felix, oral history by Rosen, 41.
42. Berkowitz and LaMountain, "Organizational Change at the NIH;" Parascandola, "Background Report."
43. *NIH Report, 1950-1951*; NIMH Organization-1950, Box 1.
44. Ralph Simon and Beatrice Shriver, "The Training Branch Program," in *An Historical Perspective on the NIMH*, 51. Similar training stipends were available for graduate students entering the psychiatry, psychiatric social work, and psychiatric nursing tracks but the stipend amount awarded in clinical psychology, psychiatric social work, and psychiatric nursing tracks never exceeded two thirds of the stipend amount awarded to those in psychiatry. (Federal Security Agency, Public Health Service, Training and Research Opportunities Under the National Mental Health Act. Mental Health Series No. 2, June 1948, U.S. Govt. Printing Office: 1948-O-793902, Box 138, NIMH, 1930-1948 Individual Institutes (Organization File), Entry 2, RG 443, NARA).
45. Philip Sapir, Jeanne Brand, and Lorraine Torres, "The Research Grants and Fellowships Branch Program," in *An Historical Perspective on the NIMH*, 30.
46. Sapir, Brand, and Torres, "Research Grants and Fellowships."
47. Cameron, oral history by Rubinstein, 10.
48. Felix, oral history by Rubinstein, 187-8.
49. NIMH Organization-1950, Box 1. Although the farms had been transferred to the Division of Hospitals of the Bureau of Medical Services, the NIMH retained a research component within the Lexington farm.
50. Sapir, Brand, and Torres, "Research Grants and Fellowships," 27.
51. *NIH Report, 1950-1951*.
52. Brand, "Antecedents of the NIMH."
53. Felix, oral history by Senn, 26.

Establishment of the National Institute of Neurological Diseases and Blindness

The oldest neurological society in the world, the American Neurological Association (ANA), was founded in 1875 with a strong grounding in European neurology.[1] The term "neuropsychiatry" first originated in the late nineteenth century but was not extensively used in the United States until World War I, when the Division of Neurology and Psychiatry within the Army Surgeon General's Office was established in 1917.[2] Although it consisted mostly of psychiatrists, the division was directed by a neurologist and was strongly dominated by members of the ANA. At the time, psychiatrists were seen as experienced hospital administrators who treated psychoses but who had little training in organic diseases of the nervous system, while neurologists exhibited the opposite pattern.[3] Neither had much experience treating psychoneuroses and, as a result, both were united under the broad label of "neuropsychiatry" and provided with the supplementary training that each specialty group lacked to treat the most pressing problem at the time: war neuroses. The use of the term "neuropsychiatry" declined after the 1930s, however, and was not revived until World War II.

By WWII, clinical neurologists' lack of emphasis on treating organic, neurological diseases solidified their reputation as diagnosticians uninterested in neurological treatment. With the rise of psychiatry and its emphasis on mental disorders resulting from emotional tensions due to interpersonal, social, and cultural maladjustments, neurological perspectives were also increasingly seen as unnecessary and perhaps even detrimental.[4] During WWII, the administrative positions of all armed services' neuropsychiatric divisions were filled by psychiatrists, not neurologists, and by the close of the war "neuropsychiatry" had become practically synonymous with "psychiatry," with medical schools requiring psychiatric or neuropsychiatric divisions for national accreditation.[5] The encroachment of neurological surgery into medical neurology also threatened to diminish or extinguish neurologists' role in the field of psychoneuroses.[6]

In order to inform the VA's Department of Medicine and Surgery on the number of neurologists available to care for and rehabilitate disabled veterans, the American Board of Psychiatry and Neurology sent out a questionnaire in 1947 to 900 diplomates in neurology and neuropsychiatry. The results identified a paucity of trained neurologists (48 compared to 456 psychiatrists), with two thirds of the neurologists compared to one third of the psychiatrists most likely to be found in teaching institutions rather than in clinical or administrative positions.[7] Such a discrepancy was attributed to the subordination of neurology to psychiatry by various medical departments of the Army, Navy, and PHS during WWII. Following the war, government agencies adopted a policy that increased full-time physicians' salaries by 25 percent if they were American Board diplomates, leading to a rush in psychiatric certification.[8]

In an effort to revive the almost extinct neurological field, Abe B. Baker, chair of neurology and psychiatry at the University of Minnesota, and a cohort of about 50 "young Turks" founded the American Academy of Neurology (AAN) in 1948.[9] In contrast to the ANA, which had a very limited membership and a participation dominated by older, established members, the AAN proved to be a boost for the field.[10] It provided an opportunity for younger neurologists, including residents, to participate in a national neurological society; it set up committees that would advance neurological training and that would influence government officials with health programs; and it provided its members with affordable continuing education during its annual meetings.[11]

Without a national institute devoted to neurological disorders, however, neurological research could not flourish. Treatment was limited, knowledge was sparse, and there was a paucity of expert physicians.[12] Citizen groups, representing research and care in multiple sclerosis, cerebral palsy, muscular dystrophy, epilepsy, and blindness, pushed for the establishment and funding of institutes relating to the particular disease with which they were concerned, but their individual attempts failed to convey the significant public health and socioeconomic impact of these organic diseases of the nervous system as a whole.[13] Even within the neurological field, there was no consensus as regards the definition and classification of neurological medicine, whether it was a branch of internal medicine, an autonomous discipline, or a part of the dominant neuropsychiatric hegemony of the time.[14]

It was not until the late 1940s and early 1950s that these voluntary health organizations–with the help of prominent ANA members such as H. Houston Merritt, Tracy Putnam, Hans Reese, and William G. Lennox, who testified before Congress on their behalf–became powerful enough to influence legislators.[15] Congressmen Robert Crosser (D), Percy Priest (R), and Andrew Biemiller (D), however, proposed minimizing duplication by creating instead a national institute dedicated to researching the entire spectrum of neurological disabilities and blindness.[16] Although blindness supporters wanted their own institute, neurology and blindness were put together in response to political pressure: Mary Lasker, Congressman Biemiller, whose mother was blind, and Senator James Murray (D), pushed to introduce blindness into the bill.[17]

President Truman's administration had growing concerns about the proliferation of disease-focused institutes within the PHS, however.[18] Although encouraging the Surgeon General to coordinate research so as to discourage such proliferation, the research need and the popular support behind the bill led Truman to sign the Omnibus Medical Research Act (Public Law 81-692) on August 15, 1950, establishing the National Institute of Arthritis and Metabolic Diseases (NIAMD; today the National Institute of Arthritis and Musculoskeletal Diseases) and the National Institute of Neurological Disorders and Blindness (NINDB; today the National Institute of Neurological Diseases and Stroke). Both institutes were formally established on November 22 of that year.[19] The NINDB would be responsible for conducting and supporting research and training in the 200 neurological and sensory disorders that affected 20 million individuals in the United States and were "the first cause of permanent crippling and the third cause of death."[20]

The most disabling conditions for the largest number of people were cerebral palsy, epilepsy, multiple sclerosis, muscular dystrophy, cerebral vascular disease, and blinding diseases. The etiology of these conditions was little understood and their manifestations complex.[21] As a result, a three-pronged approach was adopted: 1) clinical and basic intramural research on the etiology of these disorders and approaches to medication and surgery for their alleviation; 2) intramural research on "the structure, biochemistry, and physiology of the nerve cells and fibers, the nutrition and metabolism of nervous tissue and the brain, and the sensorimotor functions of the nervous system;" and 3) extramural research grants, training grants, and fellowships aimed at the entire field of neurology and blindness.[22]

Like the NIMH, the NINDB had a National Advisory Council consisting of twelve members—six professionals and six lay members appointed by the Surgeon General for four-year terms—who approved and denied research and training applications and guided the institute's policy.[23] As with the NIMH, however, Congress did not appropriate funding for the new institute—not even to appoint an institute director—so the Advisory Council meetings, approved grants, and institute maintenance and upkeep fees were covered by the Office of the NIH Director.[24]

In the summer of 1951, the NINDB received its first annual budget of $1.23 million.[25] This budget, however, was part of the Office of the NIH Director's operating expenses and was not earmarked for the creation or support of new research projects. Rather, it covered transfers of existing research projects on neurological and sensory diseases that had until then been conducted within other institutes, such as the NIMH and the National Institute of Allergy and Infectious Diseases (NIAID), into the NINDB program.[26]

Only $40,000 of this budget was used to run the institute's administration and the intramural program, including the appointment of an institute director, Pearce Bailey, as well as a secretary and administrative officer.[27] Bailey was the son of like named Pearce Bailey, one of the founders of the New York Neurological Institute, who had been president of the ANA in 1913.

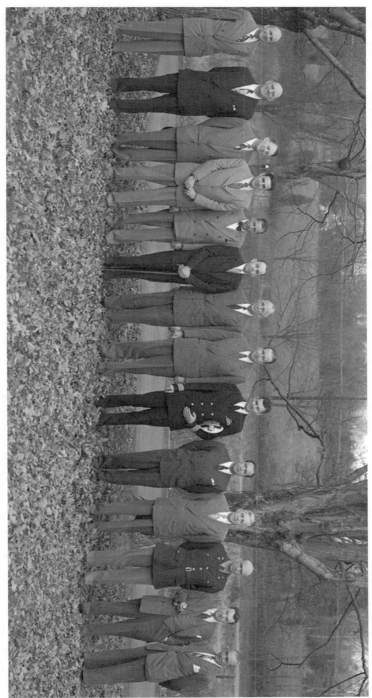

Pearce Bailey, M.D. (fifth from left) and the NINDB Council, 1950
Courtesy of the National Institute of Neurological Disorders and Stroke

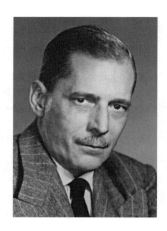

Pearce Bailey, M.D.
Courtesy of the National Institute of
Neurological Disorders and Stroke

Bailey, the son, was appointed the first director of the NINDB on October 3, 1951.[28] He had worked at the Philadelphia Naval Hospital after serving in the U.S. Navy and was at the time chief of the neurology program within the Neuropsychiatry Division, headed by psychiatrist Daniel Blain, of the VA's Department of Medicine and Surgery.[29] Bailey actively sought to "advance academic neurology through increasing facilities for training and research"[30] by creating a medical advisory committee selected by the ANA's council, and to explore ways in which "VA facilities could be supplemented to be of use to their training and research programs in neurology."[31]

An increase in the 1952 budget of the NINDB to $1.99 million still saw no money directed toward beginning any new research programs and, with the NIH Clinical Center still under construction, no laboratory or clinical space had been allocated to the NINDB either.[32] The research conducted by the institute was still supported by the NIMH and the institute's survival was unclear.[33] To address this situation, Bailey, who had been the AAN's second president in 1949-1950, appointed an AAN liaison committee to meet with the directors of voluntary health organizations and present a unified front to the Congressional appropriations committee. The National Committee for Research in Neurological Disorders (NCRND), headed by Baker, resulted from this July 25, 1952, meeting that was attended by the AAN liaison committee, also the ANA president, the organizations' directors, and the representatives of the National Society for Crippled Children and Adults.[34]

The NCRND soon presented Congress with an organized and cohesive approach to research on the broad range of neurological disabilities and the institute–like the NCI, the NHI, and the NIMH–obtained a separate line item budget and a 1953 Congressional appropriation of $4.5 million.[35] The NINDB was now able to fund its intramural program as well as its extramural research and training grants in neurology and ophthalmology.[36]

Organization of the National Institute of Neurological Diseases and Blindness

The NINDB's operating programs in the 1950s consisted of seven principal branches: an Extramural Program Branch, a Direct Training Branch, a Publications and Reports Branch, a Field Investigations and Pilot Projects Branch, a Biometrics Branch, an Epidemiology Branch, and an Intramural Research Program.

The Extramural Program Branch, headed by Gordon H. Seger, had four major objectives. The first involved providing research grants to non-governmental institutions that would conduct basic or clinical research on the brain and central nervous system that would contribute to the understanding, prevention, diagnosis, and treatment of neurological and sensory disorders.[37] The second would provide training grants to universities and medical centers in order to begin or increase their training programs in neurochemistry, neuropharmacology, neuroanatomy, neurophysiology, neuropathology, ophthalmology, otolaryngology, and sensory physiology, thereby increasing the number of qualified personnel capable of teaching or conducting research on neurological diseases and blindness.[38] The third would provide pre-doctoral, post-doctoral, and expert scientists who showed promise or expertise as researchers in neurology or ophthalmology, special research fellowships that would attract them to the field or increase their competence.[39] The last involved traineeships or training stipends awarded directly to physicians who sought advanced or special training in the diagnosis, treatment, and investigation of neurological and sensory disorders.[40] Although specific budget information is not available for every year of the first

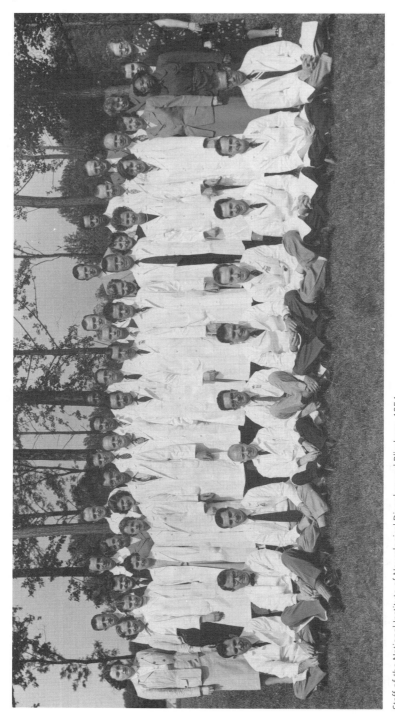

Staff of the National Institute of Neurological Disorders and Blindness, 1954
Donated to the Office of NIH History by Dr. Cosimo Ajmone-Marsan

decade, Table 3 illustrates the intramural and extramural funding allocated for 1956[11]:

Table 3. Intramural and Extramural Funding, 1956

	Intramural $2,329,000		Extramural $5,054,000	
			Research	
	Basic	Clinical	Grants	Training
	$654,150	$1,674,850	$3,900,000	$1,154,000
Neurologic Disorders	607,150	1,223,800	2,672,500	
Cerebral palsy & chronic cerebral disorders	145,000	178,000	606,000	
Epilepsy & other paroxysmal cerebral disorders	0	820,000	608,000	
Multiple sclerosis & demyelinating diseases	160,000	32,400	265,000	
Muscular dystrophy & neuromuscular disorders	177,000	149,000	262,000	
General metabolic & deficiency disorders of the nervous system	13,150	8,900	445,000	
Poliomyelitis & other infectious diseases of the nervous system	0	15,800	40,500	
Accident & injury to the nervous system	103,000	10,800	283,000	
Other nervous system disorders	9,000	8,900	163,000	
Sensory Disorders	47,000	451,050	1,227,500	
Hearing & balance	14,500	10,800	197,500	
Vision	18,500	425,000	832,500	
Cataract	0	58,300	52,500	
Glaucoma	0	46,700	144,000	
Retinopathy	0	18,300	160,000	
Retrolental fibroplasia	0	0	94,000	
Uveitis, keratitis, & other inflammatory & parasitic diseases	0	190,000	109,000	
Metabolic & degenerative diseases of the eye	0	38,200	226,000	
Strabismus & neuromuscular disorders	0	31,500	10,000	
Other ophthalmic disorders, including injuries	18,500	42,500	37,000	
Other Special Senses (taste, smell, touch, & pain)	14,000	14,750	197,500	
Training Grants				900,000
Research Fellowships				150,000
Training Stipends				104,000

Source: Compiled from *NINDB Annual Reports*

The Direct Training Branch arranged to provide training within the institute, particularly the training of younger institute scientists in particular skills needed for certain program operations.[42] In 1955 the Publications and Reports Branch was established to produce and disseminate to governmental, professional, and lay audiences scientific information pertaining to neurological and sensory disorders.[43]

The Field Investigations and Pilot Projects Branch was established in 1956. Its goal was to broaden the research program by supporting community surveys, epidemiological studies, and broad interdisciplinary and multi-institutional cooperative and collaborative studies and also to serve as the central, integrative biostatistical laboratory that would collect, correlate, and evaluate the data obtained by such studies and institutions.[44] Such a program was based on the success of earlier cooperative studies, such as the ones on retrolental fibroplasias that indicated a correlation between the administration of oxygen and the duration of the administration and blindness; kernicterus, identifying Rh factor blood incompatibilities that required multiple exchange blood transfusions; and on asparagines, found to treat successfully certain types of epilepsy.[45]

The branch's most important project was the National Collaborative Perinatal Project, involving over a dozen institutions, 150 scientists and physicians, 50,000 pregnancies, and the resulting children, who were followed up to the age of seven. This extramural and intramural joint endeavor was an attempt to collect data that would improve the classification, diagnosis, treatment, and prevention of neurological diseases, including cerebral palsy, mental retardation, epilepsy, speech defects, and reading and learning disabilities.[46]

The NINDB's Field Station of Perinatal Physiology in San Juan, Puerto Rico, was involved in a parallel study of the perinatal factors leading to cerebral palsy and mental retardation in free-ranging pregnant and infant macaque monkeys.[47]

The branch also oversaw other large scale cooperative projects on cerebrovascular diseases, specifically, intercranial aneurysms and acute subarachnoid hemorrhages (1,000 cases in 22 institutions); on the effectiveness of anticoagulants in the treatment of cerebrovascular diseases (600 cases in seven institutions); and on developing accurate screening techniques for the early diagnosis of glaucoma (four institutions).[48]

The Biometrics Branch was established in January 1957 to serve as "a focal statistical coordinating agency for the institute's collaborative field investigations and a consulting service for its intramural projects."[49] The Epidemiology Branch, closely related to the Biometrics Branch, collected and evaluated epidemiological data on selected neurological and sensory disorders.[50]

The Intramural Research Program consisted of a basic research and a clinical investigations program. The basic research program was a joint program with the NIMH basic research program and focused on the

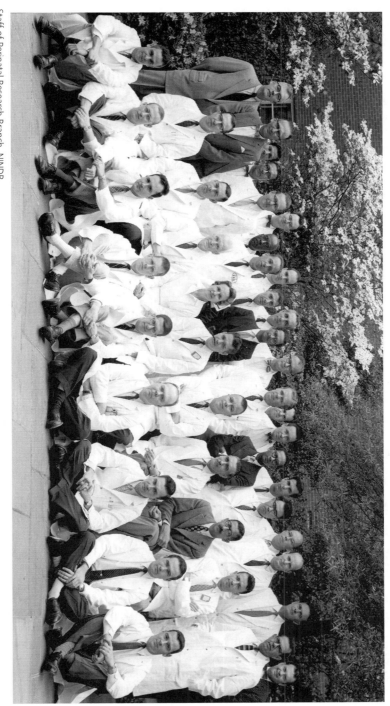

Staff of Perinatal Research Branch, NINDB
Donated to the Office of NIH History by Dr. Cosimo Ajmone-Marsan

fundamental study and understanding of the nervous system and its functions, such as the nature of the nerve impulse, the mechanism of synaptic transmission, complex lipids' routes of synthesis, and the processes of nerve regeneration.[51] Once the NIH Clinical Center opened in 1953, the clinical research program began its work on three major areas of study: epilepsy, muscle disorders, and eye diseases. Scientists of both programs collaborated not only with scientists within their own program but also with the other program, as well as with other institutes such as the NIMH, the NHI, the NCI, the NIAID, and the NIAMD, and with non-NIH institutions such as the Army and Navy Medical Centers, the Mount Alto VA Hospital, and the Physics Division of the Atomic Energy Commission.[52]

Notes

1. Pearce Bailey, "The Present Outlook for Neurology in the United States: A Factual Evaluation," *Journal of the Association of Medical Colleges* 24 (1949): 214-28. For further information on the history of neurology and of the Association, see Russell N. DeJong, *A History of American Neurology* (New York: Raven Press, 1982); William F. Windle, ed., "The Beginning of Experimental Neurology," *Experimental Neurology* 51, no. 2 (1976): 277-80; D. Denny-Brown, Adolph L. Sahs, Augustus Steele Rose, eds., *Centennial Anniversary Volume of the American Neurological Association* (New York: Springer, 1975); Lawrence C. McHenry, "The Founding of the American Neurological Association and the Origin of American Neurology," *Annals of Neurology* 14, no. 1 (1983): 153-4.
2. Pearce Bailey, "National Institute of Neurological Diseases and Blindness: Origins, Founding, and Early Years (1950 to 1959)," in *The Nervous System: A Three-Volume Work Commemorating the 25th Anniversary of the National Institute of Neurological and Communicative Disorders and Stroke, Vol. 1: The Basic Neurosciences*, eds. Donald B. Tower and Roscoe O. Brady (New York: Raven Press, 1975), xxi-xxxii.
3. "[Neurology]…, with its patient population with chronic refractory diseases, its nearly nonexistent therapeutics, and its emphasis on anatomical diagnoses, almost immediately attacked asylum psychiatry for not curing the insane, for its unscientific therapies, and for an unproductive preoccupation with diagnostics. The neurologists, largely excluded from the asylums, maintained that they could treat the insane more effectively as outpatients and that hospitalization, as suggested and practiced by asylum psychiatrists, was both unnecessary and destructive." See Jacques M. Quen, "Asylum Psychiatry, Neurology, Social Work, and Mental Hygiene–An Exploratory Study in

Interprofessional History," *Journal of the History of the Behavioral Sciences* 13, no. 1 (1977): 5.

4. Bailey, "The Present Outlook for Neurology."
5. For further information, see Gerald N. Grob, "The Inner World of American Psychiatry, 1890-1940," *Journal of the History of the Behavioral Sciences* 24, no. 3 (1988): 263-4 and Quen, "Asylum Psychiatry, Neurology, Social Work, and Mental Hygiene."
6. Bailey, "Origins, Founding, and Early Years."
7. Bailey, "The Present Outlook for Neurology."
8. Ibid.
9. Pearce Bailey, "American's First National Neurologic Institute," *Neurology (Minneap.)* 3 (1953): 321; Pearce Bailey, oral history interview by Wyndham D. Miles, October 7, 1964, transcript, Box 1, OH 149, NLM.
10. Bailey, oral history by Miles.
11. Ibid; Bailey, "Origins, Founding, and Early Years."
12. Rowland, *NINDS at 50.*
13. Bailey, "Origins, Founding, and Early Years;" Bailey, oral history by Miles.
14. Bailey, "Origins, Founding, and Early Years."
15. Ibid; Rowland, *NINDS at 50.*
16. Rowland, *NINDS at 50.*
17. William Henry Sebrell, oral history interview by Siepert and Carrigan, December 8-9, 1970, transcript, Box 1, OH 88, NLM; Rowland, *NINDS at 50.*
18. Rowland, *NINDS at 50.*
19. *NIH Almanac, 1965*; Rowland, *NINDS at 50.*
20. *NIH Report, 1951-1952*, 189.
21. *NINDB Annual Report, 1954.*
22. *NINDB Annual Report, 1954*, 1-2.
23. Bailey, "Origins, Founding, and Early Years."
24. Ibid. NIAMD received $578,000 that first year (Rowland, *NINDS at 50*).
25. *NIH Almanac, 1965.*
26. Bailey, oral history by Miles.
27. Ibid.
28. Bailey, "Origins, Founding, and Early Years."
29. Ibid; Rowland, *NINDS at 50.* In 1947, neurology's exposure and reputation was enhanced with the VA Neuropsychiatry Division's name change to Psychiatry and Neurology Service (Bailey, "Origins, Founding, and Early Years.").
30. Bailey, "Origins, Founding, and Early Years," xxiii.
31. Ibid.
32. Bailey, oral history by Miles.
33. Bailey, "Origins, Founding, and Early Years."

34. Ibid.
35. Ibid; Bailey, oral history by Miles.
36. Bailey, "Origins, Founding, and Early Years."
37. *NINDB Annual Reports, 1954* and *1955.*
38. *NINDB Annual Reports, 1954, 1956,* and *1957.* Funding information is available in the *NINDB Annual Reports*, including for clinical and pediatric neurology in the late 1950s.
39. *NINDB Annual Reports, 1954* and *1957.*
40. *NINDB Annual Reports, 1954-1957.*
41. For specific funding information on the individual extramural components, see the *NINDB Annual Reports.*
42. *NINDB Annual Report, 1960.*
43. *NINDB Annual Report, 1955.*
44. *NINDB Annual Reports, 1956* and *1957.*
45. *NINDB Annual Report, 1954.*
46. *NINDB Annual Reports, 1957* and *1960*; J. Rosser Matthews, "A Fishing Expedition: Administrative Debates about the Collaborative Perinatal Project," (paper presented at the Annual Meeting of the American Association for the History of Medicine, Kansas City, Missouri, April 26, 2002). This would eventually become its own Perinatal Research Branch.
47. *NINDB Annual Reports, 1956* and *1957.*
48. *NINDB Annual Reports, 1956, 1958,* and *1959.*
49. *NINDB Annual Report, 1957,* 2.
50. *NINDB Annual Report, 1957.*
51. *NINDB Annual Report, 1959.*
52. *NINDB Annual Report, 1957.*

Joint NIMH-NINDB Intramural Basic Research Program

Charged with creating an intramural research program, Felix was somewhat at a loss as to how to proceed. His own background included some neurophysiology but he realized he was not an expert and his career lay in administration, not science. After an unsuccessful search for three years for someone to head the program, Felix approached Norman Topping,[1] associate director of the NIH, for advice, hoping he might be able to suggest someone who had good credentials but was young enough to take a chance on becoming a scientific director.[2] Topping recommended Seymour S. Kety, a young professor in the Department of Physiology and Pharmacology at the University of Pennsylvania's Graduate School of Medicine.[3] In the summer of 1950, Felix visited Kety and discussed the plans for the program. At the end of the visit, Felix offered Kety the position of Associate Director in Charge of Research. When Kety queried him about his choice–a physiologist as opposed to a psychiatrist–Felix emphasized his preference for a scientist who would "ensure scientifically sound and rigorous research."[4]

Kety visited the Bethesda campus and saw the construction of the NIH Clinical Center already underway. He also conferred with the scientific directors of the NCI and the NHI–Harold Eagle and James Shannon, respectively–prior to making his decision. He was so impressed by Felix's tolerance of, and encouragement for, multidisciplinary research and the invaluable opportunity to direct what Felix called, "the greatest institution for the study of the brain and behavior that the world has ever seen," that he accepted the position and was appointed in May 1951.[5]

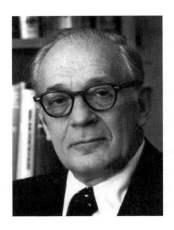

Seymour S. Kety, M.D.
*Courtesy of the National Academy
of Sciences*

At that time, the NINDB had recently been established, with Pearce Bailey as its first director. The Surgeon General had designated the NIMH to administer the NINDB's program. Felix had known Bailey from the VA and they quickly pooled their resources so that both institutes would have a large, joint basic research program under Kety's leadership. There were several reasons behind this tactical decision. It was difficult to separate basic research in neurological disease and mental illness at the time, and Kety believed that "progress in the diagnosis and treatment of nervous and mental diseases rest[ed] firmly upon a basic understanding of the [structure and function] of the nervous system through the biological and behavioral sciences."[6] His 1956 *Annual Report* highlighted this belief:

> There is a danger in the overemphasis of the purely biological aspects of illness, especially psychiatric illness… These illnesses represent an interaction between experiential and environmental factors upon a constitutional, biological substrate, and a research program which emphasizes one of these approaches to the detriment of the other is not likely fully to exploit the potentialities of science in the understanding of disease.[7]

Because of the difficulty, or impossibility, of predicting which basic research areas would yield information of greatest diagnostic or therapeutic value, Kety strongly advocated a well-balanced program that included representative research from all of the major scientific areas:[8]

> By drawing together outstanding representatives of all the relevant sciences, any new findings in one laboratory can be subjected to critical analyses by all of the other disciplines and immediate exploitation of its ramifications throughout as many different fields as possible.[9]

The institute directors also encouraged this deliberate effort to establish a combined, comprehensive basic research program, but they had more administrative reasons for such a merger, as is reflected in one of Felix's oral histories:

> We agreed that we could buy more by pooling our money than we could by each having our own intramural basic science program. There would be so much duplication we were sooner or later going to get in trouble. But I warned Pearce [Bailey] that if we did this we were going to have to be very careful to so mess up our money that nobody could find a line or cleavage or someday they would split us apart and this would be an economy move. We were so fantastically successful that we hardly knew in our own shop how to divide the money up and where it came from. Once the money was appropriated, we dumped it in and stirred it up real quick....The Bureau of the Budget time and again tried to do two things–which they never were able to do because we would always get all confused and mixed up and stupid; one was we couldn't tell them where a neurology dollar or a mental health dollar went. It just went into this program which was joint. The other [was] we could never break out research from clinical care. We were very careful that got so smeared up that we never were sure whether a dollar was

a research dollar or care dollar. Because we knew if we ever did, that [would be] the first step, then they would start directing as they are doing now. I was told by one of the people of the Bureau of the Budget that he suspected that we weren't as stupid as we appeared because if we were, we should be fired.[10]

While established and young scientists interested in research careers were delighted by Kety's appointment as the institutes' director of basic research, some psychiatrists expressed curiosity or concern, even urging him "not to drive another nail into the coffin of psychiatry."[11] Such concern, however, was misplaced, as Kety proved to be very open-minded in his approach. Given the nascent state of targeted mental illness and neurology research at the time, Kety opted for organizing the intramural research program along disciplinary, rather than disease-oriented, lines, stressing multidisciplinary cooperation between laboratories.[12] There were theoretical as well as pragmatic reasons for this approach. There were no empirically supported theories at the time concerning the etiology of most neurological and psychiatric disorders, and clinical research was mostly descriptive or anecdotal.[13] Kety also believed that by providing scientists with complete freedom to choose their own research problems, scientific discoveries were more likely to be made and young scientists would be more attracted to the program.[14]

As a result, Kety established a broad basic research program representing various disciplines. The joint intramural program centered around three kinds of research: biological, behavioral, and clinical. As Felix announced in 1954,

> Due attention is being given to keeping the broad areas of exploration–biological, behavioral, and medical–in balance. With the existing state of knowledge, we cannot afford to push one area at the expense of another. Today, most scientists are agreed that whether the primary causes of the various types of mental illness are found to be biological or psychological, there will be a close relationship between them, and treatment and prevention will need to proceed in both areas.[15]

By October 1952, Kety unveiled what he envisioned would become the NIMH-NINDB combined basic research program, consisting of the following nine laboratories (see Table 4):

Table 4. Kety's Original Concept for the Intramural Basic Research Program

Laboratory of Biophysics
> Section on Neural Transmission
> Section on Energetics
> Section on Vision and Special Senses

Laboratory of Biochemistry
> Section on Enzymology
> Section on Phosphorylation
> Section on Physical Chemistry
> Section on Endocrinology
> Section on Cerebral Metabolism

Laboratory of Neurophysiology
> Section on Cortex and Forebrain
> Section on Spinal Cord
> Section on Neuromuscular Physiology
> Section on Functional Integration

Laboratory of Pharmacology
> Section on Organic Synthesis
> Section on Cellular Pharmacology
> Section on Pharmacodynamics
> Section on Addicting Drugs

Laboratory of Anatomical Sciences
> Section on Cytoarchitecture
> Section on Functional Neuroanatomy
> Section on Developmental Neurology
> Section on Chemical Morphology

Laboratory of Experimental Neuropathology
> Section on Neuropathology
> Section on Quantitative Cytochemistry
> Section on Microbiology

Laboratory of Experimental Psychology
> Section on Aging
> Section on Animal Behavior
> Section on Human Behavior
> Section on Special Senses

Laboratory of Epidemiology
> Section on Genetics Section on Mental Disease
> Section on Neurological Disease

Laboratory of Socio-Environmental Studies
> Section on Community Studies
> Section on Family Studies
> Section on Special Studies

Source: Proposed Organization of Basic Research Program of NIMH and NINDB, August 29, 1952, RG 511, NARA

This program incorporated most of the eight already-existing sections: Developmental Neurology, Physical Chemistry, Neurophysiology, Spinal Cord Physiology, Technical Development, Aging, Drug Addiction, Endocrinology, and Socio-Environmental Studies.[16] Roger Sperry headed the Section on Developmental Neurology that was organized on September 1, 1952, at the University of Chicago while the Clinical Center on the NIH campus was being built. His section focused on the development of the nervous system, specifically, "the integrative principles operating and the respective roles of experience and maturation in the development of the visual system, and an assessment of the importance of the integument in the chemical specification of the cutaneous nerves during development."[17] Sperry's section was intended to be a section within the planned Laboratory of Anatomical Sciences[18] but he resigned to accept a position at the California Institute of Technology.[19]

The Section on Endocrinology involved Hudson Hoagland and Gregory Pincus in a collaborative project with the Worcester Foundation for Experimental Biology. Its most important contribution was the development and use of improved or new methods and techniques to determine urinary and blood steroids as well as adrenalin and noradrenalin in urine and blood.

Due to the deliberate attempt not to allocate the budget to the specific institutes or even laboratories within each institute–indeed because they also served the research interests of both institutes–the various sections of each laboratory were to be assigned to one or another institute. This assignment depended on the nature of the research conducted, which was expected to undergo revision depending on the future laboratory chiefs' appointments.[20]

Two of the proposed laboratories, the Laboratory of Neurophysiology and the Laboratory of Socio-Environmental Studies, were able to be established quickly because their chiefs had already been conducting research when the NIMH was still the PHS Division of Mental Hygiene. Physiologist Wade H. Marshall was in the Laboratory of Physical Biology within the Institute of Experimental Biology and Medicine, later absorbed by the NIAMD. When he joined the NIMH-NINDB intramural basic research program, his Laboratory of Neurophysiology became the first joint laboratory of the program. During the 1950s, it would come to have five sections, two of them within the NINDB and three within the NIMH: Spinal Cord Physiology (NINDB, Karl Frank, Chief), Special Senses (NINDB, Ichiji Tasaki, Chief), Cortical Integration (NIMH, John C. Lilly, Chief), Limbic Integration and Behavior (NIMH, Paul D. MacLean, Chief), and the Section of the Chief, under Marshall himself.[21] His laboratory focused on studying the function of the nervous system.

Sociologist John A. Clausen was a consultant in the Professional Services Branch when Kety established the intramural program. When he joined the program, the NIMH-supported Laboratory of Socio-Environmental Studies was created to study social norms and how social influences affect personality development, daily activities and relationships, and mentally ill individuals. His laboratory would come to consist of four sections during the 1950s, three in the basic research program and one in the clinical research program: Social Development and Family Studies (basic, Marian R. Yarrow, Chief), Community and Population Studies (basic, Melvin L. Kohn, Chief), Social Studies in Therapeutic Settings (clinical, Morris Rosenberg, Chief), and Clausen's own Section of the Chief.[22]

Alexander Rich was hired in August 1952 to head the NIMH-supported Section on Physical Chemistry of the second joint laboratory of the program, a Laboratory of Neurochemistry that studied the chemical structure and metabolism of the nervous system. Because the NIH Clinical Center was not yet built, his initial work was conducted at the Gates and Crellin Laboratory of the California Institute of Technology. Following the opening of the Clinical Center, Roscoe O. Brady joined the laboratory as the NINDB-supported chief of the Section on Lipid Chemistry. Kety was acting chief of this laboratory while he sought someone to head it and in doing so maintained a Section of the Chief for his own work.[23] When Rich left for MIT in 1958, he was succeeded by Sidney Bernhard. No official chief was found for this laboratory until the joint NIMH-NINDB intramural basic research program dissolved in 1960 and each institute created its own laboratory.

The remaining laboratories were established when the NIH Clinical Center opened on July 6, 1953, and as appointments were made.[24] Neuroembryologist William F. Windle arrived in January 1954 to head the Laboratory of Neuroanatomical Sciences supported by the NINDB.

Over the course of three years he created four sections and a field station that studied the structural and functional development and organization of the nervous system: Experimental Neuropathology (Jan H. W. Cammermeyer, Chief), Functional Neuroanatomy (Grant L. Rasmussen, Chief), Neurocytology (Sanford L. Palay, Chief), Field Station of Perinatal Physiology (in Puerto Rico), and his own Section on Development and Regeneration.[25]

Kenneth S. Cole's NINDB-supported Laboratory of Biophysics was established shortly afterwards, in early 1954. Research in this laboratory emphasized mathematical formulations that would predict the formation and behavior of nerve impulses under various conditions.[26]

The last laboratory to be established, in mid-1954, was the Laboratory of Cellular Pharmacology, under Giulio Cantoni. His two section chiefs–Seymour Kaufman and S. Harvey Mudd–headed the Section on Cellular Regulatory Mechanisms and the Section on Alkaloid Biosynthesis and Plant Metabolism, respectively, and Cantoni was chief of his own Section on Proteins.[27] This laboratory studied the biochemical mechanisms and action of drug and hormone synthesis.

Kety's planned program did not develop exactly as he had hoped, as he had necessarily to rely on those scientists who would accept the top positions. His appointments, however, always "demonstrated originality and conceptual ability in their choice, design, and execution of...research."[28]

Basic Research Director Transition: Kety to Livingston

By 1955, Kety's ambitious program had culminated in the establishment of eight laboratories and one field station concentrating on basic research and involving 55 scientists. These were the Addiction Research Center, Neurophysiology, Socio-Environmental Studies, Neurochemistry, Psychology, Neuroanatomical Sciences, Biophysics, Cellular Pharmacology, and Clinical Science.[29] In addition to conducting research on specific entities–as was common in the other institutes–Kety intentionally organized his program so that it would support "the principal scientific disciplines." In this way, fundamental areas of knowledge involving the "structure, function, and metabolism of the nervous system, the biochemical basis of therapy, the study of drug addiction, the development, regeneration and aging of the nervous system, perception and behavior, and human relations" were successfully represented.[30] Furthermore, a unique aspect of the program was the cross-disciplinary collaborations that occurred amongst the scientists themselves, without any administrative pressures:

> There are projects in which biochemists and biophysicists...collaborated on...the biochemical processes involved in the generation of the nerve impulse. There are...projects on the relationship between neuroanatomical and neurophysiological changes and behavior. There are...projects which interrelate pharmacology with biochemistry and physiology on [the] one hand and behavioral and clinical sciences on the other. The program of aging has been attacked from a multidisciplinary point of view ranging...from anatomical studies through biochemistry, physiology, psychology, and sociology, to clinical psychiatry and neurology.[31]

The time that Kety had to devote to administration, however, prevented him from keeping fully abreast of the latest developments in his field and from pursuing his laboratory research on cerebral circulation and metabolism. He had also become interested in psychopharmacology, specifically in monoamine neurotransmitters and the actions of psychotomimetic drugs, such as LSD, mescaline, and indole derivatives, as related to schizophrenia.[32] He thus wanted to step down from the position of director of the joint NIMH-NINDB basic research program. Robert B. Livingston was appointed in November 1956 to succeed Kety in this position and Kety became the new chief of the Laboratory of Clinical Science.[33]

Livingston had received his A.B. and M.D. degrees from Stanford University and after completing 18 months' training in internal medicine entered the Navy Medical Corps as a reserve officer.[34] He then taught at Yale University, where he worked with John Fulton. In contrast to Kety, whose chief responsibility as the first NIMH-NINDB basic research director was to create the intramural program, Livingston's

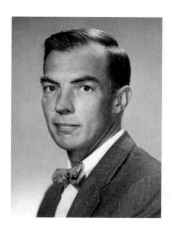

Robert B. Livingston, M.D.
Courtesy of the National Library of Medicine

tenure was marked by the establishment of a number of programs that affected the intramural scientists personally, namely, the Assembly of Scientists, sabbaticals, tenure, the Associates Training Program, and the Foundation for the Advancement of Education in the Sciences.

Assembly of Scientists

In January 1958, the NIMH-NINDB basic research laboratory chiefs sought mechanisms that would improve the "professional stature, …performance, and…long-range research development of the NIH."[35] Their aim was to "maintain the NIH as a national and international resource of important value to biomedical science and to health and welfare generally."[36] The goal was for the administration to rely more on the ideas of scientists whose responsibility and concern with the development of policies affecting them and their work as well as the mission of the institutes made them sensitive to such issues. The expectation of the laboratory chiefs was that their collective judgments with respect to such issues would be welcomed.[37] The laboratory chiefs also believed that an additional channel of communication between the scientists and the administration was necessary to ensure that the long-term philosophy of the institutes was maintained:

> the coming years will bring to bear on the NIH strong pressures to change its short-term mission and modus operandi.

The most critical changes will undoubtedly be in the direction of greater emphasis on target (sic) and contract research. Such changes may be justifiable in terms of social good, but...the Assemblies may be the only mechanism and force by which the scientific staff can act to insure that the new directions are consonant with our professional opinions as to the best way to achieve our long-term mission of understanding and curing disease.[38]

The laboratory chiefs wanted to set up an assembly of the NIMH and the NINDB intramural research scientists that would resemble a university faculty organization. It would be known as the Assembly of Scientists. Such an organization within the government was unprecedented.[39] After discussing with the NIMH and NINDB clinical branch chiefs some general principles that had evolved from the basic laboratory chiefs' discussions, several proposals emerged by early 1958. Specifically, such an assembly would be voluntary, would operate according to parliamentary principles, and would be open to all scientists above a Civil Service GS-11 rank or an Assistant Grade in the Commissioned Corps.[40] It would have "the authority to discuss and express its view upon any matter which it deems to be of general interest to the institutes, and the power to make recommendations concerning any such matters to the appropriate administrative officials at the NIH."[41]

When these principles were brought before the institute directors, they concurred that the idea had merit and encouraged further exploration of it. Although the possibility of having an Assembly drawn from the NIH as a whole was considered, it was thought prudent to explore it just with participants from the NIMH and the NINDB first. If the experience were successful, all of the other institutes could then be brought in to constitute an all-NIH Assembly.[42]

NIMH and NINDB scientists met on June 18, 1958, and proposed the beginning of the Assembly in the fall. The lack of a readily available, successful model to follow, however, prompted Kety to circulate a pamphlet published by the University of Pennsylvania about the University Faculty Senate that had been established there. During the May 1959 meeting, the 75 scientists present nominated in a temporary capacity

Haldor E. Rosvold as Chairman and Karl Frank as Secretary. Rosvold selected an interim committee that consisted of Marian Yarrow, Richard Bell, Herbert Posner, Sanford L. Palay, and Michelangelo Fuortes, which prepared a draft of a constitution for the Assembly and arranged for an election of officers.[43] In addition to the principles mentioned above, the draft also specified that the officers should include a president, a vice president, and a secretary, elected annually by the assembly members. The council would consist of these officers and eight councilors, four selected by assembly members for two-year terms and the remaining four elected annually. No administrator at the scientific director or above level was eligible for such office. The assembly meetings would be held on a yearly basis, in October.[44]

At the June 1959 meeting, Rosvold, Frank, and Palay were elected by secret ballot to be president, vice president, and secretary of the Assembly of Scientists, respectively, and Yarrow, Posner, Fuortes, Paul MacLean, John Clausen, Seymour Kety, Edward Evarts, and Giulio Cantoni were elected as the eight council members.[45]

The NIMH intramural research program chiefs, collectively and as members of the Assembly, proceeded to study NIH personnel policy

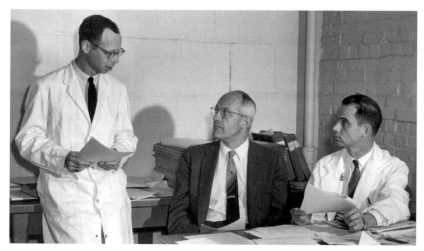

Officers of the Assembly of Scientists, 1959. Left to right: Sanford L. Palay, Secretary, from the Laboratory of Neuroanatomical Sciences, NINDB, Karl Frank, Vice President, from the Laboratory of Neurophysiology, NINDB, and Haldor E. Rosvold, President, from the Laboratory of Psychology, NIMH
Courtesy of the Office of NIH History

and prepared documents concerning the Assembly of Scientists, sabbatical policies, appointment and promotion procedures, and tenure, to be transmitted to the administration.[46]

Sabbaticals

Another feature adopted from the academic world by the NIMH and eventually the NIH as a whole was the principle of sabbatical leaves. Universities had long had the practice of allowing senior faculty members extended periods of time, at seven-year intervals, away from their regular duties in order to sustain high quality creative scholarship. Such leaves were viewed as providing scientists with "recurrent opportunities to renew their mastery of the field,…learn new technical and conceptual skills and…obtain a new perspective on scientific values relating to their work."[47] As a result, the basic research laboratory chiefs, under David Shakow's chairmanship, and with Felix's encouragement, drafted a sabbatical leave program for the NIMH and the NINDB that would allow senior scientists to benefit from such opportunities for personal intellectual growth and career development as a way of encouraging further creative work at the two institutes.[48]

Tenure

An initiative that was fine-tuned under Livingston's leadership involved the principle of tenure. Neither the Civil Service nor the Commissioned Corps distinguished between tenured and time-limited appointments, awarding employees security after only one year of probationary employment.[49] This personnel system, however, was not appropriate for a scientific research program that needed a longer period of time for the development and evaluation of junior scientists' skills.[50] Livingston foresaw three repercussions resulting from employing such a short tenure criterion: "either the institutes would have to be expanded indefinitely, or there would be inadequate space for essential research operations after only two or three years of such practice, or there would be no opportunity to provide research training for aspiring scientists."[51] As a result, a system whereby young scientists would be able to obtain research training and experience but only for a limited period of two to three years–extendable for an additional year in exceptional cases involving vacancies due to retirement or senior scientist departures–was put into place.[52] This enabled promising young scientists in the early stages of their careers to obtain a varied experience, and senior scientists could contribute to the education of a larger group of young scientists.[53] Because the NIH competed with universities for senior scientists, tenure qualifications for permanent employment were established that were equivalent to those in academia: a GS-14 or Senior Scientist level in the Civil Service or Commissioned Corps, respectively, was equivalent to an Associate Professor.[54]

Foundation for the Advancement of Education in the Sciences

In order to provide an additional educational environment that could compete with and be a model for other institutions, Livingston also spurred the creation of the Foundation for the Advancement of Education in the Sciences (FAES). The FAES was established as a non-profit corporation, sustained largely from tuition fees, by the NIH Scientific Advisory Committee.[55] This corporation took over the Graduate School Branch that the NIH had established within the U.S. Department of Agriculture, and further extended the educational opportunities available at the NIH.[56]

NIH Associates Training Program

Throughout both Kety's and Livingston's tenure, the intramural program was able to take advantage of highly qualified physicians who would arrive at the NIMH and the NINDB for two years of basic or clinical research training as part of the NIH Associates Training Program. Such a program came about as a result of Frank Berry, Assistant Secretary of Defense, devising a compromise–known as the Berry Plan–to certain provisions of the 1950 doctor's draft law.

This law allowed for the induction of medical, dental, and allied care specialists into the Army, Navy, Air Force, or PHS during the Korean War.[57] This deployment of qualified medical personnel, however, was opposed by the American Medical Association, the Association of American Medical Colleges, and the American Hospital Association which saw the need to staff the nation's hospitals.[58] The Berry Plan would allow medical personnel to defer their military obligations for a certain period of time while they continued their training. At the same time, it would provide the military services with needed trained personnel.[59] Specifically, physicians during their last year of medical school would opt for one of three possible choices: one, the physician could join the military service of his choice following internship; two, the physician could complete one year of post-internship residency, fulfill his military obligation, and subsequently return to complete his residency; or three, the physician could complete residency training in his choice of specialty prior to fulfilling his military obligation.[60] The third option turned out to be the most popular.[61]

Such deferment choices, however, were not guaranteed, so an alternative way to satisfy this military duty was by applying for service in the uniformed Commissioned Corps of the PHS.[62] Few who applied were accepted and those who were could be assigned anywhere in the world, so competition for positions in the NIH Associates Training Program was fierce.[63]

Although currently consisting of Clinical, Research, and Staff Associates, when the program began in 1953 there were only just over a dozen Clinical Associates.[64] Clinical Associates (CAs) consisted of physicians and dentists who participated in research on patients under their care at the NIH Clinical Center. The program was expanded in 1956 to include Research Associates (RAs), who participated in laboratory research but had no clinical responsibilities.[65] Associates such as Sid Gilman, Irwin Kopin, Guy McKhann, and Richard Sidman, were assigned to senior investigators at the NIMH and the NINDB upon arrival who would act as mentors and the research the Associates conducted would vary from institute to institute and would depend on their past research experience and interests.[66]

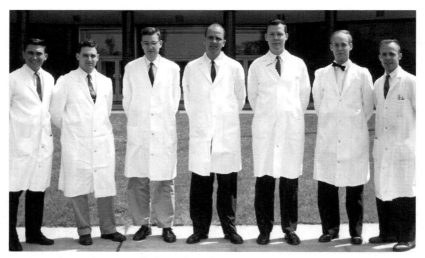

NIH Research Associates, 1958 (Left to right: Sid Gilman, Norman Bauman, Peter Huttenlocher, Edward Cohen, Donald Smiley, George Bray, and Parker Small)
Donated to the Office of NIH History by Dr. Sid Gilman

The program gained in popularity, peaking in 1973 with 229 Associates.[67] Prior to 1957, however, when the program began to require formal applications, Associates were often hand-selected and were considered the "cream of the cream" or the "Tiffanys" of the medical field.[68] Following their two-year service periods, they would return to the medical field and become the future physician-scientist leaders.[69] In the meantime, they had a lasting impact on the research conducted in the NIMH and the NINDB intramural programs.

Basic Research Director Transition: Livingston to Eberhart

By October 1959, Robert B. Livingston began discussing organizational changes and the future of the two institutes' joint basic program with the institutes' laboratory and branch chiefs as well as the NIMH and the NINDB directors.[70] As he had stated in his 1959 *Annual Report*, he wanted to step down as director of the joint institute program in basic research for several reasons. He believed that Kety had set a precedent for changing the leadership of a scientific program so that the conceptual limitations of any research group leader would not interfere with the program. He wanted to avoid being persuaded that he had the proper knowledge to make decisions only because he had the power to make them. Most important, he wanted to return to full-time research.[71]

At a December 15, 1959, meeting of laboratory and branch chiefs "a majority voted in favor of the principle that the combined [basic] program of the two institutes should be divided...[and] they recommended unanimously that an associate director for research be appointed in each institute to work closely with the institute directors and to shoulder responsibility in the entire intramural area of the clinical and basic research programs in each institute."[72]

Livingston presented the joint laboratory chiefs and both institute directors with lists of seven on the one hand and ten on the other candidates for the position of Associate Director in Charge of Research within each institute and encouraged them to suggest additional candidates for the positions (see Table 5).

Table 5. Livingston's Candidates for the Position of Associate Director in
Charge of Research, NINDB and NIMH

NINDB	NIMH
Cosimo Ajmone-Marsan	Mary A. B. Brazier
Mary A. B. Brazier	John C. Eberhart
John D. Brookhart	Joel Elkes
Jordi Folch-Pi	Jordi Folch-Pi
John D. French	Donald O. Hebb
Clark T. Randt	Harris Isbell
Theodore C. Ruch	William Lhamon
	Neal E. Miller
	Theodore C. Ruch
	Frederic C. Worden

Source: Livingston to all NIMH-NINDB Laboratory Chiefs of the Basic Research Program and the NINDB and NIMH Directors, 21 October 1959, Assembly of Scientists for NIMH and NINDB (I), M1363, AHAP

By mid-February 1960, the list had increased to 21 candidates for the NINDB and 14 for the NIMH (see Table 6):

Table 6. Candidates for the Position of Associate Director in Charge of Research, NINDB and NIMH

NINDB	NIMH
Cosimo Ajmone-Marsan	Mary A. B. Brazier
Leslie B. Arey	John C. Eberhart
H. Stanley Bennett	Joel Elkes
Mary A. B. Brazier	Jordi Folch-Pi
John D. Brookhart	Robert Galambos
Philip W. Davies	Donald O. Hebb
Hallowell Davis	Harris Isbell
Edward W. Dempsey	Seymour S. Kety
Louis B. Flexner	Lawrence Coleman Kolb
Jordi Folch-Pi	William Lhamon
John D. French	Neal E. Miller
W. R. Ingram	Eli Robins
Saul R. Korey	John T. Wilson
Robert S. Morison	Frederic C. Worden
Clark T. Randt	
Theodore C. Ruch	
James M. Sprague	
Roy L. Swank	
A. Earl Walker	
James W. Ward	
Clinton N. Woolsey	

Source: NIMH-NINDB Laboratory Chiefs of the Basic Research Program meeting: Final Recommendations for Associate Directors for Research, NIMH and NINDB, 17 February 1960, Assembly of Scientists for NIMH and NINDB (I), M1363, AHAP

Despite the recommendations of Livingston and the laboratory chiefs, however, by August 1960, G. Milton Shy had been appointed as the new Associate Director for Research at the NINDB. Maitland Baldwin took Shy's place as Clinical Director of the NINDB (see below).

The basic research laboratory chiefs at the time–Sidney Bernhard, Giulio Cantoni, John Clausen, Kenneth Cole, Seymour Kety, Wade Marshall, David Shakow, William Windle–had met informally on

December 30, 1959, to discuss opportunities that would encourage Livingston to remain at the NIH as a scientist. They expressed

> …an unanimous hope that every effort would be made to keep Dr. Livingston in the program…based upon a number of cogent considerations. These include his devotion to academic and scientific ideals and his willingness to defend them forthrightly, his breadth as a scholar of the nervous system and of behavior, the ability to utilize this knowledge in meaningful conceptualizations and the requisite competence and skill, based upon many years in neurophysiological teaching and research, [and] to organize and carry out a program of laboratory investigation.[73]

Were Livingston to remain at the NIH, sensory feedback, an area of research not well represented in the program at the time but one to which Livingston had contributed over the prior decade, would have been emphasized as a pressing research area.[74] However, the chiefs were aware that given the space limitations, pursuing such a course at the time was not feasible without taking away from existing laboratories.[75] Nevertheless, a small Laboratory of Neurobiology was established on October 18, 1960, wherein Livingston could conduct brain research using neuroanatomical, neurophysiological, biophysical, and behavioral techniques to improve understanding of perception, learning, memory, and judgment.[76] After two years, however, Livingston left the NIMH to become Chief of the General Research Support Branch, in the Division of Research Facilities and Resources. Shortly thereafter, he left NIH altogether to establish a department of neurosciences at the University of California at San Diego.[77]

In response to the recommendations of Livingston and the laboratory chiefs, however, John C. Eberhart became the NIMH's new associate director for research, succeeding Livingston.[78]

Eberhart was already well known to Felix and the NIMH scientists, having headed the NIMH's extramural Research Grants and Fellowships Branch (after Lawrence Coleman Kolb) from 1949 to 1954. In 1954, he had left to go to the Commonwealth Foundation but he returned to the NIMH in 1961 to head its intramural basic research program.

John C. Eberhart, Ph.D.
Donated to the Office of NIH History by Dr. Morris Parloff

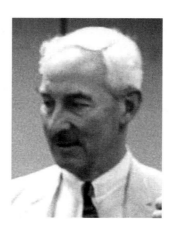

Notes

1. Topping had expected to succeed Rolla E. Dyer when the latter retired as NIH director on October 1, 1950. He left for the vice presidency of medical affairs at the University of Pennsylvania when William H. Sebrell, Jr.–formerly director of the Institute of Experimental Biology and Medicine– was appointed the new NIH director instead. (Felix, oral history by Rubinstein; Sebrell, oral history by Siepert and Carrigan). See Norman Topping, *Recollections* (Los Angeles: University of Southern California Press, 1990).

2. Felix, oral history by Rubinstein; Sebrell, oral history by Siepert and Carrigan. Several candidates were considered for the position prior to Kety, including Gregory Pincus and Hudson Hoagland. Harold Harlow was actually offered the position but turned it down when the University of Wisconsin made him a better offer (John Clausen, oral history by Eli Rubinstein, January 9, 1978, transcript, NIMH Oral History Collection, OH 144, NLM).

3. Felix, oral history by Rubinstein; Louis Sokoloff, "Seymour S. Kety, 1915-2000," *Biographical Memoirs*, 38 (2003): 1-21.

4. Sokoloff, "Seymour S. Kety," 10. One of Felix's oral histories points this out explicitly: "I was continually impressed with how utterly naïve most all psychiatrists were in research design or in research execution....And I was upset about it. We tried to get some research training started and I began to be kind of shook [sic] by the fact that our people, even those who were going to evaluate the research training programs, were not really investigators themselves." (Felix, oral history by Rubinstein, 70).

5. Seymour S. Kety, "Mental Illness and the Sciences of Brain and Behavior," *Nature Medicine*, 5, no. 10 (October 1999): 1114.

6. Kety, *NIH Report, 1951-1952*, 143.

7. Kety, *NIMH Annual Report, 1956*.

8. Kety, *NIH Report, 1951-1952*.

9. Kety, *NIMH Annual Report, 1954*, 1.

10. Felix, oral history by Rubinstein, 178-9.

11. Kety, "Mental Illness," 1114.

12. NIMH, *Research in the Service of Mental Health*; Grob, *From Asylum to Community*.

13. Kety, *NIMH Annual Report, 1955*.

14. NIMH, *Research in the Service of Mental Health*.

15. Felix, *NIMH Annual Report, 1954*, 1.

16. *NIH Report, 1951-1952*. Only Developmental Neurology and Endocrinology will be described here; the rest will be described within the respective umbrella laboratories.

17. *NIH Report, 1951-1952*, 144.

18. Proposed Organization of Basic Research Program of NIMH and NINDB, August 29, 1952, RG 511, NARA.

19. See Guth's chapter, this volume.

20. 1951-1954 and Intramural Project Reports, NIMH Central Files, Shelf 1/3, Compartment 19, row 70, Area 130, RG 511, NARA.

21. See the Laboratory of Neurophysiology review for further information and Appendices B and C for lists of all laboratory members and selected landmark papers. The Section on Cortical Integration was also known as the Section on Cerebral Cortex.

22. See the Laboratory of Socio-Environmental Studies review for further information and Appendices B and C for lists of all laboratory members and selected landmark papers.

23. See the Laboratory of Neurochemistry review for further information and Appendices B and C for lists of all laboratory members and selected landmark papers.

24. The Laboratory of Psychology and the Laboratory of Clinical Science were established in October 1953, and June 1955, respectively, but are discussed in the NIMH Clinical Research Program Section, because Dr. Robert A. Cohen, Director of Clinical Research, was most responsible for the recruitment of the chiefs of these laboratories.

25. See the Laboratory of Neuroanatomical Sciences review for further information and Appendices B and C for lists of all laboratory members and selected landmark papers.

26. See the Laboratory of Biophysics review for further information and Appendix B for a list of all laboratory members.

27. See the Laboratory of Cellular Pharmacology review for further information and Appendix B for a list of all laboratory members.

28. Sokoloff, "Seymour S. Kety," 11-12.

29. Kety, *NIMH Annual Report, 1955*. Being based in Kentucky, the Lexington Addiction Research Center will not be discussed here.

30. Kety, *NIMH Annual Report, 1954*, 2.

31. Kety, *NIMH Annual Report, 1956*, 2.

32. Sokoloff, "Seymour S. Kety."

33. See the Laboratory of Clinical Science review for further information.

34. *NIH Record, November 21, 1962* (Bethesda, MD: National Institutes of Health, November 21, 1962).

35. Cosimo Ajmone-Marsan, Maitland Baldwin, Giulio Cantoni, John Clausen, Robert A. Cohen, Kenneth Cole, Joel Elkes, David A. Hamburg, Harris Isbell, William C. Jenkins, Seymour S. Kety, Robert B. Livingston, Wade H. Marshall, Fritz Redl, David Shakow, G. Milton Shy, William F. Windle, Ludwig von Sallmann, memorandum to all intramural research scientists, NIMH and NINDB, 24 April 1959, Assembly of Scientists for NIMH and NINDB (I), M1363, AHAP.

36. Robert B. Livingston to the NIH Director, NIH Associate Director, NINDB Director, NIMH Director, and Laboratory and Branch Chiefs of the Intramural Research Program of the NIMH and NINDB, 22 April 1959, Assembly of Scientists for NIMH and NINDB (I), M1363, AHAP.

37. Agenda for the Laboratory Chiefs' Meeting, 5 November 1959, AHAP.

38. Dan F. Bradley to David Shakow, 7 December 1967, Assembly of Scientists for NIMH and NINDB (I), M1363, AHAP.

39. Ajmone-Marsan et al. memorandum, 24 April 1959, 4.

40. Assembly of Scientists pro-tem committee to unknown, letter and draft, 5 June 1959, Assembly of Scientists for NIMH and NINDB (I), M1363, AHAP.

41. Livingston letter, 22 April 1959, 2.

42. Livingston letter, 22 April 1959.

43. Pro-tem committee, letter and draft, 5 June 1959.

44. Ibid.

45. Haldor E. Rosvold, Karl Frank, and Sanford Palay to unknown, 29 June 1959, Assembly of Scientists for NIMH and NINDB (I), M1363, AHAP. By 1970, the NIMH-NINDS Assembly of Scientists had grown to include the National Eye Institute. It was not a very powerful organization, however.

46. Personnel Policy–NIMH (Intramural Program), 2 February 1961, Assembly of Scientists for NIMH and NINDB (I), M1363, AHAP.

47. Livingston, *NIMH Annual Report, 1959*, 28.
48. Livingston, *NIMH Annual Report, 1959*. Harris Isbell, of the Lexington Addiction Research Center, was the first scientist to be sent on this new program.
49. NIMH Laboratory Chiefs, Recommended Tenure Policy–NIMH (Intramural Program), 14 February 1961, Assembly of Scientists for NIMH and NINDB (I), M1363, AHAP.
50. NIMH Tenure Policy, 14 February 1961.
51. Livingston, *NIMH Annual Report 1959*, 27.
52. Livingston, *NIMH Annual Report, 1959*.
53. NIMH Tenure Policy, 14 February 1961.
54. Ibid.
55. Livingston, *NIMH Annual Report, 1959*, 29-30.
56. Ibid.
57. Buhm Soon Park, "The Development of the Intramural Research Program at the National Institutes of Health After World War II," *Perspectives in Biology and Medicine*, 46, no. 3 (summer 2003): 383-402.
58. Frank B. Berry, "The Story of 'The Berry Plan,'" *Bulletin of the New York Academy of Medicine*, 52, no. 3 (March-April 1976): 278-82.
59. Ibid.
60. Ibid.
61. Ibid.
62. Melissa K. Klein, "The Legacy of the 'Yellow Berets': The Vietnam War, the Doctor Draft, and the NIH Associates Training Program," Office of NIH History, 1998, unpublished manuscript.
63. Ibid., 4.
64. No records were kept at the time so no complete list of the program's Associates exists except for those assembled in a digitized catalogue available at the Office of NIH History. The catalogue is based on the (1957-1990) index cards that Associates submitted when they applied to the program. Prior to 1957, Associates were hand-picked and submitted no proposal.
65. To "add to the preceptor-apprentice relationship complementary means for a broad-based education in biomedical research, through the provision of course work and seminars extending into fields other than the Associate's primary specialization" (Livingston, *NIMH Annual Report, 1959*, 29-30). In the early 1960s, Staff Associates were added to the program in order to train physicians to become research administrators.
66. Klein, "Yellow Berets."
67. Ibid.
68. Donald Frederickson, oral history interview by Melissa K. Klein, 1998, transcript, ONH; J. E. Rall, oral history interview by Melissa K. Klein, 1998, transcript, ONH.
69. Joseph L. Goldstein and Michael S. Brown, "The Clinical Investigator: Bewitched, Bothered, and Bewildered–But Still Beloved," *Journal of Clinical Investigations* 99, no. 12 (June 1997): 2803-12.

70. Livingston to all NIMH-NINDB Laboratory Chiefs of the Basic Research Program, 29 October 1959, Assembly of Scientists for NIMH and NINDB (I), M1363, AHAP.
71. Livingston, *NIMH Annual Report, 1959*.
72. Livingston to NINDB Director and NIMH Director, 6 January 1960, Laboratory Chiefs–Basic Program, M1364, AHAP.
73. Sidney A. Bernhard, Giulio Cantoni, John A. Clausen, Kenneth Cole, Seymour S. Kety, Wade H. Marshall, David Shakow, William F. Windle to NIMH Director, NINDB Director, NIMH-NINDB Laboratory Chiefs of the Basic Research Program and Livingston, 7 January 1960, Laboratory Chiefs–Basic Program, M1364, AHAP.
74. Ibid.
75. Ibid.
76. Livingston, *NIMH Annual Report, 1960*; Sadie (Shakow's secretary) to Shakow, 30 August 1960, Personal-Own Personnel, M1381, AHAP.
77. *NIH Record, November 21, 1962*.
78. Sadie to Shakow letter, 30 August 1960; John C. Eberhart, *NIMH Annual Report, 1961*.

NIMH Intramural Clinical Research Program

Felix also needed to secure someone to head the clinical research within the NIMH's intramural research program. In the summer of 1952 he asked Robert A. Cohen whether he would be interested in the position. Cohen was then Clinical Director of Chestnut Lodge, a small psychoanalytic hospital in Rockville, Maryland. He was a consultant in psychiatry to the National Naval Medical Center, and on the Panel on Human Relations and Morale of the Research and Development Board of the Office of Strategic Services within the Department of Defense.[1]

Cohen had both a Ph.D. in neurophysiology, from the University of Chicago, and an M.D., was an examiner for the national psychiatry and neurology board, and was active in the early psychoanalytic movement.[2] Cohen had many misgivings about the invitation. He thought the program plan was too amorphous, that it had to be developed too quickly, that the salaries he could count on to recruit staff were too low, and that the recruitment of a large group of newly formed professionals who could work together for the first time would be extraordinarily difficult.[3] However, Cohen had personal knowledge of some members of the NIMH staff, and Felix had offered him some additional senior-grade positions to fill and had reassured him that he would have complete freedom in how he could organize the program. These incentives, combined with his own belief that the government should take responsibility for such a universal problem as mental illness, convinced him to accept the position.[4]

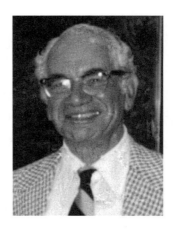

Robert A. Cohen, M.D., Ph.D.
Courtesy of the National Institute of Mental Health

After Cohen arrived at the NIH on December 31, 1952, he soon found that recruiting staff for this new governmental endeavor would prove as difficult as he had suspected. Longtime colleagues and associates who had promised to go if they were called up for service in the Korean War were not drafted and therefore did not have to leave their established positions. The comparatively lower salaries that Cohen was able to offer and the lingering fear of a McCarthyist government possibly pressuring any research agendas also worked against his recruiting efforts.[5]

When the national psychiatry and neurology specialty boards began recognizing two years of service as criteria toward certification, however, Cohen was suddenly deluged with applications from young psychiatric residents striving not to be drafted. He now had his choice among outstanding applicants and eagerly set about recruiting those with the most multidisciplinary backgrounds. He particularly sought psychiatrists who had graduate degrees or experience in other fields besides psychiatry. At the time, psychiatry did not have "a powerful theory of behavior," and Cohen believed it would be necessary to go beyond the confines of the mental hospital in order to learn more about human behavior.[6] Psychiatrists with graduate degrees in other fields, however, were not abundant, and his choices fell upon those whose interests or experience were in the areas of research he envisioned for the new program.[7]

Cohen had two overarching goals for his program: one was directed toward improving treatments for a variety of psychiatric disorders and the other was directed toward developing a better theory of normal behavior and personality development.[8] Indeed, he did not believe there could be a rational treatment for mental illness without first having an adequate theory of behavior and personality development.[9] Specifically, Cohen wanted to

> study… important types of mental illness [in order to discover] more effective methods of treatment and prevention….[apply a multidisciplinary examination of such studies in order to discover]….those experiences [that] are essential for normal personality development….[establish] a theory of personality based on objective, replicable data….[and investigate]….the anatomical structures and physiological events associated with psychological activity in order to determine how certain mental symptoms may be related to organic pathologic processes.[10]

Toward these goals, research in the NIMH intramural clinical research program was centered around three areas: one that focused on hyper-aggressive, anti-social, acting-out behaviors in pre-adolescent children; one that focused on disorders of mood and thought in adults (i.e., schizophrenia[11] and other psychoses); and one that focused on psycho-somatic disorders, each with an eye toward studying such maladaptive behaviors alongside normal controls.[12] Cohen was determined to adopt an interdisciplinary approach to such studies—including the perspectives of psychiatry, psychology, sociology, anthropology, physiology, biochemistry, and pharmacology—in which everyone was engaged in his or her specialty but also kept abreast of advances in the other areas.[13]

Cohen firmly believed that in order to evaluate behavior accurately such research had to be carried out at three levels:

> At the physical [level], to assess organic or physiologic dysfunction, at the psychological [level] to assess perceptions, affects and organization of thought, and at the sociological [level] to study behavior in relation to others and to assess the influences of the social situation in which [the patient] lives.[14]

As a result, he viewed the intramural research program's division into "clinical" versus "basic" research as misleading.[15] In contrast to the assumption that the basic research program conducted "basic" research (in laboratories) and the clinical research program conducted "applied" research, Cohen highlighted the difference in terms of the level of study. Specifically, he saw the basic and clinical research programs as both conducting basic research in the sense of "gaining an understanding of the fundamental processes involved in...development and behavior," whether this happened with animals in laboratories or patients at the Clinical Center. The clinical research program, however, concentrated "on processes which occur at the organismic level of organization [rather than] at the level of organs, tissues, and cells," as the basic research program did.[16] By having a multidisciplinary group of scientists studying patients at every level of the organization, Cohen believed the study of social, psychological, genetic, and biological variables would inevitably provide a more powerful theory of behavior than was available at the time.[17]

Clinical research required clinical facilities in which patients and researchers could be accommodated. Rather than having each institute build its own clinical center, Congress was persuaded that "several Institutes could get research space at less cost per capita Institute" if adequate appropriations were made for one large clinical center at the NIH.[18] The National Mental Health Act had authorized $10 million toward such a building, and the NCI, the NHI, and the NIMH were able to benefit from most of the clinical facilities provided by the Clinical Center because of the $62 million that the three institutes were able to procure toward the construction of the building. As the first $10 million was mental health money, the NIMH was able to secure 150 beds distributed across six wards, two on each of the first three floors of the Center, which were very favorable locations.[19] It was not easy to recruit a director for the new Clinical Center, and Felix had to offer one of the 20 advanced grade positions he had requested in the Act to bring Jack Masur to be its head.[20]

In August 1953, the first clinical NIMH ward at the Clinical Center was opened for the Child Research Branch.[21] This Branch focused on research on various therapies for hyperactive, aggressive, and pre-delinquent children and Cohen recruited Fritz Redl to be its chief. In 1955 these children were moved from the Clinical Center to a Children's Treatment Residence specifically constructed for them on campus. In 1958, Redl left the NIMH and the branch shifted its interests to studying the initial stages of family formation.

Cohen offered David Shakow the position of chief of a joint (basic-clinical) Laboratory of Psychology that was created in October 1953. This laboratory studied human and animal behavior, including normal and pathological functioning.[22] The laboratory consisted of six sections. The Sections on Aging (James E. Birren, Chief), Animal Behavior (Haldor E. Rosvold, Chief), and Perception and Learning (Virgil Carlson, Chief) were considered part of Kety's basic research program, while the Developmental Psychology (Nancy Bayley, Chief), Personality and its Deviations (Morris Parloff, Chief), and Chief (Shakow) Sections fell under Cohen's clinical research program. This would become the largest laboratory within the NIMH's intramural program.

The Laboratory of Clinical Science was established in June 1955 by an amalgamation of a Section on Clinical Biochemistry (Norman Goldstein, Chief), a Section on Clinical Physiology (Edward V. Evarts, Chief), and a Psychosomatic Medicine Branch (no Chief).[23] It sought to identify biochemical, physiological, and pharmacological correlates to psychological processes in normal and abnormal behavior. When Kety stepped down as director of basic research in late 1956, he became chief of this laboratory, the second joint (basic-clinical) laboratory of the NIMH intramural program. It consisted of seven sections. The Sections on Biochemistry (Marian Kies, Chief), Pharmacology (Julius Axelrod, Chief), Cerebral Metabolism (Louis Sokoloff, Chief), and the Chief (Kety) belonged in the basic research program and the Sections on Physiology (Evarts, Chief), Psychiatry (Seymour Perlin and later William Pollin, Chiefs), and Medicine (Roger McDonald, Chief) were part of the clinical research program.

Only a few months after the creation of the Laboratory of Clinical Science, Cohen added funds and positions to create a Section on Social Studies in Therapeutic Settings within the Laboratory of Socio-Environmental Studies, thus effectively making it the third joint basic-clinical laboratory within the NIMH's intramural research program.

The laboratory chiefs of all three joint laboratories–Psychology, Clinical Science, and Socio-Environmental Studies–attended both the basic laboratory chiefs' meetings as well as the clinical branch chiefs' meetings.

By the mid-1950s, public and professional interest in tranquilizer drugs and research studying their efficacy in relation to mental health problems was at its height. A conference on "The Evaluation of Pharmacology in Mental Illness" held in September 1956 resulted in the establishment of a Psychopharmacology Service Center within the NIMH extramural program as well as the creation of a Clinical Neuropharmacology Research Center, situated at St. Elizabeths Hospital, within the NIMH intramural clinical research program.[24] Cohen recruited Joel Elkes in September 1957 to head this center which had three sections: Clinical Psychiatry, Chemical Pharmacology (Hans Weil-Malherbe, Chief), and Behavioral Sciences (Gian Carlo Salmoiraghi, Chief). The Center's purpose was to study the action and mode of action of drugs on the mental functions of mentally ill patients.

The last branch to be added to the clinical research program was the Adult Psychiatry Branch. In December 1957, Cohen recruited David A. Hamburg to head this branch. It focused on therapy for adult schizophrenic patients in a controlled social milieu at the Clinical Center.[25] The Section on Family Studies within this branch was headed by Lyman Wynne and, in 1958, two sections, Psychosomatic Medicine and Personality Development, were added to the branch.

By 1958, the organizational phase of the clinical research program was completed. The program now consisted of three clinical branches, three joint laboratories, five wards in the Clinical Center, a children's residential treatment center, a center at St. Elizabeths Hospital, and 189 scientists and staff members.[26] The most significant outcome of the program was the interdisciplinary nature of the research conducted.[27] The intramural and extramural programs during the 1950s were small enough that there was much interaction between members of both programs.[28] Intramural research scientists also had the advantage of being able to consult their colleagues from other fields whose offices were within the same building, and often even on the same corridor. Two notable examples of such interactions involved the work of three laboratories that led to the publication of the important book *Human Aging*, as well as the collaborative work on schizophrenia in monozygotic quadruplets among five laboratories leading, among other things, to the publication *The Genain Quadruplets*. This interdisciplinary collaboration would only increase as a result of the joint laboratory and branch chief meetings established by John C. Eberhart and Robert A. Cohen when Eberhart arrived in 1961 as the new director of the NIMH basic research program.

Notes

1. Robert A. Cohen, oral history interview by Ingrid G. Farreras, January 18, 2002, transcript, ONH.
2. See Cohen's chapter, this volume.
3. Ibid.
4. Ibid.
5. Cohen, oral history interview by Ingrid G. Farreras, January 23, 2002, transcript, ONH; Cohen, *NIMH Annual Report, 1959.*
6. Cohen, *NIMH Annual Report, 1959,* 2; see Cohen's chapter, this volume.
7. Ibid.
8. Cohen, *NIMH Annual Reports, 1954-1957.*
9. Cohen, *NIMH Annual Report, 1956.*
10. Cohen, *NIMH Annual Report, 1954,* 1.
11. Ibid.: "some in whom the onset of the illness had been relatively recent and acute [and] others who had been hospitalized for many years and in whom the disease process was regarded as being relatively fixed and stable."
12. Cohen, *NIMH Annual Reports, 1953* and *1956.*
13. See Cohen's chapter, this volume.
14. Cohen, *NIMH Annual Report, 1955,* 1-2.
15. "[T]he Clinical Center Administration wished to refer to an organization which was engaged in the care and study of patients as a Branch; if it was engaged in biological research, etc. it [w]ould be termed a Laboratory" (Cohen, e-mail message to Farreras, June 29, 2004).
16. Cohen, *NIMH Annual Report, 1958,* 1-2.
17. Cohen, *NIMH Annual Reports, 1955* and *1959.*
18. Felix, oral history by Brand, 15.
19. Felix, oral history by Rubinstein. "I wanted the lower floors, because in those days it was thought...that psychiatric patients should be on the lower floors, because this way they could get out on the grounds better, and in case of fire, you'd get them out faster." (Felix, oral history by Brand, 15). The NIMH would lose 25 beds to the NCI; there was genuine pressure to use or lose the beds (Cohen's chapter, this volume).

20. Ibid. "The NIH Clinical Center was designed in the form of a Lorraine cross: one long axis cut by two shorter axes. Patients, clinical staff, and clinical researchers were located in the center of each floor. Basic science laboratories were located on the ends of the long axis and in the cross-cutting corridors. The design represented the philosophy of the facility to transfer new biomedical knowledge as rapidly as possible from the laboratory to the patient's bedside. That philosophy has never changed." (Victoria A. Harden, "A Short History of NIH," http://www.pitt.edu/~super1/lecture/lec13111/index.htm).

21. See Cohen's chapter, this volume, Richard Littmann's paper on the branch on the ONH website, and the Child Research Branch review for further information and Appendices B and C for lists of all branch members and selected landmark papers.

22. See the Laboratory of Psychology review for further information and Appendices B and C for lists of all laboratory members and selected landmark papers.

23. See Kopin's chapter, this volume, and the Laboratory of Clinical Science review for further information and Appendices B and C for lists of all laboratory members and selected landmark papers.

24. See Elkes's chapter, this volume, and the Clinical Neuropharmacology Research Center review for further information and Appendices B and C for lists of all laboratory members and selected landmark papers.

25. See Hamburg's chapter, this volume, and the Adult Psychiatry Branch review for further information and Appendices B and C for lists of all laboratory members and selected landmark papers.

26. Cohen, *NIMH Annual Report, 1958*.

27. Cohen, *NIMH Annual Report, 1959*.

28. Cohen, oral history by Farreras, January 23, 2002.

NINDB Intramural Clinical Research Program

During an American Medical Association meeting in Denver, Colorado, Pearce Bailey recruited G. Milton Shy, a young neurologist, to be director of the NINDB clinical research program (and chief of the Medical Neurology Branch within that program) and Maitland Baldwin, a neurosurgeon, to be chief of the Surgical Neurology Branch. Both men were alumni of the Montreal Neurological Institute (MNI[1]) and, at the time, had positions at the University of Colorado. They arrived at the NIH on May 1, 1953; their salaries that first year came out of the Muscular Dystrophy Association funds.[2] Once the NIH Clinical Center was opened, the NIMH had allocated some of its laboratory and clinical space to the NINDB, and the development of the NINDB intramural clinical research program became possible in late 1953. With Bailey's and Baldwin's interest in epilepsy and Shy's interest in neuromuscular disease, former colleagues and alumni of the MNI were quickly hired to build a clinical program around those two areas.[3] Four branches eventually comprised the intramural clinical research program of the NINDB: the Medical Neurology Branch, the Surgical Neurology Branch, the Electroencephalography Branch, and the Ophthalmology Branch.

The first two branches to be established were the Medical Neurology and Surgical Branches, headed respectively by Shy and Baldwin. Shy's Medical Neurology Branch focused on neuromuscular diseases, specifically their detection and abnormalities as well as the mechanisms leading to them.[4] It was one of the largest branches in the program and consisted of six sections: Clinical Neurochemistry (Donald B. Tower, Chief), Clinical Applied Pharmacology (Richard L. Irwin, Chief), Clinical Neurophysiology (Paul O. Chatfield and later José del Castillo, Chiefs),

Biophysical Applications (Shy, Chief), Neuroradiology (Giovanni DiChiro, Chief), and Shy's Section of the Chief.

Baldwin's Surgical Neurology Branch studied epilepsy, particularly in the temporal lobe, within its seven sections: Clinical Psychology (Laurence L. Frost and later Herbert Lansdell, Chiefs), Clinical Neuropathology (Ellsworth C. Alvord, Jr., and later Igor Klatzo, Chiefs), Experimental Neurosurgery (Choh-luh Li, Chief), Developmental Neurology (Anatole Dekaban, Chief), Pain and Neuroanesthesiology (Kenneth Hall, Chief), Primate Neurology, and Baldwin's Section of the Chief.[5]

An MNI colleague, Cosimo Ajmone-Marsan was recruited in January 1954 to head the Electroencephalography Branch. This branch complemented the Surgical Neurology Branch with its work on epilepsy and surgical treatments, but also provided routine diagnostic service to the other institutes at the time.[6] When Paul Chatfield, in the Medical Neurology Branch, retired in 1956, his Section on Clinical Neurophysiology was transferred to Ajmone-Marsan's branch and José del Castillo became its new chief.

The Ophthalmology Branch was not established, under Ludwig von Sallmann, until late 1954, but it quickly became a very large branch. It split off from the NINDB in 1969 to become the founding core of the National Eye Institute.[7] Sallmann's branch consisted of the Ophthalmological Disorders Services (James O'Rourke, Chief), and the Ophthalmology Pharmacology (Frank J. Macri, Chief), Ophthalmology Chemistry (Robert A. Resnik, Chief), Ophthalmology Physiology (Michelangelo Fuortes, Chief), Ophthalmology Histopathology, Ophthalmology Bacteriology, and Chief Sections. The branch complemented the intramural research program's work on neurological and sensory disorders by studying eye diseases, at that time glaucoma and cataracts in particular.

In June 1960, the joint NIMH-NINDB intramural research program was dissolved and independent intramural basic research programs were created within each institute. This naturally affected the basic research program of the NINDB more than it did the clinical program but in its reorganization, Tower's Section on Clinical Neurochemistry within the Medical Neurology Branch was abolished in favor of his becoming chief of a new Laboratory of Neurochemistry that incorporated Roscoe O. Brady's Section on Lipid Chemistry from the former joint NIMH-NINDB Laboratory of Neurochemistry.[8]

In addition, when Richard L. Masland became the new NINDB director, following Bailey's resignation to take up the position of director of International Neurological Research in Antwerp, Belgium, and Livingston stepped down as director of basic research in order to become chief of a new Laboratory of Neurobiology, Shy was appointed the new director of basic research and Baldwin became the new director of clinical research within the NINDB.

Notes

1. Founded in 1934 by the Rockefeller Foundation, the Montreal Neurological Institute (MNI)–and the National Hospital for Nervous Diseases at Queen Square in London (hereafter cited as Queen Square Hospital)–trained a great number of clinical and research neurologists under the guidance of Wilder Penfield, William Cone, Colin Russell, and others. The MNI, the VA neurology units, and later the NINDB training programs, helped bridge the academic training gap (see Tower's chapter, this volume).
2. Pearce Bailey, oral history interview by Wyndham D. Miles, October 7, 1964, transcript, Box 1, OH 149, NLM.
3. Rowland, *NINDS at 50*; see Ajmone-Marsan's chapter, this volume.
4. See the Medical Neurology Branch review for further information and Appendix B for a list of all laboratory members.
5. See the Surgical Neurology Branch review for further information and Appendix B for a list of all laboratory members.
6. See Ajmone-Marsan's chapter, this volume, and the Electroencephalography Branch review for further information and Appendices B and C for lists of all laboratory members and selected landmark papers.
7. See the Ophthalmology Branch review for further information and Appendix B for a list of all laboratory members.
8. Roscoe O. Brady, e-mail message to Ingrid Farreras, February 18, 2004.

II
Reviews of Research in the NIMH and the NINDB Laboratories and Branches

Ingrid G. Farreras

Mind, Brain, Body, and Behavior
I. G. Farreras, C. Hannaway and V. A. Harden (Eds.)
IOS Press, 2004

Adult Psychiatry Branch, NIMH

In November 1953, an NIMH ward opened at the NIH Clinical Center that was devoted to adult schizophrenic patients.[1] This was the second clinical NIMH ward opened (see Child Research Branch, NIMH). The goal was to provide intensive individual psychotherapy in a controlled social milieu. This closed psychiatric ward provided an ideal setting: one in which mental illness could be studied from a psychiatric perspective over a long period of time, in which sociological observations of the interpersonal relationships between patients and their family members could be made, and in which related physiological and biochemical phenomena could be investigated.[2]

With the ward in operation, Cohen needed to appoint a chief for the Adult Psychiatry Branch.[3] This proved difficult to do, partly because the increasing governmental funding available for extramural research in mental health led to salaries that were climbing above those in the government, and because the position imposed a restriction to full-time research (when most researchers and clinicians in the field had limited side practices).[4]

Cohen was nonetheless able to recruit psychiatrists and staff members who carried out research while he searched for a branch chief. They worked on the following early projects: 1) studying staff orientations and ward social structure to determine their impact on the treatment of the patient; 2) studying self-concept and social roles in personality development; 3) in cooperation with the Laboratory of Socio-Environmental Studies, investigating and comparing the psychopathology and therapeutic process of parents–especially mothers–and their schizophrenic children;[5] and 4) in cooperation with the Laboratory of Psychology, employing linguistic techniques and sociological role theory to analyze therapeutic interviews in order to objectify and quantify hitherto subjective interview material.[6]

By 1955-1956, the branch's interests centered around three areas: 1) studying therapeutic communities of adult schizophrenic patients; 2) involving parents in the group treatment of schizophrenic patients and comparing the families of schizophrenic patients with those of normal control subjects; and 3) studying how various types of chronic illness had an impact on personality.[7]

Finally, by December 1957, Cohen was able to recruit David A. Hamburg to head the branch. Cohen had been following Hamburg's career from the early days when Hamburg worked with David Rioch at the Walter Reed Army Institute of Research (WRAIR) in Washington, D.C., and later with Roy Grinker at the Michael Reese Hospital in Chicago,[8] to his fellowship at the Center for Advanced Study in the Behavioral Sciences at Stanford University.[9]

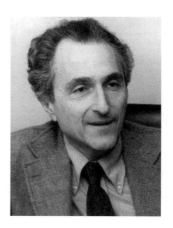

David A. Hamburg, M.D.
Courtesy of the National Institute of Mental Health

With Hamburg at the helm, the branch doubled in size and new research directions were charted. The branch adopted an increased collaborative approach, working alongside psychologists, sociologists, and physiologists from other branches. Two sections were created in 1958–Psychosomatic Medicine and Personality Development–that focused on stress and adaptation.[10] In collaboration with the WRAIR, the Section on Psychosomatic Medicine conducted research on autonomic and endocrine changes associated with psychological stress, specifically relating "fluctuations in emotional states to fluctuations in plasma and urinary levels of hydrocortisone, epinephrine, and norepinephrine."[11]

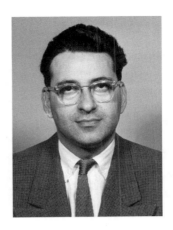

Louis S. Cholden, M.D.
Branch Member
*Courtesy of the National Institute
of Mental Health*

The Section on Personality Development focused on the problem-solving, coping behaviors of university students under stress, hoping to elucidate the mechanisms whereby some became seriously impaired while others functioned effectively in their transition through adolescence.[12] The research comparing the interpersonal relationship patterns of schizophrenic patients and their families with normal controls continued within the Section on Family Studies, headed by Wynne.

Notes

1. Cohen, *NIMH Annual Report, 1953.*
2. Ibid.
3. Formerly known as the Adult Psychiatric Services.
4. Cohen, *NIMH Annual Report, 1956.*
5. During this time, the belief that mothers' early relationships with their infants played an important role in the later development of schizophrenia was a predominant psychoanalytic tenet.
6. Cohen, *NIMH Annual Reports, 1953* and *1954.*
7. Cohen, *NIMH Annual Reports, 1955* and *1956.*
8. As Associate Director of the Institute for Psychosomatic and Psychiatric Research and Training.
9. Cohen, *NIMH Annual Report, 1957.*
10. David A. Hamburg, *NIMH Annual Report, 1958.*
11. Ibid., 13.
12. Hamburg, *NIMH Annual Report, 1958.*

Laboratory of Biophysics, NINDB

The second to last laboratory to be created within the NIMH-NINDB intramural basic research program was the NINDB-supported Laboratory of Biophysics, headed by Kenneth S. Cole, in early 1954. The Laboratory of Biophysics expanded on earlier work on the instantaneous conductivity of the nerve fiber during activity to the study of how ionic movements initiate and propagate the nerve impulse, both normally as well as under the influence of drugs and disease.[1] Specifically, it set up–via computers–complex mathematical theories in an attempt to predict the formation and behavior of the nerve impulse under various normal and pathological conditions, predictions which were then experimentally tested against a simple nerve fiber of a squid giant axon.[2]

The squid giant axon provided the first, direct measurement of the ionic movements responsible for excitation and propagation of a nerve impulse through a nerve membrane.[3] A voltage clamp allowed for the characteristics of these ion movements to be accurately, quickly, and reliably obtained.[4] Improved methods and techniques also allowed for the measurement of radioactive tracer fluxes during times of principal ionic current flows across the squid axon membranes.[5]

Some of the specific studies conducted within this laboratory involved: 1) investigating the action of synthetic cholinesterase inhibitors and their correlation with nerve action; 2) studying the effects of stereo-specifically tailored amino alcohol derivatives on the electrical activity of the single node in terms of threshold and action current parameters; 3) generating mathematical models for ionic permeability of the nodal membrane; 4) studying the effect of temperature rises on the speed of sodium and potassium processes and peak conductances; 5) assessing the effects of external calcium and magnesium ions; and 6) comparing the resting and action potentials of squid and lobster giant axons.[6]

When the joint NIMH-NINDB intramural basic research program was dissolved in 1960 and independent intramural basic research programs were created within each institute, the Laboratory of Biophysics remained within the NINDB, and the new director of basic research, Milton Shy, agreed to the laboratory's expansion, pledging 16 modules—as opposed to the six it had—in which to conduct research.[7]

Notes

1. Seymour S. Kety, *NIMH Annual Report, 1954*.
2. Ibid.
3. Kenneth S. Cole, *NIMH Annual Reports, 1956* and *1957*.
4. Cole, *NIMH Annual Reports, 1955, 1957, 1959,* and *1960*.
5. Cole, *NIMH Annual Reports, 1957* and *1960*.
6. Cole, *NIMH Annual Reports, 1956–1959; NINDB Annual Report, 1960*.
7. *NINDB Annual Report, 1960*.

Laboratory of Cellular Pharmacology, NIMH

In mid-1954 the last laboratory to be created in the NIMH-NINDB intramural basic research program was the Laboratory of Cellular Pharmacology. Biochemist Giulio L. Cantoni was chief of this new laboratory that investigated "the enzymatic and other biochemical mechanisms of drug and hormone synthesis and their action in the body."[1]

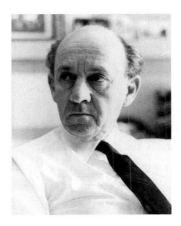

Giulio L. Cantoni, M.D.
Courtesy of the National Institute of Mental Health

The laboratory was not initially divided into sections due to its small size, and all staff instead focused on three overlapping areas of investigation: 1) biological methylation; 2) comparative biochemistry; and 3) the interrelationship between amino acid metabolism and the tricarboxylic acid cycle.[2]

The biological methylation area focused on the central role played by the amino acid methionine in enzymatic transmethylation reactions, specifically, the mechanism of reaction of the methionine-activating enzyme, the chemistry and enzymology of S-adenosylmethionine and the biosynthesis of methionine.[3] It also studied the biochemical mechanism for formation and utilization of onium compounds as well as the relationship between the enzymes thetin-homocysteine methylpherase and betaine-homocysteine methylpherase and the characteristic and structural groups of the proteins responsible for the polymerization reaction.[4]

The comparative biochemistry research was centered on understanding metabolic differences between different cells, tissues, and species in response to chemical agents and drugs, in particular the nature and mechanism of protein synthesis through the activation of amino acids.[5] The transfer of the activated amino acids to a polyribonucleotide carrier (S-RNA) and the study of its chemistry, molecular configuration, and biological characteristics was expected to elucidate a biological "coding" mechanism.[6]

The third area of research focused on the intermediary metabolism of carbohydrates and amino acids, particularly the relationship between individual amino acids and metabolites of the citric acid cycle.[7] Other research in this area also focused on the mechanism of aromatic hydroxylation reactions, especially the enzymatic conversion of phenylalanine to tyrosine and the structure and function of cofactors involved in this conversion that would elucidate the etiology of oligophrenia phenylpyruvica, a form of mental deficiency in children, as well as on the hydroxylation reaction underlying the biosynthesis of noradrenaline.[8]

In the early spring of 1959, a greenhouse research facility was constructed to conduct studies clarifying the mechanism of synthesis of alkaloids and other drugs by plants.[9] As a result, a Section on Alkaloid Biosynthesis and Plant Metabolism was established under S. Harvey Mudd that focused on: 1) mechanisms of transmethylation in higher plants, especially the role of S-adenosylmethionine; 2) the pathway and mechanisms involved in methionine biosynthesis in higher plants; and 3) the structural resemblance of certain plant alkaloids to adrenal hormones and serotonin.[10]

At this time the laboratory expanded its areas of interest to four topics–mechanisms and pathways of protein biosynthesis; biological methylation; biological oxygenation; and alkaloid biosynthesis–and created two additional sections: Proteins, under Giulio L. Cantoni, and Cellular Regulatory Mechanisms, under biochemist Seymour Kaufman.[11]

S. Harvey Mudd, Ph.D.
Courtesy of the National Institute of Mental Health

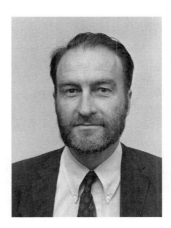

All three sections continued the work on biological methylation, but Kaufman's section focused on the roles that vitamins, folic acid, and ascorbic acid played in the phenylalanine and dopamine hydroxylating systems, and Cantoni's section studied the enzymatic biosynthesis of methionine, the properties of thetin-homocysteine methylpherase, and the nature and characteristics of S-RNA.[12]

Seymour Kaufman, Ph.D.
Courtesy of the National Institute of Mental Health

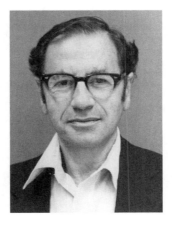

Notes

1. Kety, *NIMH Annual Report, 1954*, 9.
2. Ibid.; Giulio Cantoni, *NIMH Annual Reports, 1955-1958*.
3. Cantoni, *NIMH Annual Reports, 1957* and *1958*.
4. Kety, *NIMH Annual Report, 1954*; Cantoni, *NIMH Annual Reports, 1955* and *1958*.
5. Cantoni, *NIMH Annual Report, 1956*.
6. Cantoni, *NIMH Annual Reports, 1955, 1956*, and *1960*.
7. Cantoni, *NIMH Annual Reports, 1955* and *1956*.
8. Cantoni, *NIMH Annual Reports, 1957, 1958*, and *1960*.
9. Cantoni, *NIMH Annual Report, 1957*.
10. Cantoni, *NIMH Annual Reports, 1958-1960*.
11. Cantoni, *NIMH Annual Report, 1959*.
12. Ibid.; Cantoni, *NIMH Annual Report, 1960*.

Child Research Branch, NIMH

The Child Research Branch was the first branch created within the NIMH clinical program, a branch organized around one man: Fritz Redl.[1] Redl had a Ph.D. in philosophy and was a graduate of the Vienna Psychoanalytic Institute. He had been a student of the established psychoanalyst August Aichhorn in Vienna, who was the author of *Wayward Youth*, and a close friend and colleague of Erik Erikson. Redl had worked extensively and published two highly regarded books, *Children Who Hate* and *Controls From Within,* on the destructiveness and disorganization of hyperaggressive and pre-delinquent children with deficient behavioral controls.[2]

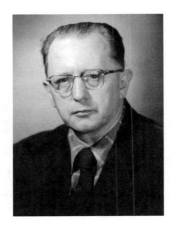

Fritz Redl, Ph.D.
Courtesy of the National Institute of Mental Health

The first clinical NIMH ward at the NIH Clinical Center opened in August 1953 and was devoted to such emotionally disturbed and destructive children. The branch focused its clinical care and research activities around three components: individual psychotherapy, milieu therapy, and remedial education in school.[3] Such a combined approach was unique at the time, allowing for a rare opportunity to integrate these different approaches and to study "the roles of the child care worker, the psychotherapist and the teacher" where ordinary psychotherapy alone had been unsuccessful.[4]

The branch consisted of scientists whom Cohen had recruited prior to Redl being appointed laboratory chief. Their early research focused on four areas: 1) the factors that determined whether rage would be expressed or controlled, and the staff's and children's attitudes toward expressed rage, destructiveness, intragroup conflict, physical settings and therapeutic interventions; 2) the identification of problems emanating from the staff when attempting to deal with such expressed rage; 3) a content analysis of the records expert and non-expert observers kept of the children's behaviors; and 4) psychological assessments of the children within the therapeutic setting in order to predict future behavior.[5]

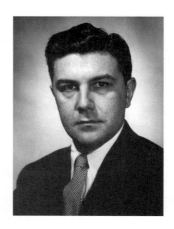

Donald A. Bloch, M.D.
Branch Member
*Courtesy of the National Institute
of Mental Health*

By 1955 it had become apparent that the Clinical Center ward was an ideal setting for the study of the biological and somatopsychic aspects of emotional disorders and the care of chronic, degenerative disease but it was not adequate for therapeutic community studies.[6] As a result, the construction of a half-way house was authorized. This half-way house provided the controlled environment of the Clinical Center ward but also allowed for a permissive, uncontrolled setting more in tune with what the children's own homes or future foster homes would entail.[7] The Children's Treatment Residence was constructed where the present day Building 37 stands. The goals of the Residence were threefold: 1) to collect research data on children who no longer needed hospital ward treatment but who were not ready to return to community life; 2) to explore the therapeutic milieu, including the social structure and staff roles, and compare it to the most conducive aspects of the closed ward treatment environment; and 3) to develop concepts and methods for the observation, description, and categorization of the children's transition or improvement from a state of pathology to one of mental health.[8]

The Child Research Branch, however, perhaps because it was created around one man, was short-lived. Redl did not feel that Felix was supportive of his work and in June 1958 returned to Wayne State University.[9] Joseph D. Noshpitz became acting chief of the branch, which was terminated in July 1959. The children receiving treatment were discharged or transferred to other institutions and the research staff stayed on until June 1960 in order to finalize writing up any data that had been collected in the various studies.[10]

Notes

1. Originally named Children's Services but, by 1954, renamed the Child Research Branch. For more information on this branch, see Cohen's chapter, this volume, Richard Littmann's paper on the ONH website, and the Child Research Branch review for further information and Appendices B and C for lists of all branch members and selected landmark papers.
2. Robert A. Cohen, oral history interviews by Ingrid G. Farreras, January 18, 23, and 29, 2002, transcript, ONH.
3. Cohen, *NIMH Annual Reports, 1953* and *1954.*
4. Cohen, *NIMH Annual Report, 1954,* 1.
5. Cohen, *NIMH Annual Report, 1953.*
6. Cohen, *NIMH Annual Report, 1956.*
7. Cohen, *NIMH Annual Report, 1955.*
8. Fritz Redl, *NIMH Annual Report, 1957.*
9. Cohen, personal communications, December 10, 2003 and January 20, 2004.
10. Joseph D. Noshpitz, *NIMH Annual Report, 1959.* During the fiscal year of 1960, a reorganized Child Research Branch was initiated under the acting directorship of D. Wells Goodrich. The aim of this new branch was to develop a "systematic longitudinal program of interlocking projects to explore the initial stages of family formation in volunteer subjects." (D. Wells Goodrich, *NIMH Annual Report, 1960,* 29). Toward this goal, three areas were explored: 1) the development of behavior in the firstborn infant from birth to 2 ½ years of age; 2) the marital bond development, from newly wed to parenthood, of different types of couples;

and 3) the relationship between these childhood interactions and later, adult interactions. Specifically, the three areas converged on an attempt to link the newlywed marriage phase to the neonatal one and the neonatal behavior patterns to the 2$\frac{1}{2}$-year-old behavior patterns (Goodrich, *NIMH Annual Report, 1960*).

Clinical Neuropharmacology Research Center, NIMH

On September 18-22, 1956, the NIMH, the American Psychiatric Association, and the National Academy of Sciences-National Research Council co-sponsored a conference on "The Evaluation of Pharmacology in Mental Illness." Over 100 investigators, including NIMH extramural and intramural scientists, participated in the conference and its proceedings were published. As a result of this conference, a Psychopharmacology Service Center in the NIMH extramural program was established, as was the Clinical Neuropharmacology Research Center (CNRC) within the NIMH's clinical research program.[1]

The CNRC was a joint project between the NIMH's clinical research program and St. Elizabeths Hospital. Felix, Kety, and Cohen had visited Overholser, superintendent of St. Elizabeths Hospital, with the hope of conducting biological research in one of the hospital's wards that would complement the research that was conducted at the NIH Clinical Center. Such a location was desirable for various reasons. St. Elizabeths provided abundant clinical material for large-scale, controlled pharmaceutical trials. It also allowed for the thorough study of individual syndromes, exposing investigators to mental illness as exhibited in a mental hospital population. And the frequent contact between scientists and hospital clinical staff was expected to engender an appreciation for each other's roles in a common research program.[2]

Overholser not only agreed to grant the NIMH a ward but, in fact, offered an entire building, the William A. White Building, in which the new Center would focus on the study of the action, and the mode of action, of drugs on mental function, particularly with reference to mental illness. Although previously unavailable to head the Psychosomatic Medicine Branch,[3] Joel Elkes, professor of experimental medicine at the

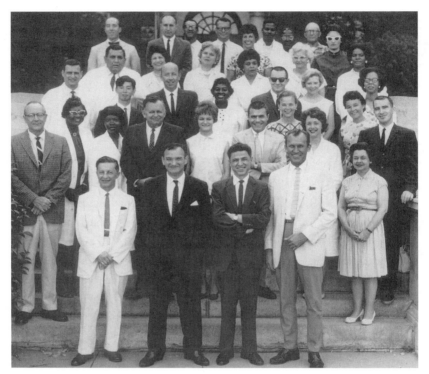

NIMH Clinical Neuropharmacology Research Center at St. Elizabeths Hospital, 1961. Left to right, front row: Hans Weil-Malherbe, Joel Elkes (Chief of Center), Gian Carlo Salmoiraghi, Stephen Szara
Donated to the Office of NIH History by Dr. Joel Elkes

University of Birmingham, in England, agreed to head the CNRC and arrived in September 1957 to plan, furnish, and equip the laboratories within the White building.

The CNRC did not move into the building until July 1958, but three research sections had been created.[4] The Section on Clinical Psychiatry focused on a survey of the existing patient population, hospital personnel, and ward conditions at St. Elizabeths Hospital, and conducted studies that determined and classified the clinical, somatic, biochemical and endocrine responses of patients to established and new drugs. Specifically, and in combination with the Laboratory of Socio-Environmental Studies, the Laboratory of Psychology, and the Biometrics Branch, this section studied the comparative effects of two

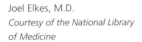

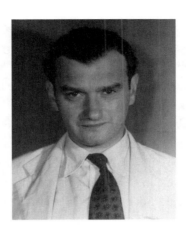

phenothiazines and a placebo with the additional goal of determining: 1) the effect of the physical environment on the responsiveness to drugs; 2) the effect of various types of nursing care on drug response; 3) the cultivation of therapeutic and research skills in ward personnel; 4) the usefulness and reliability of clinical research instruments and scales; and 5) the codification of specific patient change behavior and hospital milieu attributes, such as staff attitudes, toward the research program and the ward setting.[5] Additional research conducted by this section studied patient social interaction (i.e., association or isolation) within a chronic mental hospital ward, dependency as a factor in chronic hospitalization, the transitions of chronic schizophrenic patients into the community and the group therapeutic techniques that facilitate such transitions, and the effects of imipramine on depression.[6]

The Section on Chemical Pharmacology, headed by Hans Weil-Malherbe, focused on: 1) human and animal studies in intermediate metabolism, specifically correlating behavioral effects with biochemical structure, properties, and effects of various psychotomimetic tryptamine derivatives; 2) at the cellular level, an examination of drug effects on carbohydrate and nucleotide metabolism in the central nervous system; 3) the effects of phrenotropic drugs on the concentrations, intracellular distribution, and synthesis of catecholamines within the brain, including developing and refining reliable, sensitive, and specific methods for the routine assay of catecholamines in plasma; and 4) the effect of drugs on the operation of hormonal mechanisms, within and outside the central nervous system, with special reference to pituitary function.[7]

Finally, the Section on Behavioral Sciences, headed by Gian Carlo Salmoiraghi, conducted research in the following four areas: 1) the effect of drugs on the function of sensory pathways, specifically the analysis of mechanisms subserving the coding and transformation of information–which may be disturbed in acute mental disorder–along various levels of integration within the auditory pathway and the role of inhibitory mechanisms in this coding process; 2) the study of cat, rat, and monkey behavioral and hormonal responses to drugs and hormones applied locally to selected areas of the brain; 3) the development of baseline data of generalization gradients for reward- and punishment-controlled behavior in rhesus monkeys in order to appraise the effect of drugs on these functions in various motivational situations; and 4) the effects of drugs upon the central mechanisms governing respiration and blood pressure, specifically, identification of the location and pattern of and factors contributing to the discharge of rhythmically discharging respiratory and cardiovascular neurons in the medulla.[8]

Notes

1. See Cohen's chapter, this volume.
2. Joel J. Elkes, *NIMH Annual Report, 1957.*
3. See the Laboratory of Clinical Science review for further information.
4. Elkes, *NIMH Annual Report, 1957.*
5. Elkes, *NIMH Annual Report, 1959.*
6. Elkes, *NIMH Annual Reports, 1958-1960.*
7. Elkes, *NIMH Annual Reports, 1957-1960.*
8. Ibid.

Laboratory of Clinical Science, NIMH

The Laboratory of Clinical Science was the second joint basic-clinical laboratory in the NIMH and was an amalgamation of a Section on Clinical Biochemistry, a Section on Clinical Physiology, and a Psychosomatic Medicine Branch.[1] In keeping with his goal of studying psychosomatic disorders, Cohen hired Norman Goldstein, from the Mayo Clinic, to head the Section on Clinical Biochemistry, and Edward V. Evarts, from the Payne Whitney Psychiatric Clinic of the New York Presbyterian Hospital, to head the Section on Clinical Physiology, until the ward facilities at the Clinical Center that would allow for the study of psychosomatic patients became available.[2] Specifically, Cohen was interested in investigating how much influence emotional factors exerted on such disorders; if so, by what mechanisms and were there any specific emotions that led to specific bodily changes? What types of treatments were effective for such disorders?[3]

The Section on Clinical Biochemistry applied basic biochemical research and techniques to clinical psychiatry and investigated the metabolism of drugs that caused psychotic-like episodes in human beings (e.g., LSD) and the abnormal quantities of biochemical substances produced by neuropsychiatric disorders.[4]

Specifically, the section investigated: 1) phenolic compounds in the spinal fluid of schizophrenic patients; 2) the relationship of chymotrypsin inhibitor and anxiety in an organism responding to stress; 3) the effect of stress on anti-diuretic activity of the blood in normal and schizophrenic patients; and 4) the biochemistry of myelin and its changes accompanying breakdown.[5]

The Section on Clinical Physiology collaborated with the Section on Clinical Biochemistry and the basic Laboratory of Neurophysiology in

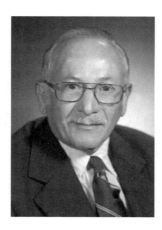

Norman Goldstein, M.D.
Courtesy of the National Institute of
Neurological Disorders and Stroke

an attempt to discover how quantifiable physiological events and behavior were related, namely, "how disordered brain function contribute(d) to the disorders of emotion and behavior," especially in major psychoses.[6]

The section investigated the effect of LSD on rhesus monkey behavior and on EEG changes in psychotic depersonalization, especially when compared to similar symptoms reported by patients with temporal lobe foci and seizures.[7] In 1954, the role of LSD as a leading tool for investigating neuropsychiatric phenomena was expanded in both the Sections on Clinical Biochemistry and that of Clinical Physiology as they investigated the electrical changes in the lateral geniculate body of the cat and the anti-diuretic action that resulted from LSD administration.[8]

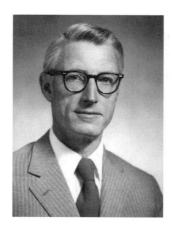

Edward V. Evarts, M.D.
Courtesy of the National Institute
of Mental Health

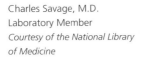

Charles Savage, M.D.
Laboratory Member
*Courtesy of the National Library
of Medicine*

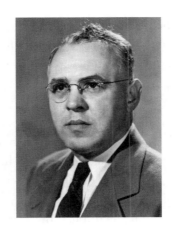

The Psychosomatic Medicine Branch did not have a chief for some time, but Cohen had nonetheless been able to recruit several investigators to begin studying the relationship between psychological and physiological phenomena in "diabetes mellitus, peptic ulcer, anorexia nervosa, bronchial asthma, and hypertension."[9] Psychological data were obtained through psychiatric interviews and psychological assessments and physiological data consisted of measured alterations in metabolic, endocrine, nervous, electrolyte, hemodynamic, and gastrointestinal functions.[10]

In June 1955, the two sections and the branch were combined to form the joint Laboratory of Clinical Science.[11] This was an organizational as well as a programmatic move, as was reflected in its seven reorganized sections: Biochemistry (basic, under Marian Kies), Physiology (clinical, under Evarts), Pharmacology (basic, under Julius Axelrod),[12] Psychiatry (clinical, under Seymour Perlin and later William Pollin), (Internal) Medicine (clinical, under Roger McDonald), Cerebral Metabolism (basic, under Louis Sokoloff[13]), and a Section of the Chief (under Kety).[14] The Section of the Chief was comprised of two units on Schizophrenia and Psychosomatics, under Elwood H. LaBrosse and Philippe V. Cardon, Jr., respectively.

The new laboratory attempted to apply biological disciplines such as biochemistry, physiology, and pharmacology to the problems of mental disease, and thus focused on seeking biological correlates to personality and psychological processes in normal and abnormal behavior.[15] Toward this aim, the new Section on Biochemistry focused on identifying and characterizing brain tissue responsible for experimental allergic encephalomyelitis as well as studying the anti-diuretic effects of LSD in normal and schizophrenic patients in order to determine the biological correlates of experimental psychosis.[16]

The Section on Physiology looked at the comparative effects on intellectual, motor, and perceptual behavior of centrally acting drugs.[17] The Section on Pharmacology, which had been an area of study within the original Section on Physiology, focused on identifying the anatomy and physiology of the psychological processes and clinical manifestations of schizophrenia through the study of the mechanisms and sites of action of LSD, demerol, seconal, and chlorpromazine.[18] The Section on Psychiatry studied the relationship between personality and psychodynamic factors and the psychological and metabolic reactions of patients taking drugs.[19] The Section on Medicine investigated the mechanisms involved in the effects of pharmacological and physiological stress on endocrine processes.[20] The Section on Cerebral Metabolism studied the mechanism of action of thyroid hormones and also developed techniques for measuring continuous blood flow. The Section of the Chief focused on the influence of emotional factors on the function of the nervous and circulatory system.[21]

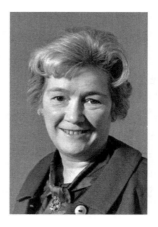

Marian Kies, Ph.D.
Courtesy of the National Institute of Neurological Disorders and Stroke

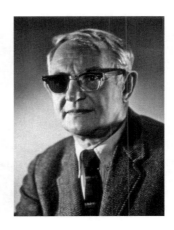

Julius Axelrod, Ph.D.
*Courtesy of the National Library
of Medicine*

With Evarts as acting chief, Cohen sought a senior research psychiatrist to head this new laboratory. He and Kety had met and been impressed by Joel Elkes, then professor of experimental medicine at the University

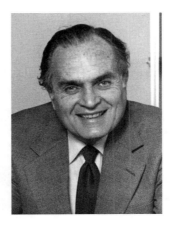

William Pollin, M.D.
*Courtesy of the National Institute
of Mental Health*

of Birmingham in England, and offered him the position. Obligations at Birmingham, however, prevented Elkes from accepting it, leaving the position unfilled until Kety stepped down as director of the joint NIMH-NINDB basic research program in 1956 and offered to fill the position.[22] After adding funds and positions from the basic program–which Kety filled with Louis Sokoloff and Jack Durell, among others–Kety became the chief of the Laboratory of Clinical Science.[23]

Roger K. McDonald, M.D.
Courtesy of the National Institute of Mental Health

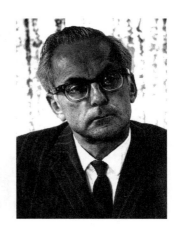

When a second ward at the Clinical Center opened up for the laboratory in July 1957, the laboratory began a series of long-range, multidisciplinary studies on the biological aspects of schizophrenia.[24] From this point on, the clinical and basic sections did not work so much as distinct sections as they did collaboratively on the following areas: 1) the metabolism of epinephrine and norepinephrine; 2) the metabolism related to the nervous system or behavior, specifically, the action of thyroxine on protein synthesis, the metabolism of histidine and other amino acids, and the enzymatic activities in blood; 3) a multidisciplinary study of possible biological factors involved in the etiology and pathogenesis of schizophrenia;[25] 4) the relationship between brain stem reticular

Louis Sokoloff, M.D.
Courtesy of the National Library of Medicine

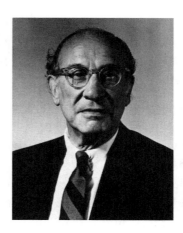

formation and physiological events occurring in a primary sensory area as elucidated by the effects of sleep, narcotic and ataractic drugs, and the interruption of sensory input; 5) the characterization and extensive purification of a brain protein acting as an antigen in the production of experimental allergic encephalomyelitis; and 6) cerebral blood flow or oxygen consumption in healthy, elderly males.[26] This last area formed part of a multidisciplinary project that also involved the Laboratory of Psychology and the Laboratory of Socio-Environmental Studies and the Biometrics Branch. The project assessed aging in 50 healthy adults over the age of 65, living in the community, by way of extensive psychiatric, psychological, physiological, and sociological measures, and published its findings in an important volume titled *Human Aging.*[27]

Notes

1. Cohen, *NIMH Annual Report, 1955.* The Psychosomatic Medicine Branch was formerly known as the Psychosomatic Service.
2. Until then the studies were conducted on outpatients or on patients hospitalized at the Clinical Center by other institutes.
3. Cohen, *NIMH Annual Report, 1953.*
4. Ibid.
5. Ibid.
6. Ibid., 20.
7. Cohen, *NIMH Annual Report, 1953.*
8. Cohen, *NIMH Annual Report, 1954.*
9. Ibid., 1.
10. Cohen, *NIMH Annual Report, 1954.*
11. Cohen, *NIMH Annual Report, 1955.*
12. See Cohen's chapter, this volume, for information on Axelrod's recruitment and his work leading to the Nobel Prize.
13. See the Laboratory of Neurochemistry review for further information.
14. The Section on Cerebral Metabolism was added after Kety became head of the laboratory in late 1956.
15. Cohen, *NIMH Annual Report, 1956.*
16. Edward V. Evarts, *NIMH Annual Report, 1956*; Kety, *NIMH Annual Reports, 1957* and *1959.*
17. Cohen, *NIMH Annual Reports, 1955* and *1956.*
18. Cohen, *NIMH Annual Report, 1955.*
19. Cohen, *NIMH Annual Report, 1956.*
20. Ibid.
21. Ibid.

22. See Cohen's chapter, this volume.

23. Cohen, *NIMH Annual Report, 1955*.

24. Kety, *NIMH Annual Report, 1957*.

25. The laboratory was involved in a collaborative endeavor with four other laboratories that involved a psychological, physiological, and biochemical study of parents and their schizophrenic children, and which included studying the etiology of schizophrenia in the monozygotic Genain Quadruplets. See the Laboratory of Psychology review for further information.

26. Kety, *NIMH Annual Reports, 1958 and 1959*.

27. James E. Birren, Robert N. Butler, Samuel W. Greenhouse, Louis Sokoloff, and Marian R. Yarrow, eds. *Human Aging* (Washington, D.C.: Government Printing Office, Public Health Publication No. 986, 1963).

Electroencephalography Branch, NINDB

To complement Baldwin's interest in seizure disorders, Shy recruited Cosimo-Ajmone Marsan from the MNI. Ajmone-Marsan arrived in January 1954 to became the Chief of the Electroencephalography (EEG) Branch within Shy's clinical research program.[1] Under Ajmone-Marsan's leadership, this branch was engaged in routine diagnostic service, research, and training in electroencephalography.

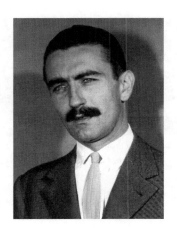

Cosimo Ajmone-Marsan, M.D.
Courtesy of the National Library of Medicine

During the 1950s, the EEG Branch was responsible for all of the electroencephalographic examinations at the NIH Clinical Center. This meant that by 1960 the EEG Branch was conducting over 1800 examinations a year, 68 percent within the NINDB, 20 percent within the NCI, and the remaining 12 percent distributed among the other four institutes, the NIMH, the NHI, the NIAMD, and the National Microbiological Institute.[2] To aid in this task, the branch would accept applicants who sought training in electroencephalography and who would often participate in the research that the branch conducted when it was not examining patients.

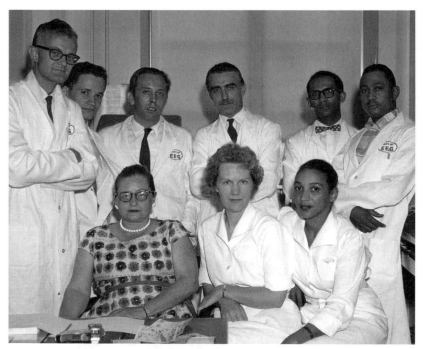

Electroencephalography Branch members, NINDB
Donated to the Office of NIH History by Dr. Cosimo Ajmone-Marsan

Some of the clinically related research conducted by the branch involved: 1) electroencephalographic correlations of metrazol-induced seizure patterns, the effects–including experimental seizures–of locally applied penicillin to thalamic nuclei; 2) studying electroencephalographic and neurological changes resulting from therapeutic Azauracil; 3) studying the relationship between epileptic patients on steroid treatment and intermittent photic activation; and 4) the electroencephalographic diagnosis of secondary brain tumors.[3]

Some of the more basic research conducted studied: 1) the relationship between cortex and scalp recordings of chronically implanted electrodes and their impact on the electrocorticography, functional morphology and diagnostic significance of the focal (i.e., temporal) epileptic seizure; 2) spontaneous and induced brain site activation where spindling occurred by chronic depth electrography; 3) the mechanism of transition from interictal spiking foci into ictal seizure discharges; 4) the mechanism for the bilateral influence of the non-specific system of the thalamus; and 5) the nature of EEG discharges considered to be typical electrographic signs of epileptic lesions.[4]

When the chief of the Section on Clinical Neurophysiology in the Medical Neurology Branch, Paul O. Chatfield, resigned for health reasons in early 1956, the section was transferred to the Electroencephalography Branch.[5] It retained its name but remained without a chief until José del Castillo was appointed as the new section chief in the fall of 1957.[6] With this new section on board, the branch's research expanded to include studying the mechanisms of excitation and conduction of nervous impulses in myelinated fibers and the mechanisms of synaptic transmission, especially at pre-synaptic terminals, and the determination of substances liberated there.[7]

The branch also collaborated in a substantial way with other units, particularly with the Surgical Neurology Branch, on the effects of hypothermia and blood pressure from cortical exposure during surgical treatment of epileptic patients or during hypophysectomies, with the Laboratory of Biophysics on nerve function, and with the Laboratory of Psychology at the NIMH on distinguishing focal from non-focal epileptic patients based on their performance on the Continuous Performance Test.[8]

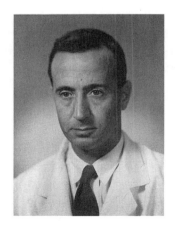

José del Castillo, Ph.D.
Courtesy of the National Institute of
Neurological Disorders and Stroke

Notes

1. For a full and detailed account of the developments in this branch, see Ajmone-Marsan's chapter, this volume.
2. Ajmone-Marsan, *NINDB Annual Report, 1960*. The number of examinations per year and per institute are listed in the *NINDB Annual Reports*.
3. Ajmone-Marsan, *NINDB Annual Reports, 1955-1959*; Shy, *NINDB Annual Report, 1955*.
4. Ajmone-Marsan, *NINDB Annual Reports, 1956-1959*.
5. Shy, *NINDB Annual Reports, 1955-1957*.
6. Ibid.
7. Shy, *NINDB Annual Reports, 1957* and *1958*.
8. Ajmone-Marsan, *NINDB Annual Reports, 1956, 1958*, and *1959*. The Continous Performance Test (CPT) requires continuous performance of simple visual recognition tasks over specific periods of time and is used to differentiate between brain-damaged individuals and those whose behavior is disturbed from other causes.

Medical Neurology Branch, NINDB

The Medical Neurology Branch within the clinical research program was headed by G. Milton Shy and focused on neuromuscular disorders such as muscular dystrophy, dystrophia myotonica, myositis, myasthenia gravis, demyelinating disorders, cerebellar ataxias, amyotrophic lateral sclerosis, and cerebral palsy.[1] The branch's research attempted to: 1) identify the basic mechanisms responsible for neuromuscular disorders; 2) detect cerebral neoplasias; and 3) study the basic abnormalities in the cerebral cortex, through neurophysiological, pharmacological, radiological, histopathological, and immunochemical techniques.[2]

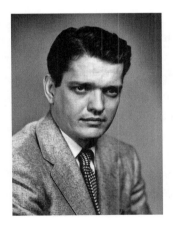

G. Milton Shy, M.D.
Courtesy of the National Library of Medicine

The branch was comprised of six sections. Shy's Section of the Chief, Neurological Disorders,[3] focused on electromyography and observation of muscle biopsies, chemistry and morphology of muscle involved in paramyotonia, and intracellular electrode recording of single muscle fibers in patients with myasthenia gravis.[4] Three other sections were established in the summer of 1953: Clinical Neurochemistry, Clinical Applied Pharmacology,[5] and Clinical Neurophysiology.

The Section on Clinical Neurochemistry was headed by neurochemist Donald B. Tower, who had been a neurochemistry research fellow at the MNI and then assistant resident in neurosurgery with Wilder Penfield before Shy recruited him for the position.[6]

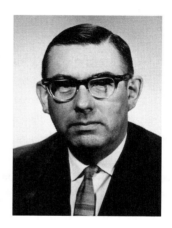

Donald B. Tower, M.D., Ph.D.
Courtesy of the National Library of Medicine

The Section on Clinical Neurochemistry was one of the largest sections of the NINDB and focused on muscle proteins, on the changes accompanying demyelinizing disorders, on the epileptic cortex and the clinical effects of glutamine and asparagines on generalized seizures, and on the amino acid, electrolyte and gamma-aminobutyric acid metabolism in normal and epileptic cortex neural tissues.[7]

The Section on Clinical Applied Pharmacology was headed by neurophysiologist Richard L. Irwin and focused on: 1) studies in "cross transfused head technique in relationship to respiratory and vasomotor response to central nervous system asphyxia;" 2) the relationship between calcium metabolism and neuromuscular blocking agents; and 3) the effects of depolarizing and competitive drugs acting upon neurotransmission.[8] The Section on Clinical Neurophysiology was originally headed by Paul O. Chatfield and studied temperature and its effect on neuromuscular transmission, specifically the myoneural junction.[9] Due to poor health, however, Chatfield resigned, and the section was transferred to the Electroencephalography Branch in 1956, with Alexander Doudomopoulous as acting chief until José del Castillo became the new section chief in early 1958.[10]

The Section on Biophysical Applications[11] was established in 1955 with Shy originally as acting chief but finally officially assuming the position as chief of the section. This section was involved in studies on the localization of cerebral tumors by isotopic detection.[12]

The Section on Neuroradiology was the last section to be established, in early 1958, within the Medical Neurology Branch. Neuroradiologist Giovanni DiChiro was chief of this section that focused on: 1) metal chelates as possible contrast media for myelography; 2) skeletal changes accompanying dystrophia myotonica; 3) the relationship between brain scanning and contrast scanning; 4) fractional encephalography; 5) encephalographic changes in the temporal lobe; and 6) radiological study of soft tissues in different muscle diseases.[13]

Notes

1. Shy, *NINDB Annual Reports, 1954, 1955,* and *1957.*
2. Shy, *NINDB Annual Report, 1960.*
3. This section was also known as the Neurological Disorders Service Section.
4. Rowland, *NINDS at 50*; Shy, *NINDB Annual Report, 1956.*
5. This section was interchangeably called the Pharmacology Section, the Neuropharmacology Section, the Clinical Pharmacology Section, and the Clinical Applied Pharmacology Section.
6. Rowland, *NINDS at 50.*
7. Shy, *NINDB Annual Reports, 1955-1957.*
8. Shy, *NINDB Annual Reports, 1955,* 3, *1956,* and *1957.*
9. Shy, *NINDB Annual Reports, 1955* and *1956.*
10. Shy, *NINDB Annual Reports, 1955-1957.*
11. This section was also known as the Applied Biophysics Section.
12. Shy, *NINDB Annual Reports, 1956* and *1957.*
13. Shy, *NINDB Annual Report, 1959* and *1960.*

Laboratory of Neuroanatomical Sciences, NINDB

Neuroembryologist William F. Windle was recruited by Kety to head the Laboratory of Neuroanatomical Sciences and his Section of the Chief, the Section on Development and Regeneration, within the NIMH-NINDB basic research program.

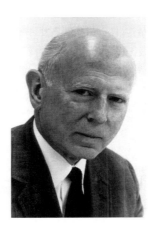

William F. Windle, Ph.D., Sc.D.
Courtesy of the National Library of Medicine

Although he arrived from Morton Grove, Illinois, on January 4, 1954, with animals he temporarily had to house in Building 14 and an ongoing research project, Windle and his staff had to remain in building T-6 until May 3, 1954, before they could begin new projects.[1] The overall focus of the laboratory was the experimental analysis of the organization of the nervous system, specifically its normal structural and functional development.[2] Within this framework, his section's research fell under four categories: 1) anatomical and physiological neurogenesis in the central and peripheral nervous system; 2) regenerative potentialities of central and peripheral neurons; 3) experimentally induced structural alterations in the central nervous system, especially

through asphyxia neonatorum, nitrogen asphyxiation, and the administration of reserpine and other drugs; and 4) technical development in
the area of tissue fixation and chemical substance preservation.[3]

Jan H. W. Cammermeyer became chief of the Section on Experimental Neuropathology on March 1, 1954.[4] His section's main objec-
tive was to determine myelopathies and, toward that aim, the studies
involved: 1) the histological and physical qualities of the brain and
spinal cord in various species at different ages that provided a baseline
for experimental myelopathy; 2) the distribution of extradural fat;
3) the development of a procedure whereby the volume and size of
the spinal cord in several species was estimated based on the animal's
size and growth; and 4) the relationship of extra- and intraspinal fluid
factors and spinal cord malfunction.[5]

Grant L. Rasmussen arrived to become chief of the Section on
Functional Neuroanatomy on November 1, 1954. The overall focus of
this section was on "nervous pathways and connections of the brain
and spinal cord, with emphasis on the neural mechanisms of auditory
and vestibular function."[6] Specifically, the section was involved in
studies looking at: 1) the effects of brain lesions and drugs on temperature regulation and metabolism and the pathways and types of
receptors involved in temperature regulation; 2) the origin, course
and termination of the various fiber constituents of the medial longitudinal fasciculus in the brain stem and spinal cord with a technique
developed within the section for selective silver impregnation of synaptic endings; 3) the auditory afferent and efferent systems, including autonomic innervation of the inner ear, especially the cochlear nucleus; 4) the
anatomical and physiological study of the ascending and descending
visceral efferent connections of brain and spinal cord; 5) the efferent
nervous component of the vestibular nerve; 6) the innervation of the
vestibular and auditory apparatus of the chinchilla; and 7) the fiber
connections of the area postrema of the medulla oblongata.[7]

In the late spring of 1956, Sanford L. Palay of Yale University joined the laboratory and became chief of the Section on Neurocytology.[8]
Pending the arrival of an electron microscope and some permanent
facilities, this section had been conducting research on cytochemical
techniques detailing the chemical analysis of single neurons, the effects

of anesthetics upon cells, and how gamma-aminobutyric acid is distributed.[9] Upon Palay's arrival, the section conducted research on: 1) the ultrastructure of nerve cells, synapses, neuroglia interrelations, and peripheral nerve fiber terminations by electron microscopy; 2) histochemical studies of cholinesterase activity distributed differently between species and GABA's role in metabolic brain reactions; 3) neurosecretory mechanisms; and 4) the normal biochemical make-up of the hypothalamus, optic tract and spinal cord.[10]

In 1957 a Field Station of Perinatal Physiology was established in Puerto Rico with a free-ranging colony of 300 rhesus monkeys and also 50 caged ones, in order to study adverse factors in monkeys' perinatal period that might lead to neurological and psychological deficits in the offspring.[11] The primary factor studied was asphyxia neonatorum. Other data on a variety of topics were also collected, however, from monkeys' menstruation and the nerve supply of the endometrium to the maturation of infants and the behavior and social organization of the colony.[12]

When Pearce Bailey left the NINDB and Richard L. Masland became the new director of the institute, Windle was appointed the assistant director of the institute. Palay became the new chief of the laboratory, Lloyd Guth became acting chief of the Section on Development and Regeneration, and the Field Station of Perinatal Physiology was transferred from the Laboratory of Neuroanatomical Sciences to the Office of the Assistant Director.[13]

Notes

1. William F. Windle, *NINDB Annual Report, 1954.*
2. Windle, *NINDB Annual Reports, 1956* and *1960.*
3. Windle, *NINDB Annual Reports, 1954-1958.*
4. Windle, *NINDB Annual Report, 1954.*
5. Windle, *NINDB Annual Reports, 1954-1958.*
6. Windle, *NINDB Annual Report, 1958,* 4.
7. Windle, *NINDB Annual Reports, 1954-1958.*
8. Windle, *NINDB Annual Reports, 1955* and *1956.*
9. Kety, *NINDB Annual Report, 1954*; Windle, *NINDB Annual Report, 1956.*
10. Windle, *NINDB Annual Reports, 1954, 1955, 1957-1959.*
11. Windle, *NINDB Annual Report, 1957.*
12. Windle, *NINDB Annual Report, 1958.*
13. Shy, *NINDB Annual Report, 1960.*

Laboratory of Neurochemistry, NIMH-NINDB[1]

The Laboratory of Neurochemistry was the second joint NIMH-NINDB laboratory within the basic research program. Kety's original concept of the laboratory included Sections in Physical Chemistry, Enzymology, Cerebral Metabolism, Phosphorylation, and Endocrinology that would study the chemical structure and metabolism of the nervous system and the biochemical processes involved in normal and abnormal mental and neurological function.[2] Only the first two sections would be realized and an official laboratory chief was never recruited.

As the laboratory's acting chief–until a chief could be found–Kety appointed Alexander Rich to be chief of the NIMH-supported Section on Physical Chemistry, on August 1, 1952. Rich began his research at the Gates and Crellin Laboratory of the California Institute of Technology, while he awaited the opening of the NIH Clinical Center.[3] His section employed X-ray diffraction and biochemical methods to study the chemical structure of molecules, specifically, the structure, properties, and synthesis of ribonucleic acid associated with protein synthesis and comparative studies of natural and synthetic polynucleotides to understand the configurations, interactions, and activity found in the ribonucleic acids (RNA).[4] Other research focused on a structural model for fibrous protein collagen and diffusion properties of lipid-containing membranes.[5]

Rich left for the Massachusetts Institute of Technology in 1958 and during David R. Davies's tenure as the acting chief of the section, Sidney A. Bernhard was recruited to succeed Rich. Bernhard had been conducting research in the Division of Physical Biochemistry of the Naval Medical Research Institute and had already been in touch with the Section on Physical Chemistry and with the Laboratory of Cellular Pharmacology.[6] When his tenure began in February of 1959,

Bernhard continued the section's work on DNA and RNA, manufacturing synthetic polynucleotides that allowed for the examination of the structure of polyadenylic acid in an attempt to understand the structure of RNA that allowed for information to be transferred from DNA to protein.[7] The time and work devoted to determining the sequence of amino acids was so substantial that, in 1959, Bernhard introduced IBM engineers and mathematicians to the concept of "breaking the code" for the nucleic acid sequencing of amino acids in genetic transmission (and all protein synthesis). He hoped the computer would markedly reduce the time required to identify the sites of genetically determined developmental and metabolic errors.[8]

Kety retained the position of acting chief of the laboratory until he could recruit a biochemist to head it, and in the meantime created an NIMH-supported Section on Cerebral Metabolism within it for his own work. When Kety had left the University of Pennsylvania to join the NIH, he had been reluctant to recruit his colleagues away from the university, but when he heard that Louis Sokoloff, with whom he had worked at the University of Pennsylvania, was about to accept a position with the Naval Air Development Center, Kety asked him in January 1954 to be the co-chief of this section.[9] The section's research focused on measurements of nutrition, circulation, and oxygen consumption of the living brain by means of the nitrous oxide technique in order to study the effects of aging, anxiety, and hallucinogenic and therapeutic drugs (e.g., LSD, Thyroxine).[10] When Kety stepped down as scientific director in late 1956, to be replaced by Livingston and to become the chief of the Laboratory of Clinical Science, the Section on Cerebral Metabolism and its members were transferred from the Laboratory of Neurochemistry to the Laboratory of Clinical Science.[11]

Kety appointed biochemist Roscoe O. Brady as chief of the NINDB-supported Section on Lipid Chemistry of the laboratory.[12] Brady had been in charge of the Clinical Chemistry Laboratory at the Naval Hospital in Bethesda, conducting research on long-chain fatty acid synthesis and also on sulfhydryl metabolism in his spare time with Earl Stadtman at the NHI. After two and a half years at the Naval Hospital, Brady arrived at the NINDB on September 1954 to investigate lipid metabolism in the central and peripheral nervous systems.[13]

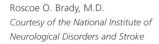
Roscoe O. Brady, M.D.
Courtesy of the National Institute of
Neurological Disorders and Stroke

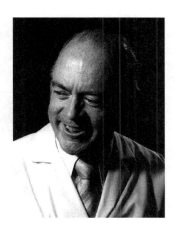

Brady's section studied the synthesis and metabolism of cerebrosides from three angles—fatty acid metabolism, sphingosine metabolism, and carbohydrate metabolism—in an effort to elucidate the etiology of Gaucher Disease as well as the metabolism of substituted derivatives of acetyl coenzyme A necessary for fatty acid and carbohydrate oxidation and fatty acid synthesis and acetyl choline formation.[14] Other section studies included: 1) the formation and concentration of nucleotides in the brain during development and under normal and pathological conditions; 2) the effect of intra axonal injection of certain key enzymes and co-factors; 3) the chemical basis of action of psychotomimetic compounds and tranquilizing agents; 4) the mechanisms of action of elements concerned with initiation and inhibition of nerve action potential; 5) the source and fate of gamma-amino butyric acid; 6) the mechanism of the formation of cholesterol and compounds which contain aromatic rings; and 7) the elucidation of the biosynthesis mechanism of inositol phosphatides.[15]

Throughout Kety's and Livingston's tenures, several attempts were made to recruit a chief for the Laboratory of Neurochemistry. By 1957, two distinguished scientists, in succession, were identified and invited to take the position. Each one was interested in joining the basic research program, even if it would bring no increase in salary. The significant handicap, however, was a lack of sufficient laboratory space. Each candidate was willing to sacrifice his existing space for the benefit of the interdisciplinary and collaborative atmosphere he would find at the

Sid Gilman, M.D.
Laboratory Member
*Donated to the Office of NIH History
by Dr. Sid Gilman*

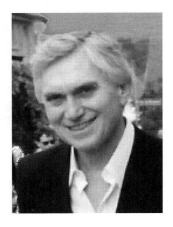

NIMH, but the space available would not have allowed them to establish even skeletal programs. After months of discussions no solutions emerged, and the recruitment of a laboratory chief and the planned establishment of two additional sections in the laboratory were dropped.[16]

In late June 1960, the joint NIMH-NINDB intramural basic research program was dissolved and independent intramural basic research programs were created within each institute. The NIMH was not much affected by this transition, but the new NINDB intramural leadership, under Milton Shy, created a Laboratory of Neurochemistry within the NINDB headed by Donald B. Tower that included Brady's Section on Lipid Chemistry.[17]

Notes

1. For further information on the history of this field, see Donald B. Tower, "Neurochemistry–100 Years, 1875-1975," *Annals of Neurology* 1, no. 1 (1977): 2-36 and Donald B. Tower, "The American Society for Neurochemistry (ASN)–Antecedents, Founding, and Early Years," *Journal of Neurochemistry* 48, no. 1 (1987): 313-326.
2. Proposed Organization of Basic Research Program of NIMH and NINDB, August 29, 1952, RG 511, NARA; Kety, *NIMH Annual Report, 1955.*
3. *NIH Report, 1951-1952.*
4. Kety, *NIMH Annual Reports, 1954-1956;* Livingston, *NIMH Annual Report, 1957.*
5. Kety, *NIMH Annual Reports, 1954-1956;* Livingston, *NIMH Annual Report, 1957.*
6. Livingston, *NIMH Annual Report, 1958;* see Laboratory of Cellular Pharmacology review for further information.

7. Livingston, *NIMH Annual Report, 1958.*
8. Livingston, *NIMH Annual Report, 1960.*
9. Louis Sokoloff, oral history interviews by Sarah Leavitt, July 10 and 31, 2001, transcript, ONH.
10. Kety, *NIMH Annual Reports, 1954-1956.*
11. As did Kety, Livingston would also keep a Section of the (Acting) Chief for his work within this laboratory.
12. After Harvard Medical School, Brady had interned at the University of Pennsylvania Hospital at the same time that Kety was on the faculty of the School of Medicine.
13. Roscoe O. Brady, oral history interview by Peggy Dillon, April 3, 2001, transcript, ONH.
14. Kety, *NIMH Annual Reports, 1954* and *1955*; Brady, oral history by Dillon.
15. Brady, *NIMH Annual Reports, 1957-1959;* Kety, *NIMH Annual Reports, 1955* and *1956*; Livingston, *NIMH Annual Reports, 1957* and *1958*; Brady, oral history by Dillon.
16. Livingston, *NIMH Annual Report, 1957.*
17. See the Medical Neurology Branch review for further information.

Laboratory of Neurophysiology, NIMH-NINDB

Wade H. Marshall, a physiologist trained at the University of Chicago by Ralph Gerard, had been conducting neurophysiological research in the Laboratory of Physical Biology within the Institute of Experimental Biology and Medicine.[1] When he joined the NIMH-NINDB's joint intramural basic research program, his became the first joint laboratory in the program. His laboratory would focus on the function of the nervous system, specifically neural transmission and neuronal interactions, the cerebral cortex, and special senses, in an attempt to understand physiological phenomena occurring in the nervous system that would mediate behavior.[2]

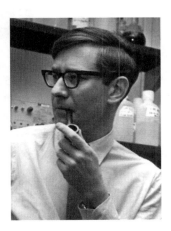

Walter H. Freygang, Jr., Ph.D.
Laboratory Member
Courtesy of the National Institute of Mental Health

Five sections were created within this joint laboratory during the 1950s: Spinal Cord Physiology and Special Senses within the NINDB, and General Neurophysiology, Cortical Integration, and Limbic Integration and Behavior within the NIMH.[3] Marshall's Section on

General Neurophysiology focused on the physiology of the cerebral cortex, especially: 1) the phenomenon of spreading depression; 2) the electrical activity of single cells in the cerebral cortex; 3) the functional activity of the lateral geniculate nucleus; 4) the effects of the blood-brain barrier on the action of certain drugs, such as LSD; 5) the action of curare on the neocortex; 6) ion exchange patterns across membranes of single muscle fiber preparations; 7) sensory discrimination in the cortex and the thalamus; and 8) extracellular and intracellular analysis of the pyramidal cells of the hippocampus.[4]

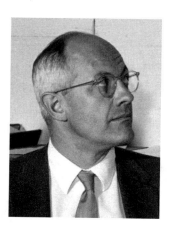

Karl Frank, Ph.D.
Courtesy of the Office of NIH History

In 1952, physiologist Karl Frank's Section on Spinal Cord Physiology joined the laboratory. The section's purpose was to elucidate the neural mechanisms operating in the spinal cord, specifically the excitation of nerve cells and the mechanisms whereby the excitation is inhibited or becomes more excitable.[5] Some of the section's work included: 1) recording electrical potentials of single nerve cells in the spinal cord with intracellular electrodes; 2) studying various types of rhythms initiated by motor neurons; 3) studying trans-synaptic events in the spinal cord; 4) recording antidromic activation; 5) developing a technique for accurate study of electrical reactions (by placing one electrode inside a neuron and another one outside of the membrane); and 6) studying sensory integrative mechanisms in the auditory system.[6]

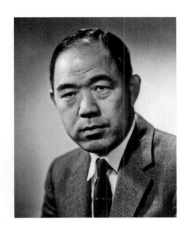

Ichiji Tasaki, M.D.
*Courtesy of the National Library
of Medicine*

Physiologist Ichiji Tasaki's Section on Special Senses focused on vision and hearing, specifically the mechanisms of nerve excitation, including impulse generation, conduction and their consequences."[7] His section studied: 1) mechanisms of production of the action potential in vertebrate nerve and muscle fiber; 2) the biochemical two stable state concept of the nerve membrane; 3) the processes underlying initiation of sensory nerve impulses in the retina, the cochlea, and the skin; 4) the application of tracer techniques to study sodium and potassium ion movements accompanying and following the action potential; and 5) how to make more accurate and less damaging measurements during passage of the nerve impulse.[8]

The Section on Cortical Integration, headed by John C. Lilly, conducted studies on: 1) unanesthetized monkeys aimed at creating a general map of spatial and temporal patterns of electrical activity on the surface of the cortex; 2) developing a method to portray and analyze activity from 256 electrodes; 3) the psychology and physiology of sensory isolation; 4) central nervous system mechanisms involved in hibernation; and 5) the electrical analysis of visual and auditory integrating mechanisms.[9]

When Kety stepped down as the director of basic research and Robert Livingston became the new director, Livingston created a new Section on Limbic Integration and Behavior within the laboratory in 1957 and recruited a former Yale University colleague to head it: Paul D. MacLean. This new section combined behavioral observation, conditioning and learning studies, electrical examination of the central nervous

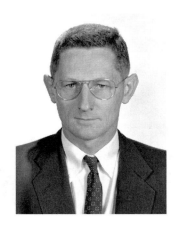

John C. Lilly, M.D.
Courtesy of the National Institute of Mental Health

system, and biochemical lesions and neuroanatomical work to study brain and behavior, particularly the limbic system. Its work focused on: 1) the hippocampus and midline nuclei; 2) the physiological and anatomical loci of genital function in the squirrel monkey; and 3) individual and social behavior of the squirrel monkey.[10]

In late June 1960, the joint NIMH-NINDB intramural basic research program was dissolved and independent intramural basic research programs were created within each institute. The Laboratory of Neurophysiology remained a joint laboratory until a new basic research building became available for the Sections on Spinal Cord Physiology and Special Senses to form the nucleus of a new Laboratory of Neurophysiology within the NINDB.[11] The NIMH-supported sections of the laboratory remained intact within the NIMH.

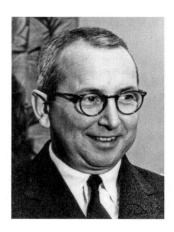

Paul D. MacLean, Ph.D.
Courtesy of the National Library of Medicine

Detlev Ploog, Ph.D.
Laboratory Member
*Donated to the Office of NIH History
by Dr. Sid Gilman*

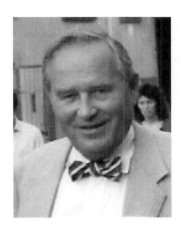

Notes

1. The Institute of Experimental Biology and Medicine was established November 1, 1948, but was absorbed by the NIAMD when the latter was created on August 15, 1950, through the Omnibus Medical Research Act.
2. Kety, *NIMH Annual Report, 1954.*
3. Walter H. Freygang, Jr., headed his own Section of Membrane Physiology by October 1960.
4. *NIH Report, 1951-1952*; Wade Marshall, *NIMH Annual Reports, 1955-1960.*
5. *NIH Report, 1951-1952.*
6. Ibid.; Kety, *NIMH Annual Report, 1954*; Marshall, *NIMH Annual Reports, 1955, 1958,* and *1960.*
7. *NINDB Annual Report, 1960,* 57.
8. Kety, *NIMH Annual Report, 1954*; Marshall, *NIMH Annual Reports, 1955-1960.*
9. Kety, *NIMH Annual Report, 1954*; Marshall, *NIMH Annual Reports, 1955-1958.*
10. Marshall, *NIMH Annual Reports, 1958-1960.*
11. *NINDB Annual Report, 1960.*

Ophthalmology Branch, NINDB

The Ophthalmology Branch was the last one to be established within the NINDB intramural clinical research program but grew to be one of the largest. It eventually separated from the NINDB and became the founding core of the National Eye Institute.[1] Ludwig von Sallmann was recruited in 1955 to head the Ophthalmology Branch, which had been unofficially headed by William Hart and Ralph W. Ryan since 1953 during the ongoing search for an official chief.[2] The Ophthalmology Branch launched a broad program on the causes and mechanisms underlying eye diseases, with special attention paid to glaucoma, cataract, and inflammatory diseases of the orbit.[3]

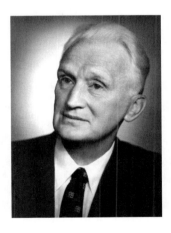

Ludwig von Sallmann, M.D.
Courtesy of the National Library of Medicine

Von Sallmann's Section of the Chief oversaw many of the specific projects. With respect to glaucoma, it: 1) studied thalamic and hypothalamic nuclei, peripheral receptors, the formation and outflow of the aqueous humor of the eye, and the effects of muscle relaxants, all in relation to internal ocular pressure; and 2) developed tests to diagnose glaucoma and determine the adequacy of glaucoma therapy.[4] It also studied the origin of cataracts by manipulating ionizing radiation, diet, and different drugs, in addition to studying the metabolism and growth of the lens.[5] Uveitis, its relation to toxoplasmosis, and its treatment by steroids, was also a major area of study.[6]

The Ophthalmological Disorders Service, headed by James O'Rourke, was involved in the detection of ocular tumors by radioisotope tracer methods, especially differentiating between melanomas and other intraocular tumors.[7] Some research it conducted also involved studying the effects of the endocrine glands, especially the thyroid, upon exacerbations of uveal tract inflammatory disorders, the multiple remissions of uveal infections, and the effects of steroid therapy in patients with uveitis.[8]

The Section on Ophthalmology Pharmacology, headed by pharmacologist Frank J. Macri, focused on the physiology and pathology of intraocular pressure and its relationship to glaucoma.[9] It also studied the effects external ocular muscle tension had on intraocular pressure (i.e., inflow and outflow mechanisms) and the effects of various muscle relaxants on the extraocular striate and skeletal muscles.[10]

Robert A. Resnik was chief of the Section on Ophthalmology Chemistry which was part of the broader research program on the etiology and mechanisms underlying cataracts.[11] Resnik's section focused on the enzymatic systems present in the lens, cornea, and aqueous humor, specifically the fractionation of lens proteins into homogenous components through base ion exchange resin and ultracentrifuge and electrophoresis.[12] Enzyme interactions with normal and pathologic eye tissues were expected to increase understanding of the growth, degeneration, and form of cataracts.[13]

Two sections were established in the fall of 1956: Ophthalmology Physiology and Ophthalmology Histopathology. Physiologist Michelangelo Fuortes was recruited for the position of chief of the Section on Ophthalmology Physiology. Until Fuortes arrived in the fall of 1956, Hans Bornschein had been working as acting chief on the lengths, intensity, and rate of rise of photopic stimuli in order to study accommodation in the optic nerve.[14] This scotopic and photopic electroretinogram (ERG) would allow for the differential diagnosis and prognosis of congenital anomalies or hereditary degenerations and retinal or nerve disease.[15] Combined with adaptometry, which allowed for the determination of visual field thresholds, such physiological testing was highly significant in the diagnosis of complex diseases.[16] When Fuortes became chief of the section, the section focused on cellular microelectrode techniques for studying the electrical activity of retinal elements, especially those of the horseshoe crab, the frog, and fish, in an attempt to understand transducer action whereby external energy (i.e., light) is perceived at a retinal level and then transmitted as a nerve impulse.[17] The Section on Physiology had a physicist by the name of Ralph Gunkel who assisted in these endeavors by developing and constructing many of the necessary ophthalmic instruments and screening methods.[18]

The Section on Ophthalmology Bacteriology did not have an official section chief throughout the 1950s, but the scientists within the section, focused their efforts on inflammatory diseases of the eye (i.e., orbit), especially the trachoma virus and the relationship between adenoidal-pharyngeal-conjunctival (APC) and epidemic keratoconjunctivitis (EKC) viruses with hela cell suspensions.[19] Another major aspect of the research program involved the etiology and differential diagnosis of uveitis patients, whose hormonal state, particularly the thyroid function, they also evaluated.[20] Finally, the section also studied toxoplasma precipitating antibodies and radioisotope uptake of intraocular tumors.[21]

Notes

1. See Frederick C. Blodi, "The History of the National Eye Institute," *American Journal of Ophthalmology* 115 (1993), 420-5, and Ruth Harris, "Brief History of the National Eye Institute," *Government Publications Review* 12 (1985), 427-48.
2. National Institutes of Health Telephone and Service Directories, September 1953–June 1955, ONH.
3. Shy, *NINDB Annual Report, 1954.*
4. Shy, *NINDB Annual Reports, 1955-1959.*
5. Shy, *NINDB Annual Reports, 1955-1958.*
6. Shy, *NINDB Annual Reports, 1954* and *1956.*
7. Shy, *NINDB Annual Reports, 1955, 1956,* and *1958*; Ludwig von Sallmann, *NINDB Annual Report, 1957.*
8. Shy, *NINDB Annual Reports, 1955, 1956,* and *1958.*
9. Shy, *NINDB Annual Reports, 1957* and *1959*; Von Sallmann, *NINDB Annual Reports, 1957* and *1959.*

10. Von Sallmann, *NINDB Annual Report, 1956.*

11. Shy, *NINDB Annual Report, 1955.*

12. Shy, *NINDB Annual Reports, 1955, 1957,* and *1958*; Von Sallmann, *NINDB Annual Report, 1956.*

13. Von Sallmann, *NINDB Annual Report, 1957.*

14. Shy, *NINDB Annual Report, 1956*; Von Sallmann, *NINDB Annual Report, 1956.*

15. Shy, *NINDB Annual Reports, 1956* and *1958*; Von Sallmann, *NINDB Annual Report, 1956.*

16. Shy, *NINDB Annual Report, 1958*; Von Sallmann, *NINDB Annual Report, 1957.*

17. Shy, *NINDB Annual Reports, 1957-1959*; Von Sallmann, *NINDB Annual Report, 1956.*

18. Shy, *NINDB Annual Reports, 1955* and *1958*; Von Sallmann, *NINDB Annual Report, 1956.*

19. Shy, *NINDB Annual Report, 1955*; Von Sallmann, *NINDB Annual Report, 1956.*

20. Shy, *NINDB Annual Report, 1957.*

21. Ibid.

Laboratory of Psychology, NIMH

The original plan was to have two separate psychology laboratories, one in the basic research program and one in the clinical research program. Kety had envisioned a basic Laboratory of Psychology consisting of four sections–Aging, Animal Behavior, Human Behavior, and Special Senses.[1] Cohen had hoped to address the more clinical and developmental aspects of the field of psychology. While Kety relied on Bobbitt, Program Planner, and Eberhart, Extramural Program Director, for advice on possible psychologists, Cohen consulted with Shakow, then a member of the National Mental Health Advisory Council, and relied on the fruitful collaborations and relationships with psychologists that had stemmed from his earlier work in the Department of Defense.[2]

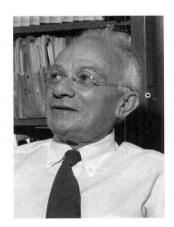

David Shakow, Ph.D.
Donated to the Office of NIH History
by Dr. Morris Parloff

After several unsuccessful hiring attempts for chiefs in both laboratories, Cohen suggested to Kety that the clinical and basic resources be combined and a joint laboratory offered to Shakow. Kety agreed, but

Shakow's acceptance in 1953 was delayed for a year while he recovered from a heart attack. In the meantime, Richard Bell, a psychologist already in the PHS, acted as chief, organizing the laboratory and hiring psychologists until Shakow arrived. The Laboratory of Psychology quickly became the NIMH's largest laboratory.[3]

The first members of the laboratory arrived on the scene in October of 1953. Because some of the hiring of new intramural scientists occurred prior to the completion of the NIH Clinical Center, these scientists were temporarily located in Building T-6.[4]

The laboratory consisted of six sections–Aging, Animal Behavior, and Perception and Learning (within the basic division), and Developmental Psychology, Personality and its Deviations, and the Section of the Chief (within the clinical division)–reflecting the breadth of the field of psychology and the NIMH's expansive mission.[5] In addition to Building T-6, these sections were also located in the Clinical Center, once it opened, as well as in Building 13 and Building T-9–which later became Building 9–where the Section on Animal Behavior housed its animals.

The Section on Aging had actually been created prior to the establishment of the laboratory.[6] Its chief, James E. Birren, had been a member of Nathan Shock's Gerontology Unit within the NHI at the Baltimore City Hospitals. The heavy medical orientation led Birren to approach the NIMH about creating a more behaviorally oriented section. As the Clinical Center was not yet ready to open, he was temporarily assigned to the University of Chicago for three years. When he returned to Bethesda in the summer of 1953, he had recruited an unusually multidisciplinary team–physiologists, neuroanatomists, and psychologists–to work with him in the Section on Aging. The overall purpose of the section was "to identify the primary factors leading to decline in the function and structure of the nervous system with advancing age."[7]

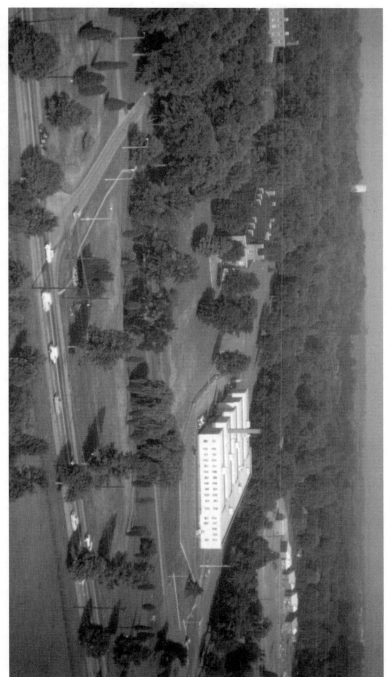

Aerial view of Building T-6 and Building 6
Donated to the Office of NIH History by Dr. Earl Feringa

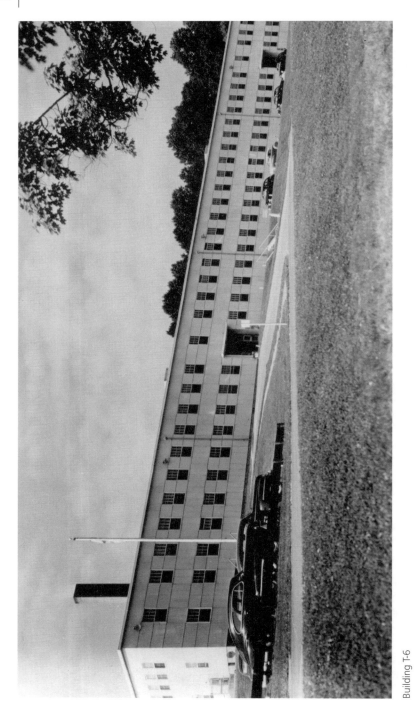

Building T-6
Courtesy of the Office of NIH History

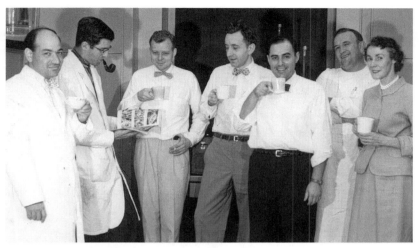

Section on Aging, Laboratory of Psychology, NIMH, late 1950s (left to right: Eugene Streicher, Joseph Brinley, Joel Garbus, James E. Birren, Jack Botwinick, unknown animal caretaker, and Mrs. Oeast, secretary)
Donated to the Office of NIH History by Dr. Jack Botwinick

As a result, its research focused on: 1) behavioral and physiological age-related changes in rats, such as in drive states, nervous tissue, and learning rates; 2) age-related changes in intelligence test performance, specifically with Wechsler Adult Intelligence Scale scores; 3) the relationship of aging to higher cognitive processing; and 4) the research for which the Section is most known, the 1963 book *Human Aging* that resulted from a collaborative effort across three laboratories.[8]

Haldor E. Rosvold, Ph.D.
Donated to the Office of NIH History
by Dr. Mortimer Mishkin

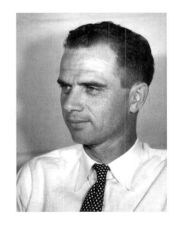

The Section on Animal Behavior consisted of Rosvold, from Yale University, as chief, and its research focused on: 1) the prefrontal cortex in problem-solving and the effects of frontal lobe damage on delayed-response, discrimination, and learning-set tasks; 2) the dorsal and ventral streams in visual information processing, specifically, the relationship of the inferior temporal cortex to the striate cortex in visual discrimination learning; 3) behavioral deficits following brain damage through the Continuous Performance Test; 4) EEG correlates of sustained attentive behaviors in humans; 5) behavioral effects of centrally-acting drugs; 6) cerebral mechanisms underlying functional plasticity; and 7) the neural regulation of appetitive behavior.[9]

Allan F. Mirsky, Ph.D.
Donated to the Office of NIH History by Dr. Mortimer Mishkin

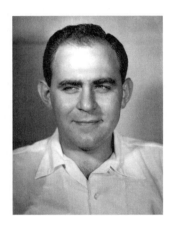

Mortimer Mishkin, Ph.D.
Donated to the Office of NIH History by Dr. Mortimer Mishkin

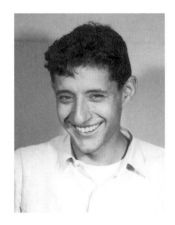

The Section on Developmental Psychology was first led by Nancy Bayley, who had arrived from Berkeley where she had worked on the Berkeley Growth Study evaluating maturational and environmental determiners of personality and development in infancy. This section's research focused mostly on: 1) the development of measures that would quantify parent-child interactions and correlate parent and child personalities with the behavioral, emotional, and intellectual development of children; 2) the intellectual stimulation of culturally-deprived infants; 3) the shaping of an infant's social and exploratory behavior; 4) social deprivation and satiation; and 5) emotional dependence in early childhood.[10]

Virgil "Ben" Carlson had been recruited from the Johns Hopkins University by Bell to head the Section on Perception and Learning. This section's research included: 1) the effects of LSD on visual functions (threshold, constancy, and illusions); 2) the satiation theory of perception; 3) discriminative visual learning (constancy and adaptation) in humans and pigeons; 4) processes involved in stimulus control and stimulus generalization in pigeons; 5) developing a technique for recording eye movements and eye position electronically; and 6) the naturalistic observation of rat behavior such as crowding, sleeping, eating, and exploring in large colonies housed at Poolesville, Maryland.[11]

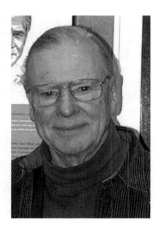

Virgil R. Carlson, Ph.D.
Courtesy of the Office of NIH History

The Section on Personality and its Deviations, soon thereafter shortened to Section on Personality, was led by Morris B. Parloff, whom Cohen recruited from the Johns Hopkins University. This section focused on

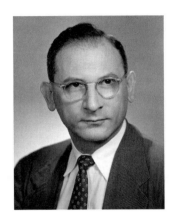

Morris B. Parloff, Ph.D.
*Donated to the Office of NIH History
by Dr. Morris Parloff*

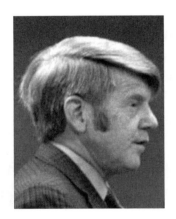

Donald S. Boomer, Ph.D.
Laboratory Member
*Donated to the Office of NIH History
by Dr. Morris Parloff*

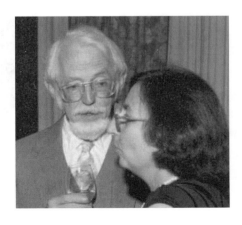

Allen T. Dittmann, Ph.D.
and Irene Waskow, Ph.D.
Laboratory Members
*Donated to the Office of NIH History
by Dr. Morris Parloff*

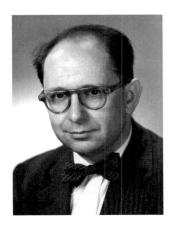

Herbert C. Kelman, Ph.D.
*Donated to the Office of NIH History
by Dr. Morris Parloff*

six areas of research: 1) creativity research, identifying the personality characteristics of creative young scientists; 2) psychotherapy research, including assessing the impact of patient-therapist relationships on the therapeutic outcome, distinguishing specific from common factors in psychotherapy, assessing the role of therapist characteristics in treatment outcome, assessing the therapists' ability to recognize and respond to nonverbal cues, studying the impact of psychotherapy research on health policy, and comparing the efficacy of treatments for major depression; 3) working with the Section of the Chief in videotaping and analyzing a course of psychoanalysis; 4) assessing the therapeutic dynamics and mechanisms of group therapy; 5) measuring the impact of the Clinical Center's and Chestnut Lodge's ward milieus on patients

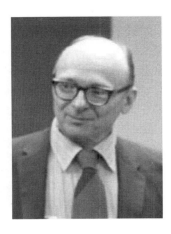

David Rosenthal, Ph.D.
*Donated to the Office of NIH History
by Dr. Morris Parloff*

and staff; and 6) studying the uses and abuses of small group dynamics in family therapy.[12]

Finally, the Section of the Chief and the laboratory as a whole were headed by David Shakow. He had been recruited by Cohen from the Illinois Neuropsychiatric Institute and College of Medicine-University of Illinois. He had previously had a 20-year long career in schizophrenia research at Worcester State Hospital in Massachusetts. This section's research centered mostly on Shakow's interests and focused on three areas: 1) the nature and etiology of schizophrenia, specifically the psychological deficits, the psychophysiological characteristics, and genetic factors contributing to the disorder; 2) the psychotherapeutic process for which Shakow created a psychotherapy sound-movie program, also known as Shakow's Folly, in which a course of psychoanalysis was recorded on film as a resource for individuals interested in research on the therapeutic process; and 3) the psychological aspects of illness, in which self-concept and body image were studied as related to disease susceptibility and resistance and organ choices.[13]

In addition to the Section on Aging's work resulting in the book *Human Aging*, another significant example of the scientist-initiated collaborations at the time was a study among the Laboratory of Psychology's Section of the Chief and four other NIMH laboratories and branches. This study investigated the genetic factors involved in monozygotic quadruplets with schizophrenia, resulting, among many other publications, in the important edited volume, *The Genain Quadruplets*.

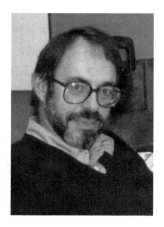

Theodore P. Zahn, Ph.D.
Donated to the Office of NIH History
by Dr. Theodore Zahn

Notes

1. Proposed Organization of Basic Research Program of NIMH and NINDB, August 29, 1952, RG 511, NARA.
2. Cohen, oral history by Farreras, January 18, 2002, transcript, ONH.
3. Upon Shakow's retirement in 1966, this laboratory was renamed the Laboratory of Psychology and Psychopathology, under David Rosenthal. Upon Rosenthal's death in 1975, Allan Mirsky succeeded him as Chief and in 1997 the Laboratory was renamed the Laboratory of Brain and Cognition, under its current chief, Leslie Ungerleider.
4. Morris B. Parloff, oral history interview by Ingrid G. Farreras, January 3, 2002, transcript, ONH.
5. This laboratory was the first joint basic-clinical laboratory established at the NIMH. Although three of its sections were part of the larger basic research program headed by Kety, and the other three were within the clinical research program headed by Cohen, the entire laboratory is described here because Cohen–not Kety–recruited Shakow.
6. See James E. Birren, oral history interview by Ingrid G. Farreras, March 22, 2002, transcript, ONH.
7. *NIH Report, 1951-1952.*
8. See the Laboratory of Clinical Science review for further information.
9. In 1975, this section would become its own laboratory, the current Laboratory of Neuropsychology.
10. David Shakow, *NIMH Annual Reports, 1955-1960.*
11. Shakow, *NIMH Annual Reports, 1956-1960.*
12. Parloff, oral history interviews by Farreras, January 3, 9, and 17, 2002, ONH; Shakow, *NIMH Annual Reports, 1955-1960.*
13. Shakow, *NIMH Annual Reports, 1955-1960.*

Laboratory of Socio-Environmental Studies, NIMH

Prior to the establishment of the intramural research program, John A. Clausen had been a consultant to the NIMH's Professional Services Branch, surveying national attitudes toward mental illness and psychiatry.[1] His research program for the Laboratory of Socio-Environmental Studies (SES) was initiated in 1951 with a project at St. Elizabeths Hospital that investigated factors in family life that influenced the rehabilitation of mental patients.[2] When Kety established the intramural basic research program, the Laboratory of SES was incorporated into it. According to Clausen, the laboratory was based on three propositions about the relationship between mental health or illness and the social order: 1) that life circumstances and relationships with family and friends affect an individual's vulnerability to certain types of mental illness, the precipitation of mental illness, and the duration of such illness; 2) that social organization of mental institutions and the beliefs, attitudes, and behaviors of the staff influence patients' desire and ability to interact with others and cope with their illness; and 3) that the stigma society attaches to mental illness adversely affects the onset of and recovery from the illness as well as an individual's ability to be involved in normal social relationships.[3]

As a result, Clausen envisioned the laboratory's goal to be the study of social norms and processes which influence the development of personality, how they affect a person's ability to carry out normal family, occupational, or community responsibilities and activities, and the way mentally ill individuals are perceived, defined, and dealt with.[4] For this he recruited a multidisciplinary staff consisting of sociologists, social psychologists, and social anthropologists that produced a multiplicity of methodologies, including sample surveys, controlled experiments, participant observation, unstructured interviews, and epidemiological studies.[5]

Toward that goal, the laboratory was made up of four sections, three in the basic research program—the Section of the Chief, the Section on Social Development and Family Studies, and the Section on Community and Population Studies—and one in the clinical research program—the Section on Social Studies in Therapeutic Settings. The Section of the Chief, headed by Clausen, analyzed theoretical and methodological issues in the sociology of mental health and illness and the relationship between social structure and personality. It also studied the impact of mental illness on the family and the adaptation of the mentally ill patient to his or her family upon release from the hospital.[6]

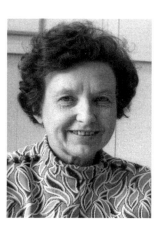

Marian R. Yarrow, Ph.D.
Courtesy of the National Institute of Mental Health

The Section on Social Development and Family Studies was headed by Marian R. Yarrow and focused on the psychosocial factors that influenced an individual's mental health as well as an individual's personality at various stages of development, with an emphasis on childhood and old age. Specifically, some of its studies included: 1) the development of observational techniques to supplement and cross-validate interview techniques assessing interpersonal relationships within the family; 2) assessing the validity of retrospective data on early parent-child relationships and family conditions; 3) assessing how children perceive, evaluate, and respond to others, especially their awareness and sensitivity to the psycho-social characteristics and motives of others; 4) children's development of self-identity and later formation of peer relationships;

5) the influence of maternal employment upon a mother's attitudes about and performance of the maternal role; and 6) the impact of mental illness upon the family, especially of husband-wife communication and interaction in the period preceding hospitalization of either for mental illness.[7]

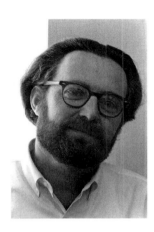

Melvin L. Kohn, Ph.D.
Courtesy of the National Institute of Mental Health

Clausen recruited sociologist Melvin L. Kohn from Cornell University in June 1952 and assigned him to a field research unit in Hagerstown, Maryland, to assess the local distribution of mental illness and social backgrounds of schizophrenic patients hospitalized there.[8] Kohn became head of the Section on Community and Population Studies, which focused on the relationship between the broader aspects of community organization, social structure or cultural dynamics and mental health, personality development and behavior. This involved analyzing important aspects of life in distinct populations, such as socio-economic strata, ethnic origin or community of residence, or common stresses, as can be seen in some of the studies conducted by this section: 1) the relationship between social class and family structure in child-rearing values and practices, personality development, and development of schizophrenia; 2) patient characteristics, treatment with tranquilizing drugs, and duration of hospitalization as predictors of successful release from mental hospitals among first-time functional psychotic admissions; 3) the cultural differences in utilization of community mental health resources; 4) mental deficiency in twins; and 5) the ways in which the meaning of a person's job and career is related to his or her values and emotional and physical health.[9]

Robert A. Cohen, the director of the clinical research program, was interested in having a sociology section within the clinical program as well and thus offered to fund and add clinical positions to the laboratory, making it, in late 1955, the third joint basic-clinical laboratory in the NIMH intramural program.[10] The resulting Section on Social Studies in Therapeutic Settings, headed by Morris Rosenberg, was concerned with the influence of social factors on the forms and effectiveness of treatments provided in mental hospitals, including the patients' adaptation to the hospital world and of the consequences of this for rehabilitation. Specifically, the section studied: 1) the interactions and relationships among patients and between patients and staff in mental hospitals; 2) the adoptions of, attitudes toward, and responses to traditional patient and nursing roles; 3) the social life of the mental hospital patient; 4) the lines of communication and patterns of decision-making in the hospital; 5) the values, norms, and behaviors of administrators, physicians, nurses, attendants, and patients; 6) the relationship between various psychological and social background factors and the chronic schizophrenic's reluctance to affiliate with others; and 7) birth order in schizophrenia.[11] Rosenberg stepped down as section chief in 1959 to join Kohn's Section on Community and Population Studies and pursue research on adolescent self-image and self-ideals and their relationship to tension, depression, and neuroticism as well as values, attitudes, and interpersonal relationships. Anthropologist William Caudill, who joined the laboratory in July 1960, replaced him and studied cultural factors involved in the occurrence and treatment of psychiatric illness in Japan.[12]

The Laboratory of Socio-Environmental Studies was very involved in collaborative research with other branches. In conjunction with the Laboratories of Psychology and of Clinical Science, the section actively studied the interrelationships between psychosocial and physiological conditions in an elderly population. The section also collaborated with four other laboratories and branches in the self-identification, social relationships, and family-community influences in monozygotic quadruplets. The section worked with the Child Research Branch observing and recording acting-out behavior on a ward. Finally, the section was also involved in collaborative research with the Clinical Neuropharmacology Research Center on the social organization and impact of St. Elizabeths Hospital, as well as with the Adult Psychiatry Branch on how normal students successfully cope with stressors.

When Clausen left the NIMH in 1960 to become professor of sociology and Director of the Institute of Human Development at the University of California at Berkeley, Melvin L. Kohn became the new laboratory chief.[13]

Notes

1. National Institutes of Health Telephone and Service Directories, 1949-1951, ONH.
2. *NIH Report, 1951-1952.*
3. John A. Clausen, *NIMH Annual Report, 1955.*
4. Clausen, *NIMH Annual Report, 1959.*
5. Clausen, *NIMH Annual Reports, 1956* and *1959.*
6. Clausen, *NIMH Annual Reports, 1956-1959.*
7. Ibid.
8. See Kohn's chapter, this volume.
9. Clausen, *NIMH Annual Report, 1956-1959.*
10. Clausen, *NIMH Annual Report, 1955*; see Cohen's chapter, this volume.
11. Clausen, *NIMH Annual Report, 1956-1959.*
12. Melvin L. Kohn, *NIMH Annual Report, 1960.*
13. Kohn, *NIMH Annual Report*, 1960. Melvin L. Kohn and Glen H. Elder, "Obituary: John Adam Clausen, 1914-1996," *Society for Research in Child Development Newsletter* (Spring 1996).

Surgical Neurology Branch, NINDB

The Surgical Neurology Branch's major emphasis was on the study of epilepsy and the convulsive process. A multidisciplinary team involving medical and surgical neurologists, clinical psychologists, clinical neuro-physiologists, neuropathologists, and neurochemists approached this study in two ways. One focused on brain physiology and pathology and its relation to epilepsy, specifically looking at the function of the temporal lobe, the etiology of temporal lobe epilepsy, autonomic changes in temporal lobe seizures, and the language and psychological abnormalities that resulted from such seizures.[1] The other focused on the surgical treatment of epileptogenic lesions, in particular, the anatomical effects of temporal lobectomy.[2]

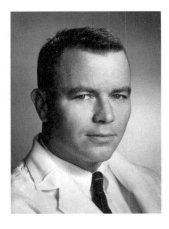

Maitland Baldwin, M.D.
Courtesy of the National Library of Medicine

Neurosurgeon Maitland Baldwin, former student of Wilder Penfield at the MNI, was hired by NINDB institute director Pearce Bailey to head this branch. His Section of the Chief (the Neurosurgical Disorders Service), in addition to the above topics, also studied: 1) neoplasias within the central nervous system and their effect upon visual, autonomic,

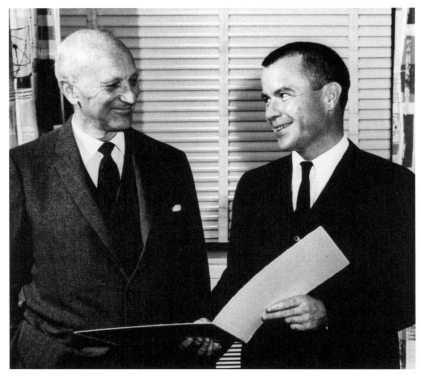

Wilder Penfield, M.D. (left) and Maitland Baldwin, M.D.
Courtesy of the National Institute of Neurological Disorders and Stroke

and physiological anatomical relations; 2) hypophysectomies; 3) function-al anatomy and pathology of the human and visual system, especially the effect of temporal lobectomy on the visual field; 4) altered physiology and treatment of involuntary movements; and 5) electrical stimulation of frontal, temporal, occipital, and parietal cortices.[3]

The branch would come to consist of six more sections by the end of the decade. In 1953 the Section on Clinical Psychology was established, with psychologist Laurence L. Frost at its head. Frost observed patients with temporal lobe seizures in an attempt to determine the effect of seizures on memory, attention, concentration, perceptual behavior, attitude, language, and speech. He also studied the effects of anti-epileptic agents on intelligence. When Frost left the NINDB in 1958 to accept the position of psychologist to the Washington, D.C., Juvenile Court, he was replaced by Herbert Lansdell. Landsell continued the section's research on psychological evaluations of temporal lobe seizure patients as well as on the effect of fear-provoking stimuli on visual discrimination in primates.[4]

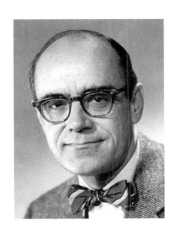

John M. Van Buren, M.D.
Courtesy of the National Institute of Neurological Disorders and Stroke

The Section on Clinical Neuropathology was established in November 1953 with Shy's appointment of Ellsworth C. Alvord, Jr. During the two years that Alvord was chief of the section, he looked at X-ray induced lesions of the central nervous system, at artificial demyelization, and at the "necessity of the sensory-motor area to startle response under light chloralose."[5] When Alvord left for Baylor University in 1955, John M. Van Buren was acting chief until Igor Klatzo arrived in 1956 to replace him as chief of the section. The section, under the new leadership, focused its research on: 1) the analysis of histological and histochemical changes in epileptogenic lesions; 2) the demyelization that followed hypothermia to injured and normal brain tissue; 3) the study of muscles with fluorescent antibody techniques; 4) pinocytosis of labeled proteins in tissue culture; 5) the localization of myosin in human striated muscle; and 6) characteristics of Kuru disease.[6]

Choh-luh Li was chief of the Section on Experimental Neurosurgery, established in 1954 and responsible for research on the functional properties of cortical neurons.[7] More specifically, this section conducted studies involving: 1) the response of motor neurons and denervated muscle to micro-stimulation; 2) microelectrode, intracellular potential

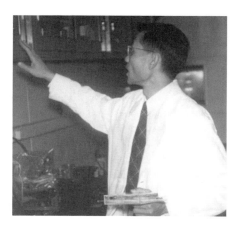

Choh-luh Li, M.D.
Donated to the Office of NIH History by
Dr. Cosimo Ajmone-Marsan

recordings in the epileptic cortex and cells grown in tissue culture of normal and tumor cerebral and cerebellar and muscle tissue; 3) the effects of hypothermia upon the central nervous system and cerebral edema; 4) inhibitory interneurons of the cerebral cortex in the soma-tosensory and visual areas; and 5) stimulation of the cortex by remote radio frequency.[8]

The Section on Developmental Neurology was established in late 1955 to study the developmental anatomy of congenital and early acquired cerebral lesions.[9] Headed by Anatole Dekaban, this section conducted large-scale investigations, in collaboration with local hospitals and using both animal and human subjects, into the abnormalities occurring in the perinatal period.[10] The primary research areas addressed by this section included studying: 1) the site, type, and extent of central nervous system lesions in cerebral palsy; 2) the pathological central nervous lesions that occurred during the prenatal, intranatal, and early postnatal life found in postmortem examinations; 3) the neurological abnormalities in infants born to mothers with diabetes and other conditions; 4) sex differences in external and internal orbital distances throughout life; and 5) the embryology of the mouse brain.[11]

The Section on Pain and Neuroanesthesiology was established in 1956 under the leadership of Kenneth Hall. Its primary emphasis was to study respiratory and blood volume patterns of patients undergoing major intracranial surgery, specifically isolating cerebral hypothermia while leaving the rest of the body under normal temperature.[12] Other research within this section also focused on using Fluothane as an anesthetic agent, anesthesiology and surgical technicology involved in the separation of the craniopagus, and the use of succinyl choline in awake craniotomy.[13] In 1958, Hall resigned and left for an associate professorship in anesthesiology at Duke University.[14] The section remained within the Surgical Neurology Branch although no official chief was appointed thereafter.

Finally, the Section on Primate Neurology was also established in 1956 to study: 1) the effects of specific temporal and frontal excisions on communication capabilities in chimpanzees; 2) the effects of hallucinogenic agents upon higher primates after removal of specific areas of brain; 3) the effects of low temperature on epileptic discharges in the limbic system and on frontal and central cortex electrical activity; 4) deep nuclei of temporal lobe; and 5) the effects of radio frequency energy on primate brain mechanisms.[15]

Notes

1. Shy, *NINDB Annual Reports, 1954-1956, 1958,* and *1959.*
2. Shy, *NINDB Annual Reports, 1954-1956,* and *1958*; Maitland Baldwin, *NINDB Annual Report, 1958.*
3. Shy, *NINDB Annual Reports, 1955-1958* and *1960*; Baldwin, *NINDB Annual Report, 1956.*
4. Shy, *NINDB Annual Reports, 1955, 1958,* and *1959*; Baldwin, *NINDB Annual Reports, 1956, 1958,* and *1959.*
5. Shy, *NINDB Annual Report, 1955,* 5.
6. Shy, *NINDB Annual Reports, 1957-1959*; Baldwin, *NINDB Annual Reports, 1956* and *1958.*
7. Shy, *NINDB Annual Report, 1955.*
8. Shy, *NINDB Annual Reports, 1955* and *1957-1959*; Baldwin, *NINDB Annual Reports,* 1956 and 1959.
9. Baldwin, *NINDB Annual Report, 1956*; Anatole Dekaban, *NINDB Annual Report, 1955.* This Section was originally named the Section on Embryological Neuropathology.
10. Shy, *NINDB Annual Report, 1956.*
11. Baldwin, *NINDB Annual Reports, 1957* and *1958.*
12. Shy, *NINDB Annual Reports, 1956-1958.*
13. Shy, *NINDB Annual Reports, 1957* and *1958*; Baldwin, *NINDB Annual Report, 1958.*
14. Baldwin, *NINDB Annual Report, 1958.*
15. Shy, *NINDB Annual Reports, 1958* and *1959*; Baldwin, *NINDB Annual Reports, 1956, 1958,* and *1959.*

III
Scientists' First-Person Accounts

Mind, Brain, Body, and Behavior
I. G. Farreras, C. Hannaway and V. A. Harden (Eds.)
IOS Press, 2004

Clinical Neurophysiology and Epilepsy in the Early Years of the NINDB Intramural Program*

Cosimo Ajmone-Marsan

A detailed description of the events leading to the creation of a neurological institute within the National Institutes of Health (NIH) in the early fifties, as well as a recounting of the original organizational decisions, professional staffing, and research program outlines through 1959, were provided by the first institute director, Pearce Bailey.[1] Historical data on the development and growth of the institute were contributed by the subsequent institute directors: Richard L. Masland[2] for the years 1959 to 1968 and Edward F. MacNichol, Jr.,[3] for the period from 1968 to 1973.

To summarize briefly Bailey's chronicles, the creation of the original National Institute of Neurological Diseases and Blindness was officially authorized in 1950 and its first director was nominated in the fall of 1951. The institute entered the active planning stage in 1952 with an original budget of less than 2 million dollars. In 1953, there was a sensible increase in the financial appropriations, and clinical and laboratory space were allocated in the new Building 10, the NIH Clinical Center. The institute was officially opened at the end of that calendar year, making it possible to inaugurate a program of intramural clinical investigations.

The philosophical basis of this intramural program–and essentially of analogous programs in all other NIH institutes–was unique and original. The Clinical Center was not a primary or even a specialized care center.

---

* This account is a revised version of the article "National Institute of Neurological Diseases and Stroke, NIH: Clinical Neurophysiology and Epilepsy in the First 25 Years of Its Intramural Program," *Journal of Clinical Neurophysiology* 12 (1995): 46-56, reprinted with the permission of Lippincott Williams & Wilkins.

It was not a structured, teaching institution, as its junior professional staff–consisting of Ph.D.s or M.D.s–had at least completed their residency and, very often, their fellowships. It was a center where basic research was closely integrated with high-level clinical research. Patients were admitted solely as referrals from practitioners around the country, being accepted only if they met certain criteria, i.e., if they were affected by ailments or diseases that happened to fit the field of research interest of each principal investigator at any given time, at the specific institute, or if their disease was included among the current "targets" of the main institute research programs. Patients were offered–free of any charge–the best and most up-to-date care available, but at admission they were asked to sign a very complete informed consent form, outlining a battery of tests, procedures, and treatments, including those that were still in the experimental phase that they were expected to undergo in the course of their hospital stay.

The scientific directors headed the basic research of the intramural program. In the early years of the NINDB, the scientific directorship, under Seymour S. Kety and then Robert B. Livingston, was shared with the National Institute of Mental Health (NIMH). In 1960, when the two institutes became completely independent, the intramural program of NINDB was run by several such scientific directors including, up to 1979, G. Milton Shy, Karl Frank, Henry G. Wagner, and Thomas Chase. Some of them were well-recognized authorities in their fields, leaving a substantial mark on the institute's output; some were also, or mainly, reasonably good administrators.

Shy headed and managed the intramural NINDB clinical research program. Shy and Maitland Baldwin were also selected as the respective chiefs of the Medical Neurology and Surgical Neurology Branches. Both of these investigators had obtained their basic scientific-neurological formation at the Montreal Neurological Institute (MNI). Shy had additional exposure to the British "cradle" of neurology thanks to a year's clerkship at the National Hospital for Nervous Diseases at Queen Square in London. His main interest and expertise was in muscles and peripheral neurology. Baldwin's main training and interest had always been in the surgical treatment of seizure disorders. Both had spent a brief period at the University of Colorado before their NIH recruitment.

Baldwin's heading the Surgical Neurology Branch of the institute illustrated Bailey's intentions to make epilepsy, with an emphasis on this special form of treatment, one of the major areas of research within the intramural program.

In keeping with this specific goal, related branches were established at the end of 1953, such as my Electroencephalography (EEG) Branch. Beginning in 1950, I had spent 18 months collaborating with Herbert H. Jasper, at the MNI, on a number of experimental research projects including a successful *Stereotaxic Atlas of the Cat Diencephalon*.[4] I learned clinical EEG and electrocorticography and actively participated in the selection and work-up of epileptic patients who were potential candidates for surgical treatment. At the end of my fellowship, I accepted a permanent position at the MNI, which I held until the end of 1953 when I accepted Milton Shy's invitation to move to the NIH in January 1954. Shy and Baldwin were familiar with my expertise in epilepsy and surgical treatment, and Laurence L. Frost—the first neuropsychologist who was originally with them in Colorado and had some experience in EEG—was the temporary chief of the branch until I arrived.[5] I remained at the NIH through June 1979, when I left to join the Department of Neurology at the University of Miami.

We were soon joined in 1955 by other MNI alumni with a more or less direct interest in the field of epilepsy. They included, among others: Choh-luh Li, associate neurosurgeon of the Surgical Neurology Branch, Igor Klatzo in the Surgical Neurology Branch's Section on Clinical Neuropathology, and John M. Van Buren, associate neurosurgeon of the Surgical Neurology Branch.

To complete the original NINDB intramural nucleus of scientists with a more or less direct interest in the field of seizures, additional faculty members were recruited who did not come from Montreal. These included Giovanni DiChiro (trained at the then famous neuroradiological School of the Serafinerlazarettet in Stockholm, Sweden), who was invited from Naples to head the Section on Neuroradiology within the Medical Neurology Branch in late 1957; and Paul O. Chatfield, who had worked with Alexander Forbes and Dominick Purpura, to head the Medical Neurology Branch's Section on Clinical Neurophysiology (however, with only a marginal interest in seizure disorders).

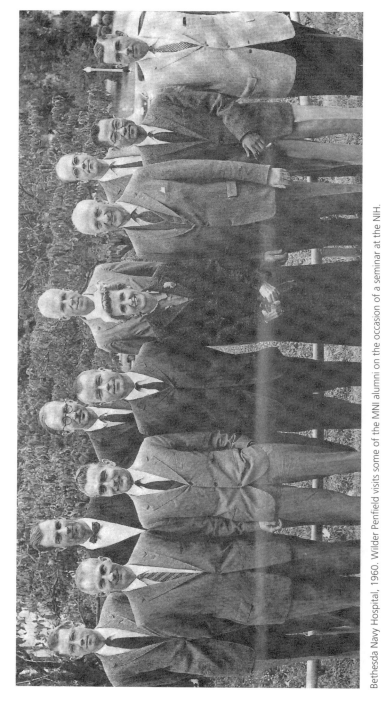

Bethesda Navy Hospital, 1960. Wilder Penfield visits some of the MNI alumni on the occasion of a seminar at the NIH. Left to right, front row: Anatole Dekaban, Cosimo Ajmone-Marsan, Maitland Baldwin, unidentified social worker, Wilder Penfield, Choh-luh Li, and Donald B. Tower. Back row: K. Engel, Robert B. Livingston, Igor Klatzo, Richard L. Masland (second NINDS director), and John Van Buren.

Donated to the Office of NIH History by Dr. Cosimo Ajmone-Marsan

For these relatively young and also for well-established investigators, the greatest advantage of working at the NIH in those early years was the unquestionably high level of the professional scientific surroundings. To a neurophysiologist in particular, the caliber of such specialists, not only at the NINDB but at the NIMH and other institutes, was exceptional. Any researcher needing help had simply to walk a few floors up or down, or just across the corridor from his or her laboratory to find illustrious world authorities like Ichiji Tasaki, Kenneth Cole, Michelangelo Fuortes, Seymour S. Kety, Louis Sokoloff, Wade H. Marshall, Eric Kandel, Karl Frank, Walter H. Freygang, Jr., José del Castillo, Robert B. Livingston, Robert Galambos, Edward V. Evarts, Mortimer Mishkin, Patricia Goldman (later Goldman-Rakic) and Allan F. Mirsky, available and willing to provide advice, guidance, or criticism. Furthermore, the NIH is located at walking distance from the National Naval Medical Research Center and a short drive away from the Walter Reed Medical Center, Georgetown University, and the Johns Hopkins University, the latter also, at that time, a true mecca for neurophysiologists.[6]

Returning to more specific information about investigators closely related to the scientific activities of my branch, Baldwin, in the course of his residency at the MNI, had become one of the preferred pupils and a protégé of Wilder Penfield, pioneer in the surgical treatment of seizure disorders and director of the MNI. Baldwin himself had the greatest admiration for his teacher and made no secret that he aimed to emulate him–albeit it with uneven success–in many endeavors. These included Baldwin's major interest in temporal lobe epilepsy and its surgical treatment, as well as the strict discipline he required of his staff, technicians, and clinical associates, and his highly structured approach to research plans. The fact that he was also a dedicated Marine in the inactive reserve, with exhaustive physical training every weekend, must have contributed to his quasi-militaristic attitude to clinical investigation.

In any case, Baldwin transferred a very similar organizational approach to the field of surgical management of epilepsy from the MNI to the NIH. This approach emphasized a detailed analysis of epileptic seizures, mostly through a careful history and/or a detailed description by patients, their family, and hospital staff,[7] and a close collaboration with electroencephalographers, neuropsychologists, and neuroradiologists. Radiographs consisted mainly of plain X-rays, pneumoencephalographs, and, occasionally, angiograms (these were pre-CT and pre-MRI years!). Final discussion of a case with the presentation of specific findings from each of the various team members took place at weekly "EEG Conferences" in the presence of the patient. As was the case in Montreal, acute electrocorticography monitoring in the course of cortical exposure was routinely performed (see photo below).

This technique played an important role in the outline of the regions to be excised and, in particular, to check for completion or, if necessary, to extend the ablation of such regions after the main excision had been performed. The surgical procedure itself included a protracted period of cortical stimulation studies (with the patient awake and alert), not only to identify important functional areas but also to extend Penfield's original investigations on cortical localization of secondary motor and sensory areas.[8]

Baldwin and his group's interest in the surgery of temporal lobe seizures (the terminology of "partial complex" seizures would be introduced

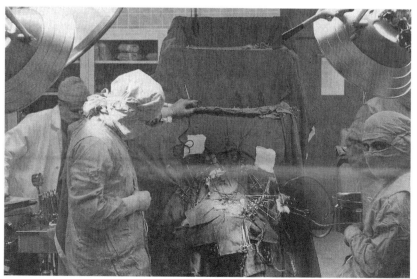

NIH Clinical Center, 1954. The first neurosurgical operating room. Surgeons are Maitland Baldwin (left) and Bruce L. Ralston. Photograph is taken from the window separating the OR unit from the ECoG monitoring room (similar to the original outline at MNI).
Donated to the Office of NIH History by Dr. Cosimo Ajmone-Marsan

a few years later) generated renown among epileptologists in the United States and abroad. As a consequence, Henry Gastaut and Earl A. Walker, respectively president elect and president of the International League Against Epilepsy in late 1954, recommended that the next Temporal Lobe Epilepsy Colloquium (following the first one held in Marseilles in that year) be held at the NIH, hosted and organized by the NINDB. This took place in the spring of 1957 and the proceedings were published soon after.[9]

Another close associate of mine in the investigation of epilepsy mechanisms and treatment was John Van Buren. Van Buren had an excellent clinical preparation and a very solid basis in research.[10] Besides thorough training in neurosurgery with Arthur Eldvidge and Penfield in Montreal and as a senior fellow at the Lahey Clinic in Boston, he had also spent an elective year (1949-50) in experimental neurophysiology with Boris Babkin at the MNI,[11] several months with Jasper in clinical electroencephalography, a six-month clerkship in neurology at the Queen Square Hospital in London, and, after joining the NIH, another year in basic neuronal physiology (intracellular recording) with Karl Frank, chief of the Laboratory of Neurophysiology's Section on Spinal Cord Physiology. Van Buren also possessed a strong scientific and technical background in both microscopic and gross neuroanatomy, obtaining a Ph.D. in this specialty at George Washington University in 1961, and authoring three important books. Ironically, it was rumored that later in the course of his career, an unfair criticism was brought against him by one of the scientific advisors reviewing the activity of his branch. The advisor apparently suggested that he was too much of a neuroanatomist. Clinical Associates who were trained with him during his tenure at the NIH included D. A. Maccubbin, J. G. Ojemann, R. A. Ratcheson, and N. Mutsuga.

Soon after joining the NINDB, Van Buren and I began to utilize this invasive method of investigation in combination with the use of cortical strips or grids whenever justified in the work-up of diagnostically complex patients with intractable seizures, who were otherwise potential candidates for surgery. Part of these results was presented at the above mentioned 1957 colloquium. The use of depth electrography for both recording and stimulation in humans had been pioneered in Boston, the

Mayo Clinic, and Tulane University in the early 1950s. At about the same time the use of permanently implanted leads began at the Johns Hopkins University with Walker and Curtis Marshall[12] and a few years later at the Ste. Anne Hospital in Paris,[13] and eventually at numerous other centers in the United States and abroad. The French investigators, in particular, came to attribute such a crucial role to this invasive, diagnostic method that they used it routinely in practically every epileptic patient who might be a surgical candidate. Many of the present surgical epilepsy centers, such as those at Yale University, Toledo (Ohio), Notre Dame Hospital (in Montreal), and Zurich University medical school have been founded and/or are still directed by investigators who were trained in Paris and who share a similar philosophy.

The activity of the Electroencephalography Branch (later renamed the Clinical Neurosciences Branch) included both clinical and experimental aspects. The clinical aspect of the branch was subdivided into service and research activity. It was the only branch on the NIH campus suitable to provide EEG consultation services to all of the patients of the various institutes located within the NIH Clinical Center. About 50 percent of the referrals originated outside the Surgical Neurology Branch; they included research subjects from the NIMH, the National Cancer Institute, the National Heart and Lung Institute (now National Heart, Lung, and Blood Institute), the National Institute for Arthritis and Metabolic Diseases (now National Institute of Diabetes and Digestive and Kidney Diseases and National Institute of Arthritis and Musculoskeletal and Skin Diseases), and the National Institute of Child Health and Human Development. The branch's research activity included projects originating primarily in the branch itself, and those in collaboration with the main project of surgical epilepsy treatment. The branch, for its first 25 years, was under my continuous direction, the only tenured professional. The other branch members, as indicated above, consisted of Clinical or Research Associates (actually fellows and visiting scientists) who would spend from two to four years at the institute, either collaborating with the branch chief or carrying out independent research under his supervision. The scientific caliber of many of these Research Associates was exceptionally high, as attested by the standard of their publications and, for many, their subsequent careers and current academic positions. Some, among the numerous Associates, are listed, alphabetically, in Table 1 (see also photos on pages 160 and 161).

Table 1. National Institutes of Health, National Institute of Neurological Diseases and Blindness: Electroencephalography Branch Clinical and Research Associates (1950s)

> Kristof Abraham (Hungary)
> D. C. Bienfang
> T. Francis Enamoto (Japan)
> Paul Gerin (France)
> Robert G. Gumnit
> John R. Hughes
> Darrel V. Lewis
> W. R. Lewis
> Gordon R. Long
> Hideo Matsumoto (Japan)
> Arturo Morillo (Colombia)
> Bruce L. Ralston
> Nelson G. Richards
> R. G. Scherman
> Charles E. Wells
> Lennart Widen (Sweden)
> D. L. Winter

Much of the clinical research activity of the EEG Branch was carried out in close cooperation with the Surgical Neurology Branch, utilizing the patient material from the main project of surgery of epilepsy. It had already been stressed by Penfield that the correct localization and delimitation of the functional epileptogenic process were of critical importance in selecting those patients who were the most likely candidates for this type of treatment. Of equal importance was the assessment and identification of the site of onset of ictal episodes, commonly indicated by type and location of aura(s). In an attempt to analyze in greater detail the development of the entire seizure and its variable patterns of spread, a systematic investigation was undertaken, first with Bruce L. Ralston, a young neurosurgeon who was in the very first group of Baldwin's Clinical

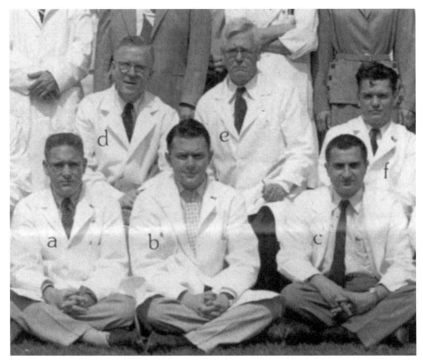

Three members of the earliest group of Clinical Associates, NIH campus, 1955: Charles E. Wells (a), K. Magee (b), and Bruce L. Ralston (c), together with the first clinical director of the NINDB, G. Milton Shy (f) and the first two visiting professors: neuropsychologist D. O. Hebb (d) from McGill University and neuropathologist J. G. Greenfield (e) from Queen Square Hospital
Donated to the Office of NIH History by Dr. Cosimo Ajmone-Marsan

Associates and who was spending an elective year in the branch (see photos on pages 156 and 160), and then with Kristof Abraham, a bright neurologist who had just escaped from the 1956 uprising in Hungary (see photos on pages 161 and 162). This endeavor together with similar sporadic studies carried out in Marseilles at about the same period can be considered the precursors of the so-called epilepsy intensive monitoring.

Lacking the personnel and equipment for a continuous, 24-hour or longer monitoring of a spontaneous epileptic attack, most ictal episodes were initially induced by slow pentylenetetrazol (Metrazol) intravenous injections. This method had become quite popular at that time (beginning around 1949) to induce seizures and/or activate the resting EEG. The technique described by Jasper and Guy Courtois in 1953 was especially popular.[14] The method had obvious advantages but also unquestionable

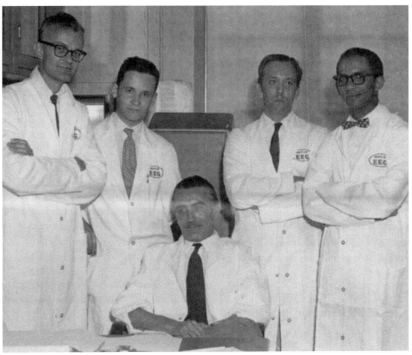

Electroencephalography and Clinical Neurophysiology Branch, NINDB, 1960
Left to right: Research Associates are Lennart Widen, Paul Gerin, Kristof Abraham, and
Arturo Morillo, with the Branch Chief, Cosimo Ajmone-Marsan
Donated to the Office of NIH History by Dr. Cosimo Ajmone-Marsan

disadvantages. Most important was the risk that the procedure might induce a nonspecific seizure (after all, the test had originated as shock therapy to provoke *grand mal* seizures in non-epileptic, psychiatric subjects) or a seizure with different characteristics from those of the spontaneously occurring ictal episodes. Analogously, the drug was likely to produce EEG changes also of a nonspecific, paroxysmal type that could mask the focal features or lead to misinterpretation. At variance from the viewpoint of a number of investigators at that time, the procedure was never considered as a valid one for the *diagnosis* of epilepsy (e.g., by utilizing threshold data or induced EEG changes), but rather it was accepted as a potentially useful procedure to gain additional information of a topographic-localizing nature in an otherwise well-established epileptic patient.

In any case, to increase confidence that the Metrazol-induced seizure was indeed a valid reproduction of those occurring spontaneously in any

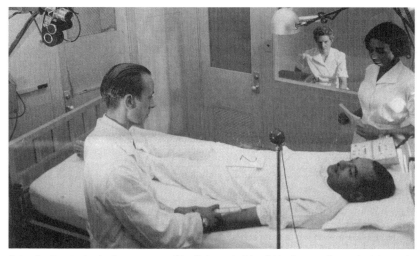

Setup for the study of seizure patterns (details in text). Kristof Abraham performs the Metrazol activation while EEG technologist Barbara Lightfoot assists. In the background is chief EEG technologist Maureen Benson-DeLemos (also trained at the MNI), at the camera control and EEG recording equipment (not shown)
Donated to the Office of NIH History by Dr. Cosimo Ajmone-Marsan

given patient, a careful comparison study was carried out to confirm such an assumption.[15] For this purpose, the patterns of each ictal episode (spontaneous and induced) and their temporal sequence were transformed into "formulas" for a better qualitative and quantitative comparison. By this method, it was possible to accept as quite reliable and specific the large majority of induced seizures. No examples of incorrect lateralization were encountered. The main difference between the two types of seizures was the higher tendency for the induced ones to generalize quickly into major tonic-clonic episodes. The occasional induction of a purely *grand mal* convulsion only led to the conclusion that the activating technique had been of no use for localizing or lateralizing purposes in that patient.

On the basis of these studies it was possible to analyze the variety of seizure patterns and the characteristic pathway of spread from different original foci (see fig. 1), in a large number of subjects with more or less faithful scalp or direct cortical or depth EEG correlations.[16] Beginning in 1955, these studies were carried out, when specifically indicated, in parallel with the use of invasive recording procedures (see above).

The long-suspected limitations of scalp EEG were readily confirmed by simultaneous recording from the various levels.[17] Convincing quantitative and morphologic differences could be demonstrated between the scalp and the cortical or subcortical levels regarding apparent site(s) of origin of the epileptiform discharges. These differences could be quite variable and unpredictable.[18]

Monitoring of the (induced) clinical seizures (see page 162) was performed using a single-frame camera adapted with an electric motor to make it possible to shoot automatically up to 1 frame/s (in practice it was enough to use 1 frame/2 s). The camera was furnished with a 50-foot capacity film magazine so that the entire seizure episode could be photographed without interruption.[19] It is obvious that with this single-frame method certain types of rapid movement were likely to be missed. On the other hand, this method had the great advantage of easy and faithful reproducibility of pictures for detailed analysis and high quality publication, something not easily obtainable with either movie or video techniques. A good correlation with the concomitant electrographic events was facilitated by a simple, properly regulated electronic timer with automatic control of the camera shutter and with a simultaneous

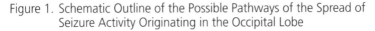

Figure 1. Schematic Outline of the Possible Pathways of the Spread of Seizure Activity Originating in the Occipital Lobe

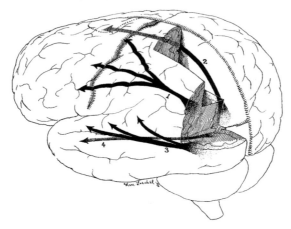

Donated to the Office of NIH History by Dr. Cosimo Ajmone-Marsan

input to the amplifier of one EEG recording channel. This provided a signal that would permit the identification and synchronization of each single frame with the corresponding event in the tracing.[20] Furthermore, because the seizures were induced, the investigator who performed the activation test could continuously dictate all clinical observations. Both the dictation and the patient's answers, or lack thereof, to questions were recorded on the same audio tape for later analysis. This permitted the monitoring of subjective feelings, sensations, aphasic signs, etc., that may have been missed in video monitoring when the observer was not always present.

In the research project dealing with the pre-operative workup for the selection of potential surgical candidates, Van Buren and I placed great importance on the electrographic manifestations of the ictal episode for the correct localization and lateralization of an epileptogenic process. On the other hand, with either scalp or direct electrography, the interictal phenomena were never ignored, and were considered significant, not so much for reaching the correct diagnosis, but rather to decide on prognosis or possible contraindication to surgery. Thus, in the common situation in which there was extensive interictal evidence for bilateral, active and independent epileptogenic processes, a patient might eventually be classified as a poor candidate or as a noncandidate for local temporal ablation, even if the onset of seizures was proven to be consistently only on one side.

Of those involved in surgical treatment of epilepsy, Van Buren et al. were among the first to emphasize the need for a reasonably long post-operative follow-up period, before reliable conclusions can be drawn on the potentially successful results of surgery.[21] Still, at the present time, most published data, with the exception of the MNI school, include a predominance of cases with post-operative follow-ups of from six months to less than two years. The NINDS experience, derived from the study of over 120 temporal lobe epileptics, seems to suggest that a minimum of four years of follow-up is required, before concluding the surgical procedure was a "total success." Indeed one may find up to 63 percent of patients seizure-free during the first post-operative year. However, this percentage may fall to less than 25 percent after 10 years or longer of follow-up.

The experimental aspect of the Electroencephalography Branch included some interesting studies on the physiology of the visual system, on callosal interactions, and on thalamocortical mechanisms, but the main investigative goals were focused, from the very beginning, on the basic neuronal mechanisms underlying the electrographic changes that are considered the expression of epileptic activity. Through the years, starting in 1954, and in collaboration with many of the Research Associates whose names are listed in Table 1, various experiments were designed using models to mimic acute seizure disorders in the cat and the monkey, with emphasis on: (a) models that would reproduce the interictal and ictal manifestations of focal cortical epileptogenic processes; (b) models that might throw some light on possible subcortical mechanisms for primary generalized seizure disorders; and c) models to analyze patterns of electrographic seizure activity and those at the basis of seizure onset, or transition from interictal phenomena. Most of these investigations utilized extra- and intracellular microelectrodes for recording cortical and subcortical structures. In addition, several chemical substances were either systemically administered, topically applied, or iontophoresed to reproduce epileptiform phenomena. Repetitive electrical stimulation leading to after discharges was also utilized.

The results from these various studies were published between 1955 and 1980. Studies by T. Francis Enamoto and I[22] and Hideo Matsumoto and I,[23] dealing with analysis of the neuronal events underlying the occurrence of the so-called "EEG spike," demonstrated that in an acute epileptogenic focus produced by topical application of strychnine or penicillin, there is a high degree of synchronization in the firing of most neurons within the local population affected by the epileptogenic agent, in correspondence with, and obviously resulting in, the surface cortical EEG spike. This confirmed Jasper's "hypersynchronization" theory. However, this "spike," is not a simple "envelope" of action potentials, but rather the summation of large, and relatively long-duration shifts of depolarization undergone paroxysmally by the membrane of the individual neurons (see fig. 2), often followed by considerable hyperpolarizing shifts.

This was the first systematic analysis and description of these characteristic membrane modifications and cellular events within the (acute) epileptogenic process. Some of these phenomena had been described by

Goldensohn and Purpura at about the same time[24] and had been hy-pothesized by Bremer in the early forties as part of the strychnine effects.[25]

Figure 2. Paroxysmal Depolarization Shift

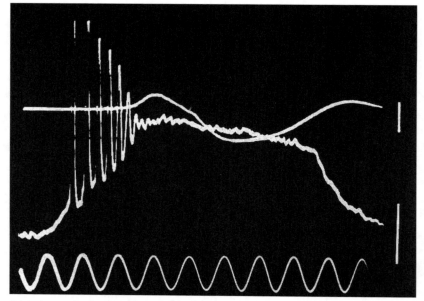

Original example of "paroxysmal depolarization shift" (lower channel), obtained from intracellular recording of a cortical neuron in a cat, following surface topical application of penicillin. (Calibrations: 1&10 mV and 100 c/s).
Donated to the Office of NIH History by Dr. Cosimo Ajmone-Marsan

Notes

1. Pearce Bailey, "National Institute of Neurological Diseases and Blindness: Origins, Founding, and Early Years (1950 to 1959)," in *The Nervous System: A Three-Volume Work Commemorating the 25th Anniversary of the National Institute of Neurological and Communicative Disorders and Stroke, Vol. 1: The Basic Neurosciences,* ed. Donald B. Tower and Roscoe O. Brady (New York: Raven Press, 1975), xxi-xxxii.

2. Richard L. Masland, "National Institute of Neurological Diseases and Blindness: Development and Growth (1960-1968)," *Ibid.,* xxxiii-xlvi.

3. Edward F. MacNichol, Jr., "National Institute of Neurological Diseases and Stroke (1968-1973)," *Ibid.,* xlvii-lii.

4. Herbert H. Jasper and Cosimo Ajmone-Marsan, *A Stereotaxic Atlas of the Diencephalon of the Cat* (Ottawa: National Research Council of Canada, 1954).

5. Frost was also chief of the NINDB Surgical Neurology Branch's Section on Clinical Psychology.
6. Ernst Niedermeyer, "EEG and Clinical Neurophysiology at the Johns Hopkins Medical Institutions: Roots and Development," *Journal of Clinical Neurophysiology* 10 (1993): 83-8.
7. Video monitoring was not yet fully developed in the early 1950s.
8. In 1965, after Shy left the NIH to become chairman of the Department of Neurology at the University of Pennsylvania and then–for a too-brief period–at Columbia University, Baldwin became clinical director of the NINDB intramural program. He assumed greater administrative duties and delegated progressively more and more surgical activity and responsibilities to John Van Buren, who had joined the NIH in 1955.
9. Maitland Baldwin and Pearce Bailey, eds., *Temporal Lobe Epilepsy: A Colloquium* (Springfield, Illinois: Charles C. Thomas, 1958).
10. In 1970, after Baldwin's sudden, premature death, Van Buren was named acting chief of the Surgical Neurology Branch, and in 1972 became chief in his own right. Van Buren continued Baldwin's main research interests, while extending the surgical approach to other forms of focal cortical (i.e., extratemporal) seizures, as well as to the management of involuntary movements, in keeping with the fashionable interest of that time, especially popularized by Irving Cooper of St. Barnabas Hospital in New York. Although the latter type of surgical activity was relatively short-lived, it provided a good opportunity for gathering information on stereotactic localization of anatomical targets. It allowed extensive investigations on thalamus and other subcortical structures in humans and on their topographical variations (see, e.g., the impressive two-volume monograph by Van Buren and Borke: John M. Van Buren and R. C. Borke, *Variations and Connections of the Human Thalamus* (New York: Springer-Verlag, 1972)), and yielded interesting information on the results of electrical stimulation of many such structures and their interconnections. Stimulation was carried out during simultaneous recording, prior to the coagulation of specific targeted structures.

    Of primary significance for the surgery of epilepsy, however, this therapeutic investigation in the field of involuntary movements allowed Van Buren to develop a practical type of stereotactic apparatus, and to identify reliable and consistent anatomic/radiologic landmarks that could be utilized for the placement of chronically implanted deep electrode sets. In collaboration with Ajmone-Marsan, he also demonstrated, by the same approach, that there was no evidence of interictal epileptiform activity in any of the records derived from multiple insertions of such electrodes in a number of different cortical and subcortical structures of over 40 patients affected by abnormal movements but *without* seizure disorders. It was thus apparent that the suspected acute "injury" effects, by insertion of needle electrodes into the brain, do not commonly mimic electrographic epileptiform phenomena, at least within *nonlimbic* structures.

11. William Feindel, "Brain Physiology at the Montreal Neurological Institute: Some Historical Highlights," *Journal of Clinical Neurophysiology* 9 (1992): 176-94.

12. Michel Ribstein, "Exploration du Cerveau Humain par Electrodes Profondes," *Electroencephalography and Clinical Neurophysiology* Suppl 16 (1960): 1-129.

13. J. Bancaud, J. Talairach, A. Bonis, et al., *La Stéréo-Electroencéphalographie dans l'Epilepsie* (Paris: Masson, 1965).

14. Herbert H. Jasper and Guy Courtois, "A Practical Method for Uniform Activation With Intravenous Metrazol," *Electroencephalography and Clinical Neurophysiology* 5 (1953): 443-4.

15. Cosimo Ajmone-Marsan and Bruce L. Ralston, *The Epileptic Seizure: Its Functional Morphology and Diagnostic Significance* (Springfield, Ill: Charles C. Thomas, 1957).

16. Ibid.

17. Cosimo Ajmone-Marsan and John Van Buren, "Epileptiform Activity in Cortical and Subcortical Structures in the Temporal Lobe of Man," in Baldwin and Bailey, eds., *Temporal Lobe Epilepsy: A Colloquium.*

18. Kristof Abraham and Cosimo Ajmone-Marsan, "Patterns of Cortical Discharges and Their Relation to Routine Scalp Electroencephalography," *Electroencephalography and Clinical Neurophysiology* 10 (1958): 447-61.

19. Video TV recording would not be developed until several years later.

20. Cosimo Ajmone-Marsan and Kristof Abraham, "A Seizure Atlas," *Electroencephalography and Clinical Neurophysiology* Suppl. no. 15 (1960).

21. John M. Van Buren, Cosimo Ajmone-Marsan, N. Mutsuga, and D. Sadowsky, "Surgery of Temporal Lobe Epilepsy," in *Neurosurgical Management of the Epilepsies*, eds. D. P. Purpura, J. K. Penry, and R. D. Walter (New York: Raven Press, 1975), 25-33.

22. T. Francis Enamoto and Cosimo Ajmone-Marsan, "Epileptic Activity of Single Cortical Neurons and Their Relationship With Electroencephalographic Discharges," *Electroencephalography and Clinical Neurophysiology* 11 (1959): 199-218.

23. Hideo Matsumoto, Cosimo Ajmone-Marsan, "Cortical Cellular Phenomena in Experimental Epilepsy: Interictal Manifestations," *Experimental Neurology* 9 (1964): 286-304; Hideo Matsumoto and Cosimo Ajmone-Marsan, "Cortical Cellular Phenomena in Experimental Epilepsy: Ictal Manifestations," *Experimental Neurology* 9 (1964): 305-26.

24. 1963.

25. Frédéric Bremer, "Le Tétanos Stychnique et le Mécanisme de la Synchronization Neuronique," *Archives of International Physiology* 51 (1941). See also Daniel Pollen and Cosimo Ajmone-Marsan, "Cortical Inhibitory Post-Synaptic Potentials and Strychninization," *Journal of Neurophysiology* 28 (1965): 342-58.

Mind, Brain, Body, and Behavior
I. G. Farreras, C. Hannaway and V. A. Harden (Eds.)
IOS Press, 2004

The Section on Aging of the Laboratory of Psychology in the NIMH During the 1950s

James E. Birren

These are my personal observations about the history of the 1950s at the National Institute of Mental Health (NIMH) with some documentation about the context of research on aging. In 1946 I had received a year's fellowship from the National Institutes of Health (NIH) to complete my Ph.D. at Northwestern University. What was curious about it was that I was asked to make an appointment in the spring of 1946 to meet the NIH director. Imagine today, with the volume of fellows, having a predoctoral candidate calling on the NIH director! I recall the director asked me why I described myself as an experimental psychologist since he assumed all researchers were experimentalists. My answer must have been plausible since I received the fellowship.

In the fall of 1947, I joined the staff of the Gerontology Center at the Baltimore City Hospitals under the direction of Nathan Shock. Nathan Shock told me he arrived in Baltimore to start the gerontology research program on Pearl Harbor Day, December 7, 1941. He had been doing research for ten years on child development at the University of California at Berkeley. It is relevant that he had both a psychologist and a biologist on his Ph.D. Committee at the University of Chicago–Lewis Thurstone and A. Baird Hastings–who later joined the faculty at the Harvard University Medical School.

The program in gerontology was quickly derailed on behalf of war-related research until the end of the war. Then Nathan Shock recruited me as a psychologist along with other staff members to carry out research on aging. I was at the Baltimore unit for three years and, among other research on aging, I studied the rate and level of adaptation to the dark in relation to age. I borrowed the dark adaptation equipment from a staff member of the Institute of Experimental Biology and Medicine at the NIH, an institute that no longer exists. The findings were that the rate of dark adaptation did not change with age although the level did. I became interested in adaptation to the dark because a member of the Naval Research Staff had used the same equipment and had used me as a young control subject when I was in my late 20s in the Navy. The question being asked then was whether a nasal spray of vitamin A, or its precursor, beta carotene, would enhance the night vision of combat troops. The head of the project found that the nasal spray was not effective.

I wanted to broaden my perspective on the effects of aging on behavior and the nervous system and asked to be transferred to the NIMH. This was done in 1950, and I was assigned to do research on aging at the University of Chicago during the time that the research facilities of the NIMH were being built. The massive Building 10–the NIH Clinical Center—was being constructed that would house both laboratory and clinical research from all of the institutes. In 1953, I arrived at the new NIMH facilities and was assigned to the Laboratory of Psychology, as chief of the Section on Aging. Looking back, I see that my model of the organization of research on aging was multidisciplinary and was somewhat different than that of many of my contemporary colleagues.

The Context of Research on Aging in the 1950s

At that time there was a shifting emphasis in the Public Health Service (PHS) from the infectious diseases of the 1930s to the chronic diseases in the 1950s. This change put the human organism in the role of a contributor or a cause of illness rather than as a host to an invading foreign agent. This emphasis was expressed in the efforts of the Josiah Macy, Jr., Foundation, particularly in its support of the publication of E. V. Cowdry's influential volume, *Problems of Ageing*.[1] The Josiah Macy, Jr., Foundation later supported the PHS's conference on "Mental Health in Later Maturity" in May 1941. The conference, addressed by the Surgeon General, was attended by biologists, physicians, psychiatrists, psychologists and other disciplines, reflecting the growing awareness that problems associated with aging involve many scientific disciplines and many professions. This emerging broad orientation toward the processes of aging was later reflected in a publication of the Social Science Research Council:

> The study of the biological processes involved in the decline of functions through tissue aging or disease is not the task of the social scientist but of the biochemists, the physiologist, and the medical or psychiatric research worker. However, the effect of these biological processes of aging on the individual's capacities for participation in various activities is the concern of the student of social adjustment. It is evident that the understanding and correction of problems of adjustment arising from declining physical and mental powers call for the application of knowledge of both biological and social science.[2]

This view reflected a growing organismic perspective about the biological, environmental, and behavioral factors contributing to aging. Recognition of the nervous system as the primary regulatory organ of the body was also emerging, a regulatory role that could influence the health of an aging organism in many ways. When the Section on Aging was developed, it had a physiologist, a neuroanatomist, and several psychologists reflecting a multidisciplinary view of aging. Perspectives surrounding research on aging were somewhat broader than those of other problem areas.

The NIMH Climate of Growth in the 1950s

The subjective side of research productivity is often overlooked as the methods and products of research are focused upon. When I joined the NIMH, I was impressed with the optimistic climate. The three senior staff of the NIMH were Robert H. Felix, Joseph Bobbitt, and Seymour D. Vestermark. In a humorous vein they were known as the Id, the Ego, and the Super Ego, in that order. Their personal qualities complemented each other and their effectiveness as a team contributed to the progress of the institute. The clinical intramural research was the domain of

Robert A. Cohen and the basic intramural research was the domain of Seymour S. Kety.

In general, the clinical climate was not overly favorable to encouraging research on aging since there was a dominant psychoanalytic perspective that personality and character were laid down in the first few years of life and adult life was an acting out of the scenario laid down in those early years. Freud did not believe that psychotherapy was useful for persons over the age of 50 since so much material had to be recalled and digested. However, another psychoanalyst, Jung, held that an individual did not have enough experience to review effectively until 50 or more years had passed. In the early 1960s, Robert Butler and I presented a proposal to the intramural NIMH research program that a Laboratory on Aging be created. The proposal was turned down and we were left with the impression that perhaps the psychoanalytic perspective was the reason, although other considerations may have influenced the decision.

The National Institute of Child Health and Human Development was then created in 1963, with research on both early development and aging on its agenda. This indicated that research on aging was emerging as a priority area. In 1975, the National Institute on Aging was created as a further expression of the growing awareness that the study of aging was of both scientific and public importance.

The NIMH Study of Healthy Elderly Men

A major research project developed from an informal conversation Louis Sokoloff and I had while we were walking from Building 10 to Building 1 for another purpose. He mentioned his interest in finding out what changes there were in healthy, older men in their cerebral blood flow and cerebral metabolism. Having the techniques in his laboratory to measure them, it was possible to develop a project that would recruit healthy, older men to participate in a broad range of measurements of physiological, intellectual, motor, and social psychological variables. With the active interest of other colleagues in the NIMH, the project evolved into a significant multi-laboratory and multidisciplinary research project on human aging. Healthy men over the age of

65 were recruited as volunteers to be residents in the NIH Clinical Center for two weeks each. During the two weeks, numerous laboratories made physical, physiological, psychological and social assessments of the volunteers. This was one of the earliest attempts to distinguish healthy aging in contrast to the debilitating effects of specific diseases associated with advancing age. The comprehensive report of the completed research project included the details of the many measurements that were made on the sample of healthy older men and was well received.[3]

Of the many findings of the project, an important one was that cerebral circulation and metabolism were not significantly lower in the healthy older men compared with what was normal for younger men.[4] Earlier studies that reported reductions with age were likely influenced by use of residents of facilities for the aged who were not representative of the healthy, elderly population. Another finding was that psychosocial losses experienced by the healthy, elderly subjects were reflected in their physiological status. This finding corroborated the view that not only do biological influences affect the mental well being of aging individuals but also that psychosocial events influence health and physical well being.[5]

Section on Aging Research

In addition to participation in the comprehensive study of the healthy, elderly men, the Section on Aging conducted numerous other research projects in humans and also in rats. The section maintained a rat colony, the Fisher strain, throughout the life span of the rats. This colony provided the basis for conducting behavioral and biological studies of aging in the rats and also for following up features of human aging that might have related processes or analogues in the rat population.

William Bondareff, a neuroanatomist, examined many features of the rat's aging nervous system, including the deposit of pigment in the cells of the spinal ganglia.[6] His research is summarized in his chapter on the morphology of the aging nervous system in the volume edited by me.[7]

Eugene Streicher, a physiologist, did pioneering research on the aging of the nervous system of aging rats. He studied the distribution of mineral content in the brains of aging rats. Later, with Joel Garbus, he explored the role of the mitochondria in the cells of aging rats. This topic is still in the forefront of research on the physiology of aging since the mitochondria are the sources of energy for an organism.

Jack Botwinick, a psychologist, introduced the study of the role of mental set in learning. He found that older adults had a lower anticipatory set or expectancy for a stimulus.[8] In another of his studies he found that in conditioning and extinction of the galvanic skin response, older subjects conditioned less readily but also extinguished more quickly than young subjects.[9] This suggests a lower level of arousal in the older subjects. Edward Jerome conducted a series of learning experiments in an attempt to identify differences in human learning behavior with aging.[10]

One of the four main interests of the section's research program was investigating the slowing of behavior widely observed in older persons. Early investigators tended to attribute the slowing to either sensory input deficiency or to motor output mechanisms. Such views tended to minimize the role of changes in the central nervous system itself as a source of the slowing. Summarizing a large amount of research conducted in the Section on Aging, findings showed that the major source of the slowness was in the nervous system itself and not in the peripheral nerve conduction velocity or in sensory or perceptual input. The research came to be recognized as a major contribution to the understanding of the behavioral changes of aging and the linking of brain function with specific intellectual and psychomotor behaviors.

One of the technical developments was the design and construction of an instrument in the then pre-computer age for measuring the difference in the speed of response to the complexity of stimuli. The instrument was designed and built within the NIMH facilities. It was called the Psychomet and it made it possible to hold constant the response conditions while altering the complexity of the stimuli to which the subject had to react. Based on the use of the Psychomet, experiments by myself, Klaus Riegel and Donald Morrison[11] added to the growing recognition that there was a general psychophysiological factor of speed in the functioning of the central nervous system that became slower with advancing age. From the viewpoint of the neurophysiology of the aging nervous system, it suggested that a property of the brain was changed resulting in a generalized slowing that was involuntary and not under the control of the individual. A later review article suggested that the slowing in behavior could be attributed to changes in the basal ganglia. This included the slowing of initiation and execution of movements as well as intellective processes.[12]

Visiting Scientists

During the 1950s and the early 1960s, there were several visiting researchers who spent a year in residence at the NIMH in the Section on Aging doing research. Two of them were professors from British universities, Patrick M. A. Rabbitt, and Harry Kay. They both returned to Britain and continued their interest in research on aging, with Patrick Rabbitt specializing in cognitive aging. Asser Stenback, a psychiatrist from Helsinki, Finland, was interested in mental health and aging in relation to physical disease. Klaus and Ruth Riegel, both psychologists from Germany, were also visiting scientists and were active in research on both the speed of behavior and other aspects of behavioral changes associated with aging. In addition to his empirical research, Klaus Riegel did an analysis of the growth of research on aging. His analysis of the literature showed that during the decade of the 1950s as much literature was published on the psychology of aging as had been published in the prior one hundred

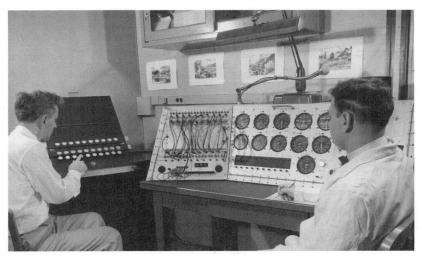

James Birren and Joseph Brinley, 1958, with the Psychomet
Donated to the Office of NIH History by Dr. James E. Birren

years.[13] Clearly the 1950s initiated a dramatic growth era of research on the psychology of aging and the Section on Aging played an active role in the emerging era and the defining of important research issues. After he left the Section on Aging, Klaus Riegel became professor of psychology at the University of Michigan and both he and Ruth Riegel remained active in research on the behavioral aspects of aging.

The Gerontology Discussion Group

An informal Gerontology Luncheon Group was formed with initiative from the Section on Aging. Its first meeting was February 18, 1954, in the snack bar of the NIH Clinical Center. About forty NIH scientists requested that their names be on the mailing list. As it evolved, its name was changed to the Gerontology Discussion Group. It met every two weeks and both intramural and extramural personnel attended (see Appendix 1). The topics ranged from cellular phenomena of aging to the aging of insects and the social issues of human aging (see Appendix 2). The Discussion Group provided an informal pathway for the exchange of information about aging across institutes and between intramural and extramural staff members. An indication of the openness of information exchange is seen, for example, in the fact that, on June 1954, Richard Williams, of the extramural division of the NIMH, presented a draft paper to the discussion group on "Preliminary Planning of Program Development on Mental Health Aspects of Aging."

The Gerontology Discussion Group encouraged personnel contacts across laboratories and institutes at the NIH and also contacts with outside scientists at a time when the published literature was still relatively small and there were not many national meetings on the subject matter. The Gerontology Discussion Group began to invite scientists from outside the NIH who were visiting Washington, D.C., including some from abroad, to present their specialized views of aging and their findings. Appendix 2 contains the names of presenters and the titles of their talks at many of the meetings held between 1954 and 1958. The discussion group met twice a month until 1957, when the director of the Center on Aging of the National Heart Institute, G. Halsey Hunt, suggested that it meet once a month.

Relations with Extramural Activities

Research publications on aging were increasing as interest was shifting from the earlier period of dominance of interest in infectious diseases because of the impact on children to an emphasis on chronic diseases common to middle aged and older adults. The NIMH extramural program sponsored a conference on the "Psychological Aspects of Aging" that was organized by the American Psychological Association. It was held in 1955 at the Stone House on the NIH grounds. Both intramural and extramural personnel were involved. In a sense, the conference marked the emergence of a new generation of researchers on aging whose entire careers were devoted to the study of aging, in contrast to the few earlier investigators who began in other fields of study.

It is of interest that several of the pioneers in the area of research on child development attended and were influential in determining the agenda: for example, John Anderson, University of Minnesota; Raymond Kuhlen, Syracuse University; Harold Jones, University of California, Berkeley; and Sydney Pressey, Ohio State University. They were expanding their concepts of change during the adult years in relation to the processes of development in childhood they had studied. John Anderson, one of the leaders in research on child development, chaired the conference and was editor of the report.[14]

A further step in the expansion of interest in research on aging was the 1957 conference on aging supported by the National Institute of Neurological Diseases and Blindness (NINDB). It was also held on the grounds of the NIH with attendance of both intramural and extramural personnel. The editors of the conference report were from both the NINDB and the NIMH.[15]

Political Climate of the 1950s

With the rise of Joseph McCarthy's influence in the U.S. Senate there were reverberations at the local level. As an example, I received a telephone call from the NIMH personnel office asking me if one of the staff scientists of the Section on Aging had belonged to the National Association for the Advancement of Colored People (NAACP) when he was an undergraduate student. Presumably, this was suspicious activity in the political climate of the era. When I inquired of my colleague, he said that, yes, he had been a member and that the university chaplain had recruited students to the NAACP. He joined up but said he had not been active in the association since he left Syracuse University. I was puzzled by the request and its status, so I inquired of a lawyer who was familiar with the courts, what I should do about a telephone inquiry of this character. He suggested that I ask the personnel officer to put his request in writing and then say I would put my reply in writing. When I phoned the personnel officer to tell him of my position, he said "That is a great idea." I never heard any more about it. Presumably, the hierarchical system did not want to go on record asking questions of this sort in writing since it would be an apparent invasion of privacy.

A second episode of this sort in the 1950s involved a psychologist I knew who was employed by the military. When I phoned him, he said, "Don't call me, my phone is being tapped." He was later discharged from government service. This was attributed to the fact that he refused to testify about the political background of his wife's first husband when called before a hearing by McCarthy. The psychologist recovered from the loss of his government position and later became professor of psychology at Yale University, but the disruption resulting from the termination of his government employment was very unsettling.

Conclusion

The 1950s were years of expansion of research in the NIMH, and the Section on Aging was active contributing research findings to a growing literature on aging. The productivity of the Section on Aging was encouraged by the climate of optimistic support of research by the NIMH and its leadership. The section's research contributed to the replacement of earlier simplistic assumptions about the nature of aging through its many publications. The section's research also contributed to modifying the idea of an inevitable and universal pattern of decline with age in mental capacities. What was coming to be apparent was that aging was a complex set of processes, one of the most complex areas of research facing science in the 21st century.

Appendix 1
Gerontology Luncheon Group Members (February 12, 1954)

James E. Birren (Building 10)
Kathryn Knowlton (Building 3)
James Hundley (Building 4)
Thelma Dunn (Building 8)
Alexander Symeonidis (Warwick Clinic)
David Scott (Building 4)
Eugene Streicher (Building 10)
Richard C. Arnold (Building 3)
Harold Dorn (Building 1)
Leon Sokoloff (Building T-6)
Richard Williams (Building T-6)
Olaf Mickelson (Building 4)
Nathan Shock (Section on Gerontology,
    Baltimore City Hospitals, Baltimore, Maryland)
Joseph Bunim (Building 10)
Wilton Earle (Building 6)
Wilhelm Hueper (Building T-6)
James Watt (Building 3)
Leroy Duncan (Building 10)

William Carrigan (Building 1)
Donald Watkin (Building 10)
Eleanor Siperstein (Building 6)
Monte Greer (Building 10)
Harold M. Fullmer (Building T-6)
Evelyn Anderson (Building 10)
Robert Resnik (Building 10)
Albert Russell (Building T-6)
Joseph Bobbitt (Building T-6)
David Shakow (Building 10)
Seymour Perlin (Building 10)
Charles Huttrer (Building T-6)
Nancy Bayley (Building 10)
Seymour S. Kety (Building 10)
Wade H. Marshall (Building 10)
John Calhoun (Building 10)
Haldor E. Rosvold (Building 10)
Harold Halpert (Building T-6)

Appendix 2
Gerontology Luncheon Group Speakers

January 6, 1954
Jan Cammermeyer, Chief, Section on Experimental Neuropathology, Laboratory of
Neuroanatomical Sciences, NINDB
"Informal Discussion on Neuropathological Changes of Aging"

January 20, 1954
Seymour S. Kety, NIMH
"Age Changes in Brain Circulation and Metabolism"

March 3, 1954
Evelyn Anderson
"Discussion of chapters in Cowdry's *Problems of Ageing*, 3rd ed., 1952, on endocrine aspects
(chapters 15, 16, 17)"

March 17, 1954
Katherine Snell, NCI
"Discussion of Pathological Changes in Aging Rats"

April 7, 1954
Laurence Frost, Chief, Section on Clinical Psychology, Medical Neurology Branch, NINDB
"Some Physiological and Psychological Aspects of Aging"

April 21, 1954
Joel Garbus, Section on Aging, Laboratory of Psychology, NIMH
"A Discussion of the Literature of the *In Vitro* Metabolism of Aging Tissues"

April 22, 1954
James E. Birren, Chief, Section on Aging, Laboratory of Psychology, NIMH
"Age Changes in Mental Organization"

May 6, 1954
Kathryn Knowlton
"Anabolic Response to Testosterone at Various Ages"

October 7, 1954
Albert Lansing
"A Biologist Looks at Aging of the Nervous System"

October 21, 1954
James E. Birren, Chief, Section on Aging, Laboratory of Psychology, NIMH
Nathan Shock, NHI (Baltimore City Hospitals)
"A Report on the International Gerontological Congress, held in London, July 19-23"

November 4, 1954
Nancy Bayley, Section on Developmental Psychology, Laboratory of Psychology, NIMH
"A 30-year Follow-up Study of Termen's Gifted Children"

November 18, 1954
Eugene Streicher, Section on Aging, Laboratory of Psychology, NIMH
"Age Changes in the Physiology of the Nervous System"

December 2, 1954
Paul Stevenson, NIMH
"Informal Discussion of Some Major Problems in the Field of Aging"

December 16, 1954
James Hundley, NIAMD
"Nutritional Aspects of Aging"

February 3, 1955
John Calhoun, Laboratory of Psychology, NIMH
"A Panel Discussion on Maturational and Aging Problems in Animals"

March 18, 1955
Drs. Duncan and Watkins
"Metabolism of Aging"

April 26, 1955
Herbert Landahl, Associate Professor of Mathematical Biology, University of Chicago
"Biomathematical Studies of the Nervous System and Some Implications for the
Investigation of Aging"

November 3, 1955
J. W. Still, Department of Physiology, George Washington University
"A Theory of Aging"

November 17, 1955
Leon Sokoloff, NIAMD
"Aging of Articular Tissues in Rats"

December 1, 1955
Barry G. King, Medical Division, CAA
"Problems of Aging in Commercial Airline Pilots"

December 15, 1955
Nathan Shock, NHI
James E. Birren, Chief, Section on Aging, Laboratory of Psychology, NIMH
"Perspectives on Scientific and Professional Meetings in Gerontology during 1955"

February 9, 1956
Robert Havigmurst, Professor of Education, University of Chicago
"Social Roles of Middle-Aged People"

March 15, 1956
William G. Banfield, Laboratory of Pathology, National Cancer Institute
"Age Changes in Collagen"

April 12, 1956
Leonell C. Strong, Director, Roswell Park Memorial Institute, Springville, New York
"The Genetic Approach to Gerontology"

April 19, 1956
Else Frenkel-Brunswik, University of California
"A Description of Psychological and Physiological Studies of Aging in the Industrial
Relations Center and the Donner Laboratory of the University of California."

October 4, 1956
Torben Geill, Director "Old Peoples Town"
"Gerontological Research in Denmark"

March 21, 1957
Halsey Hunt–Introductory Statement
Eugene Weinbach, LTD, NIAID
Joel Garbus, Section on Aging, Laboratory of Psychology, NIMH
"Age and Oxidative Phosphorylation

April 25, 1957
F. Bourlière, Faculty of Medicine of Paris, France
"Research Problems in the Comparative Physiology of Aging"

Notes

1. E. V. Cowdry, ed. *Problems of Ageing: Biological and Medical Aspects* (Baltimore, MD: Williams & Wilkins, 1939).
2. Otto Pollak. *Social Adjustment in Old Age: A Research Planning Report* (New York: Social Science Research Council, 1948), 48.
3. James E. Birren, Robert N. Butler, Samuel W. Greenhouse, Louis Sokoloff and Marian R. Yarrow, "Interdisciplinary Relationships: Interrelations of Physiological, Psychological, and Psychiatric Findings in Healthy Elderly Men," in *Human Aging*, eds. James E. Birren, Robert N. Butler, Samuel W. Greenhouse, Louis Sokoloff, and Marian R. Yarrow (Washington, D.C.: Government Printing Office, Public Health Publication No. 986, 1963), 283-305.
4. Darab K. Dastur, Mark H. Lane, Douglas B. Hansen, Seymour S. Kety, Robert N. Butler, and Louis Sokoloff, "Effects of Aging on Cerebral Circulation and Metabolism in Man," in *Ibid.*, 59-76.
5. Marian R. Yarrow, Paul Blank, Olive W. Quinn, E. Grant Youmans, and Johanna Stein, "Social Psychological Characteristics of Old Age," in *Ibid.*, 259-79.
6. William Bondareff, "Genesis of Intracellular Pigment in the Spinal Ganglia of Senile Rats: An Electron Microscope Study," *Journal of Gerontology* 12 (1957): 364-9.
7. William Bondareff, "Morphology of the Aging Nervous System," in *Handbook of Aging and the Individual*, ed. James E. Birren (Chicago: University of Chicago Press, 1959), 136-72.
8. Ibid.
9. Jack Botwinick and Conan Kornetsky, "Age Differences In the Acquisition and Extinction of the GSR," *Journal of Gerontology* 15 (1960): 83-84.
10. Edward A. Jerome, "Age and Learning-Experimental Studies," in *Handbook of Aging and the Individual*, 655-99.
11. James E. Birren, Klaus F. Riegel, and Donald F. Morrison, "Age Differences in Response Speed as a Function of Controlled Variations of Stimulus Conditions: Evidence of a General Speed Factor," *Gerontologia* 16 (1962): 1-18.
12. L. H. Hicks and James E. Birren, "Aging, Brain Damage, and Psychomotor Slowing," *Psychological Bulletin* 74 (1962): 377-96.
13. Karl F. Riegel, "History of Psychological Gerontology," in *Handbook of the Psychology of Aging*, ed. James E. Birren (New York: Simon & Schuster, 1977), 70-102.
14. John E. Anderson, ed. *Psychological Aspects of Aging* (Washington, D.C.: American Psychological Association, 1956).
15. James E. Birren, H. A. Imus, and William F. Windle, eds. *The Process of Aging in the Nervous System* (Springfield, Illinois: Charles C. Thomas, 1959).

Mind, Brain, Body, and Behavior
I. G. Farreras, C. Hannaway and V. A. Harden (Eds.)
IOS Press, 2004

The Early Years of the NIMH Intramural Clinical Research Program

Robert A. Cohen

Late in the summer of 1952, Robert Hanna Felix, the first director of the National Institute of Mental Health (NIMH), asked whether I would be interested in developing the NIMH intramural clinical research program. The NIH Clinical Center was scheduled to open in March 1953. There would be 100 beds on six wards, two on each of the three floors designated to mental health, as well as associated laboratories and offices. Patients and normal control volunteers would be admitted without charge for the entire duration of the studies in which they participated. When I asked what studies were planned, Felix replied that the decision would be entirely up to me; there were no preliminary conditions. The NIMH-NINDB basic research program would be directed by Seymour S. Kety, appointed in 1951, who also served in that capacity in the National Institute of Neurological Diseases and Blindness (NINDB).[1] The budget for the clinical research program would be one million dollars; nurses or social workers would be hired out of the hospital budget. My salary would be $15,000–the top of the Civil Service scale. I would have complete freedom in the choice of a reasonable number of associates but all of them would be at a lower salary level. Felix took me on a tour of the Clinical Center, which was still under construction, flicked on the lights in the auditorium that had already been completed and remarked prophetically, "Here's where we will introduce our Nobel Prize winner." We went on to meet Norman Topping, then associate director of the National Institutes of Health (NIH), John R. Heller (director of the National Cancer Institute),

Floyd Daft (director of the National Institute of Arthritis and Metabolic Diseases), and James Shannon (then scientific director of the National Heart Institute[2]). There was no flexibility with respect to the opening date; Congress had been promised that research would begin in March.

After serving five years in the Navy and completing my own psychoanalysis–which had started before the war–I was serving as clinical director of Chestnut Lodge, a small psychoanalytic hospital in Rockville, Maryland. There were 15 physicians on the staff, several of whom I had recruited. Felix, then president of the American Psychiatric Association, was a friend of the director of the Lodge, Dexter M. Bullard, and occasionally visited our staff conferences, sometimes accompanied by members of his staff. For over six years I had been a consultant at the National Naval Medical Center and I had also been a member of the Panel on Human Relations and Morale of the Research and Development Board of the Department of Defense.

Felix agreed with me that ideally it would be preferable for the program to grow more slowly, to have time to find several senior staff, and to develop with them the program that would be instituted. But he was certain that we would have complete freedom and full understanding from experienced administrators. I knew one former and several current members of the NIMH staff. Lawrence Coleman Kolb and I had taken Adolf Meyer's brain modeling class at the Johns Hopkins University in 1937, and we had worked together for over a year at the Norfolk Naval Hospital. We shared an office during a brief venture in part-time, private practice, and were both members of Francis Braceland's[3] examining team on the American Board of Psychiatry and Neurology.[4] Kolb had joined the NIMH staff immediately after release from active duty and had taken part in all of the early planning for the new institute. He had been the secretary for the meeting of the first National Mental Health Advisory Council.[5]

John Eberhart, a social psychologist, had come as Kolb's associate in 1947. I had met Eberhart when he was serving as director of the extramural research program of the NIMH. He made a searching site visit to Chestnut Lodge when Alfred Stanton and Morris Schwartz applied for support for a sociological study of a mental hospital ward. They received the 51st grant awarded by the institute.[6]

I had attended several meetings with Morton Kramer, chief of the Biometrics Branch, and was deeply impressed by the pertinence and quality of his reports. Donald Bloch, from the Lodge staff, had enlisted in the PHS's Commissioned Corps and was working in the office of Joseph Bobbitt, chief of the Professional Services Branch.

Wade H. Marshall, chief of the NIMH-NINDB Laboratory of Neurophysiology, his wife Louise Hanson, my late first wife, Mabel Blake, and I had worked together for more than four years in the Physiology Department of the University of Chicago, and we had taken Ph.D.s within several months of each other in the mid-1930s.

I knew of the early work of John Clausen from the Illinois Institute for Juvenile Research in Chicago, where I had served as Senior Fellow in 1939-1940. He was now chief of the NIMH's Laboratory of Socio-Environmental Studies, working out of the Public Health Center in Hagerstown, Maryland.

And everyone with even a remote interest in physiology knew of Seymour S. Kety's development of a method to measure directly the metabolism of the human brain.

My sole reservation about the NIMH offer was the restriction of supergrade appointments. I believed that the government's taking responsibility for a widespread human problem was socially very desirable but I did not relish the prospect of rushing to create a functioning, world-class 100-bed research institute with only one senior person supervising a newly formed group of young men and women who had never worked together before. This was to be within the larger setting of a 500-bed hospital similarly constituted. I called Felix and declined his offer.

But my conflict was obvious. A week later Felix called to say that he could offer me three additional senior, supergrade positions. In addition to their studies at the Washington Psychoanalytic Institute–where by fiat only M.D.s could participate–all of the Lodge's senior staff were engaged in taking and/or presenting courses with social and biological scientists in the Washington School of Psychiatry. Prominent in this group was David McKenzie Rioch who had left his position as professor of neuropsychiatry at Washington University in St. Louis to come to the Lodge because of his interest in the work of Frieda Fromm-Reichmann and

Harry Stack Sullivan in the Washington School of Psychiatry. He was a fellow consultant at the Naval Medical Center and, in addition, was engaged in building a behavioral research program at the Walter Reed Army Medical Center. The aforesaid studies were partly supported by offering accredited courses to mental health workers and partly through relationships established by the most senior teachers. The Washington School of Psychiatry also established a journal, *Psychiatry-Interpersonal and Biological Processes*, that has been published without interruption since 1938, and is now under the direction of its fifth editor. The opportunity to carry on such studies with the full-time participation of a multidisciplinary staff was like a dream come true. I hoped to assemble such a staff and believed it would work better if the heads of each major division were of equal rank and received equal pay. I accepted Felix's offer and arranged to report on December 31, 1952.

It took me three months to disengage from my clinical obligations. During that period I tried to find at least one senior clinician to join me in operating the clinical program and I consulted widely concerning ideas for the development of a meaningful research operation. My search for an associate was completely unsuccessful. I called upon and/or wrote to everyone I knew, to many I did not know but whose papers I regarded as significant and stimulating, and to all those whose master's and doctoral degrees indicated interest in or commitment to research. All the people I reached who were actively engaged in research were committed to their current positions. In some instances, my invitation came too late; they or their departments had received unsolicited funds from the NIMH extramural program and they were fully engaged in studies already under way.[7] Three exceptionally well-qualified women could not even contemplate such a move since it involved a change for husbands and children. Some otherwise qualified persons found the full-time research requirement unacceptable; most preferred appointments that placed primary emphasis on teaching and practice.[8] Some who believed the supergrade salary was too low predicted I would continue to have difficulty assembling a research staff; I was the only one who ever came for less than he was making. Working for the government was also not regarded as necessarily a good thing because of the intrusion of Congress into the operations. Congress did not have any great influence, but one or two people had been turned down because they might have been involved in liberal causes, and the memories of Senator McCarthy were vivid. So there was some concern over the government or Congress giving orders, but there was also concern over the stability and funding on an annual basis.

As the end of December 1953 approached, I realized I would have to begin with a staff largely composed of men called up for military duty who chose assignment to the PHS in preference to the armed services. I planned to assign the staff members to branches and/or laboratories for which the chiefs had not yet been recruited. Although the final content of the program would be determined by the staff who operated it, I envisioned three main divisions in the clinical branches: one that studied behavior disorders in children; one for disorders of mood and thought (i.e., manic depressive psychosis and schizophrenia), and one for psychosomatic disorders, while in every instance taking advantage of our freedom to study and compare patient behavior and physiological processes with those of normal controls. The disciplines represented would include psychiatry, clinical and developmental psychology, sociology, anthropology, physiology, biochemistry, and pharmacology. An essential difference between the program I envisioned and that of any psychiatric organization of which I had been a part was that studies of the clinical condition would consider the relevance of interdisciplinary collaboration, and that whatever was studied in the pathological would be studied in the normal. I hoped that many of the multidisciplinary staff would maintain a modest acquaintance with the operations of the entire program, and that out of such relationships useful ideas might come.

My entry date had been set for December 31, 1952, but when I arrived at Building T-6 its only occupant was Hector Ragas, an administrative officer, who fortunately knew that I was expected. He seated me at the only available desk, that of Pearce Bailey,[9] who would be away for a week. He gave me a folder of PHS regulations, a pad of paper and some pencils, and disappeared. In mid-afternoon Edward V. Evarts and Josephine Semmes wandered by. They had come to visit Marshall's laboratory in the building and were pleased to find me, but not nearly as glad as I was to see them. They were actually excited about the prospect of a full-time research program, wanted to know our plans, and told me of theirs. Evarts was in the middle of the second year of residency at the Payne Whitney Psychiatric Clinic (New York Presbyterian Hospital); Semmes had an NIMH fellowship at a New York University laboratory. They had both worked at the Yerkes Laboratory of Primate Biology and had visited the Queen Square Hospital in London. They hoped we would have positions for them in 1954.

I returned after the New Year holiday to find a sheaf of letters and a list of telephone numbers from men who wished to serve their obligated duty in the PHS. Since our program could not provide only one year of credit toward board certification, I had decided to accept no one with fewer than two years of residency. An M.A. or a Ph.D. would be a strong recommendation; for others I would depend on my evaluation and records of clinical competence. Three psychiatrists met the first criterion: Louis S. Cholden with an M.S. in psychology from the Menninger Clinic in Topeka, Kansas; Lyman Wynne with Ph.D. prelims in sociology and psychiatric training at Harvard University; and Norman Goldstein with an M.S. in biochemistry who had worked in both the internal medicine and psychiatry division of the Mayo Clinic. Cholden and Wynne were assigned to the Adult Psychiatry Branch and Goldstein was assigned to the Psychosomatic Medicine Branch. A colleague from Chestnut Lodge, Jarl Dyrud, refused my invitation but arranged a meeting with Morris B. Parloff (then at the Phipps Clinic at the Johns Hopkins University) and Roger McDonald (then a PHS officer). Happily, both accepted the appointments—Parloff in the Laboratory of Psychology and McDonald in the Psychosomatic Medicine Branch. Richard Bell, a psychologist in Bobbitt's Professional Services Branch interviewed all applicants interested in psychology and was himself appointed to the Laboratory of Psychology.

As my roster of appointments was almost completed, Evarts called from New York to report that he had been called up for obligated service and had been rejected by the PHS because of a heart murmur, but he had been accepted by the Army. The Administrative Officer was able to obtain a reversal of that decision. Evarts and Semmes came to the NIMH—he to the Psychosomatic Medicine Branch and she to the Laboratory of Psychology. Philippe V. Cardon had been a resident at Bellevue Hospital and had worked with both Harold and Stewart Woolf at New York Hospital. He and Charles Savage, from the Naval Medical Center, came to the Psychosomatic Medicine Branch. Robert Pittenger, who had been Chief Resident at Yale University, Juliana Day from the Johns Hopkins University, and Irving Ryckoff from Chestnut Lodge came to the Adult Psychiatry Branch. Donald Bloch from Chestnut Lodge and D. Wells Goodrich from Harvard University came to the Child Research Branch. A late appointment was that of Robert N. Butler; I appointed him to the Psychosomatic Medicine Branch, where he joined Seymour Perlin from Columbia University.

The Clinical Center's opening date was postponed from March to July 7, 1953. Before that date, I recruited Fritz Redl as chief of the Child Research Branch. He accepted the appointment even though most of the staff positions available to him had been filled. He was Distinguished Professor of Behavioral Science at Wayne State University. Since his student days, he had been a close friend and colleague of Erik Erikson. Redl was widely known for his studies of the disorganization and breakdown of behavior controls, and he had a degree of success in developing treatment programs for hyperaggressive and antisocial children. Two of his books, *Children Who Hate* and *Controls From Within*, were almost required reading for those engaged in primary and secondary education. Redl settled in quickly after his arrival, met with the professional and support staff who had already been assigned to the Child Research Branch, and began the development of the branch with Bloch, Goodrich and Earle Silber. For the first project, they gathered a group of NIH staff children. They became our first normal volunteers. These children helped staff get acquainted with each other and with the institution in which they would work. Then they admitted a group of children who had been uncontrollable in primary school.

In the first six months of operation of the clinical program, the following self-selected studies were undertaken. Wynne, Savage and Cholden were interested in ward organization and psychotherapy. Day and Ryckoff treated the mothers of each other's child patients. Evarts and Savage studied the mechanisms by which emotional disturbance and biochemical processes led to identical psychopathology. Cardon and Goldstein compared epinephrine and norepinephrine blood levels in response to various types of stress. Schaeffer, Bell, and Parloff examined the relationship between parental attitudes and the personality development of their children. Parloff, Boris Iflund, and Goldstein investigated the process of communicating therapy values between therapist and schizophrenic patients: specifically, the conditions associated with shifts in patient-therapist concordance and awareness of each other's treatment values. Virgil Carlson and Ralph Ryan, an ophthalmologist at the NINDB, studied perceptual learning. Goldstein, Marian Kies, and Evarts determined the level of phenolic compounds in the spinal fluid of schizophrenic patients at Spring Grove State Hospital in association with Leonard Kurland at that institution. Goldstein and Kies determined the effects of stress on antidiuretic activity of blood in normal controls and schizophrenic patients. Evarts and Savage described the effects of LSD on the behavior of monkeys.

In my search for a laboratory chief in psychology, I consulted with David Shakow for help in finding investigators in clinical and developmental areas. In the 1920s, the McCormick family, disheartened by the lack of progress of a schizophrenic family member in conventional therapy had consulted Walter Cannon, professor of physiology at Harvard University, about establishing a research center devoted to the development of an endocrine treatment for the illness. In its nineteen years (1927-1946) of operation, the center, established at Worcester State Hospital in Massachusetts, had made notable contributions both to the study of schizophrenia and to the disciplines represented by its staff. Shakow had been chief of psychology during that period. Seven men suggested by Shakow as worthy candidates made individual visits to the NIH; each of them was impressed by the setting and our plans and assured us they would be watching our progress with interest but not with their participation. Kety had been equally unsuccessful in finding a psychologist to head the basic research laboratory in psychology. It was clear that Shakow had felt that psychology should be strongly represented in the institute. It occurred to me that he might join us if he were asked to develop psychology in both the clinical and basic programs. After some consideration, Kety agreed to this proposal. Shakow consented, and came to head our first joint laboratory.

Evarts was responsible for the next important development in the program. At the time, we thought that LSD might induce a model for psychosis and that if we could find out what was going on in the brain with LSD, we would know what was going on in schizophrenia. Evarts and Conan Kornetsky had expanded their study of the effects of LSD by developing a 47-item questionnaire which they administered to a large group of subjects in order to define as precisely as possible the subjective nature of the subjects' experience. Then Evarts went to Marshall's laboratory to study the effects of LSD on the performance of tasks by a monkey he had trained, and with Marshall, William Landau and Walter Freygang, Jr., he administered LSD to a cat. Utilizing a Horsley-Clarke apparatus, it was found that transmission of the visual impulse was blocked at the external geniculate body. Then Evarts went to the National Heart Institute, where he and Julius Axelrod, Roscoe O. Brady, and Bernhard Witkop studied the metabolism of LSD. Evarts then sent me a letter when I was in Paris in 1954 visiting research centers, strongly urging the appointment of Julius Axelrod as a pharmacologist in the Psychosomatic Medicine Branch. He enclosed supporting letters from Shakow and William Jenkins, chief of clinical care in our program. Axelrod was a GS-12[10] chemist who had joined Shannon's program at Goldwater Memorial Hospital in New York in 1946, and had come down to continue his work at the National Heart Institute in 1949. Axelrod expected to receive a Ph.D. from George Washington University by the end of the year (1954) and I wrote back to Evarts and agreed to offer him a position.[11] Axelrod's fourth paper from the NIMH was the first of the series that led to his Nobel Prize award in 1970.[12]

I turned to locating a senior research psychiatrist and chief to head the Psychosomatic Medicine Branch. I visited research centers in Europe on a trip planned by the World Health Organization (WHO). Among others I had visited Joel Elkes, professor of experimental medicine at the University of Birmingham. His ideas and operations were very congenial with ours and I believed he would be an ideal person to head the Psychosomatic Medicine Branch.[13] Kety agreed that Elkes would bring desirable strengths to our programs and we invited him for a visit in 1956 that proved mutually stimulating and in which we offered him the position of chief of the Psychosomatic Medicine Branch. However, he had obligations at Birmingham that had to be met before he could move. We received Elkes's letter of regret, but I was astonished and elated when Kety said he wished to step down as scientific director and fill the place we had offered to Elkes as laboratory chief. Evarts, Axelrod, Cardon, Kies, Perlin, Butler, McDonald, Kornetsky, William Pollin, Irwin Feinberg, and Irwin Kopin were already members of the laboratory. Kety brought with him Louis Sokoloff and Jack Durell, added funds and positions from the basic program, and the Laboratory of Clinical Science became the second joint basic-clinical laboratory in the NIMH intramural laboratory.

Since John Clausen had already established a productive sociology group, I asked him to consider adding positions from my budget. He agreed and thus the Laboratory of Socio-Environmental Studies became the third joint laboratory.

In 1956, Kety and I had been appointed to a committee with Ralph Gerard,[14] Jonathan Cole[15] and Jacques Gottlieb[16] to plan and organize a Conference on the Evaluation of Pharmacology in Mental Illness. The conference was co-sponsored by the NIMH, the American Psychiatric Association, and the National Academy of Sciences-National Research Council, and was held on September 18-22, 1956. Over 100 investigators took part; both the extramural and intramural programs of the NIMH were strongly represented in the meeting. The proceedings were published in a 650-page volume: *Psychopharmacology: Problems in Evaluation*, (Publication 583) under the auspices of the National Academy of Sciences-National Research Center in 1959.

One immediate result of the conference was the establishment of the NIMH Psychopharmacology Service Center under Cole's direction in the extramural program. Another was the establishment of the Clinical Neuropharmacology Research Center at St. Elizabeths Hospital under the direction of Joel Elkes. Elkes—who by 1957 was able to come to the

United States—had published one of the early papers on the use of chlorpromazine and reserpine in the treatment of psychotic patients. He had been one of the organizers of a WHO conference that had been attended by Morton Kramer, chief of the Biometrics Branch, who brought back reports of the significant studies in European centers. Elkes was invited to chair one of the sessions at our conference and was an active participant in the proceedings of the meeting in September 1956. Felix, Kety, and I had recently met with Winfred Overholser, superintendent of St. Elizabeths Hospital, about the possibility of having one of the wards assigned to us for studies that would complement and extend those in which we were engaged at the NIH Clinical Center. Overholser suggested that we take over the William A. White Building. Felix enthusiastically seized the opportunity, and thus we were committed to carrying out studies in an institution typical of those in which perhaps 95 percent of psychotic patients were confined and treated.

As 1958 approached, the organizational phase of the clinical research program neared completion. For several years I had been trying to bring David A. Hamburg into the program. I had served as referee on a paper he submitted to the journal *Psychiatry* in which Hamburg described the organization and study of a ward for Army burn victims. It was thorough, resourceful, and effective. David Rioch had visited the Army hospital, had arranged for Hamburg's transfer to his research program at the Walter Reed Army Medical Center, and had introduced him to the staff at Chestnut Lodge. He was already committed to join Roy Grinker's program at Columbia Michael Reese Hospital and Medical Center in Chicago and soon became his principal associate. Hamburg had expressed an interest in the NIMH clinical program but felt he was not prepared to make the move. As he climbed up the professional ladder, he finally came to the NIMH in December 1957, as chief of the Adult Psychiatry Branch after he finished a fellowship at the Center for Advanced Study in the Behavioral Sciences at Stanford University.

In 1963, each NIH clinical director was asked to list ten significant achievements from his institute's program. The group of clinical directors then selected one achievement from each program which was to be presented at a meeting with President John F. Kennedy on the tenth anniversary of the opening of the Clinical Center. The plans for this meeting were quietly cancelled, but the ten achievements of the NIMH's clinical research program's first decade of research, plus several more of equal merit, were as follows:

- the discovery of catechol-o-methyl transferase and the elucidation of the processes involved in the neurotransmitter role of the catecholamines
  (Julius Axelrod; this led to his Nobel Prize in 1970)[17]

- family studies and communication deviance in schizophrenia
  (Lyman Wynne and Margaret Thaler Singer)

- social variables and the development of schizophrenia
  (Melvin Kohn)

- the impact of mental illness on the family
  (John Clausen and Marian Yarrow)

- hormones and depression
  (David A. Hamburg, John Mason, William Bunney)

- a comprehensive, multidisciplinary study of the factors involved in human aging
  (James E. Birren, Robert N. Butler, Samuel Greenhouse, Louis Sokoloff, and Marian Yarrow)

- the functional anatomy of the visceral brain
  (Paul MacLean)

- the biochemical lesion in phenylpyruvic oligophrenia
  (Seymour Kaufman)

- genetic factors in the development of schizophrenia
  (David Rosenthal, Seymour S. Kety, and Paul Wender)

- the organization of the Clinical Neuropharmacological Research Center
  (Joel Elkes)

- the comprehensive delineation of the psychological features of schizophrenia
  (David Shakow)

- advances in systematic process and outcome psychotherapy research
  (Morris B. Parloff)

- the primary role of thyroxin in protein synthesis as revealed by mental retardation in cretinism
  (Louis Sokoloff)

- the crucial involvement of brain catecholamines in the manifestations of affective disorders
  (Joseph Schildkraut et al. and William Bunney et al.)

- psychoactive tryptamine derivatives
  (Stephen Szara)

Three important reports presented at the monthly NIH Clinico-pathological Case conferences also emerged from this first decade of research and were published in the *Annals of Internal Medicine*:

- The Metabolism of the Catecholamines: Clinical Implications
  (Robert A. Cohen, William Bridgers, Julius Axelrod, Hans Weil-Malherbe, Elwood LaBrosse, William Bunney, Philippe V. Cardon, and Seymour S. Kety)[18]

- Some Clinical, Biochemical and Physiological Actions of the Pineal Gland
  (Robert A. Cohen, Richard Wurtman, Julius Axelrod, Solomon Snyder)[19]

- False Neurochemical Transmitters
  (Robert A. Cohen, Irwin Kopin, Cyrus Creveling, José Musacchio, Josef Fischer, J. Richard Crout, John Gill)[20]

When Kety stepped down as scientific director of the joint NIMH-NINDB basic research program to head the Laboratory of Clinical

Science, Robert B. Livingston took his place as the new scientific director of the NIMH-NINDB basic research program. Livingston had worked with John F. Fulton at Yale University and brought Paul MacLean to the NIH with him when he accepted. Livingston had even less contact with my clinical research program than Kety had had. I had met with a small committee of scientific directors, including DeWitt Stetten, Jr., Robert Berliner, and G. Burroughs Mider, to discuss complaints about the way the National Institutes of Health was being administered from downtown. I ended up establishing a good relationship with them.[21] When Livingston left, John Eberhart emerged as a good candidate to replace him as scientific director, given his experience with the extramural program of the institute from the very early days.

Looking back, the plan I developed for the intramural clinical research program could be considered grandiose, but there was a sense of urgency, a belief that this was to be a one-time opportunity not subject to growth and gradual development. The NIMH budget in 1952 was close to $12 million. Felix talked to the intramural scientists once a year and he would tell them, "I need to have a gimmick when I go before Congress; if any of you ever have an idea or, particularly, some little discovery that I can tell them, it'll be very helpful." An example of his foresight in those days was that when Felix testified before Congress at the time the budget was about $15 million, Senator Lister Hill asked, "How much do you think you'll eventually come ask me for?" Felix took a deep breath and responded, "Senator, I can foresee the day when I will ask you for $25 million." We speculated that in some far distant day the government might support two or even possibly three institutes like the NIH in different parts of the country because this was such a fantastic opportunity to do full-time research. We believed we had already reached the limit of workable size. As I look back, some of that was gratifyingly successful, but I believe, in balance, we did not find the men and women as much as they found us.[22]

Acknowledgments

This paper grew out of the extensive series of interviews by Dr. G. Ingrid Farreras of all current and many past staff members, and her preparation of a superb history, of the Laboratory of Psychology. She stimulated all of us to recount the ideas which motivated us as we struggled to establish the intramural research program of the NIMH over fifty years ago. She called our attention to items gleaned from her perusal of the *Annual Reports*, clarified and tactfully resolved obscurities and inconsistencies.

There are two others who must be mentioned. Kety came to establish the intramural research programs of the NIMH and the NINDB in 1951. He represented the two institutes in all of the deliberations by which the NIH operates, established the basic research programs for both institutes, and then undertook the direction of a highly productive laboratory. For over two years, he and I attended Felix's biweekly staff conferences, and met weekly with John Eberhart and Joseph Bobbitt. The formulation and operation of our respective research programs were critically discussed in these settings. His 1960 paper, "A Biologist Examines Mind and Behavior," is a classic which is still relevant and worth reading today. Even after he left the NIH for Harvard University, his associates maintained a close relationship with him, and welcomed his return in emeritus status.

Dr. John C. Eberhart served seven years as director of the extramural research program in the early days of the institute. In that capacity he visited over 50 universities to stimulate the establishment of training programs in clinical psychology. After seven years with the Commonwealth Fund, he returned to the NIMH as director of the intramural research program. He knew and was respected by major figures in all the foundations engaged in the support of medical research. He came to be one of the most influential of the group of scientific directors who governed the NIH for almost 20 years. He once remarked that the early NIH leaders had limited personal but strong organizational ambition. That was certainly true of him. He erased the gap between the basic and clinical divisions. He and I began each morning in his office or mine; for the first time, all of the laboratory chiefs met as a group.

Finally, I want to express my personal appreciation to Dr. Morris Parloff. He is one of the first who came to the program in 1953. We worked together on a study of psychotherapy before he went to the extramural program to develop and lead a nationwide study and evaluation of the various psychotherapies. I have long valued his judgment and sought his opinion on organizational issues. When Dr. Farreras called to talk about the early days, I immediately called him to join us.

Notes

1. Today the National Institute of Neurological Disorders and Stroke (NINDS).
2. And subsequently the NIH director from 1955-1968.
3. Braceland occupied many important positions: Chief of the Navy's Neuropsychiatry Branch, President of the American Psychiatric Association, Head of Psychiatry at the Mayo Foundation, and Medical Director of the Hartford Retreat.
4. When I began residency training in September 1937, psychiatry was not a widely accepted specialty. My 1935 class at the University of Chicago did not have a single lecture in the subject. The American Board of Psychiatry and Neurology, however, had just been established in 1936–many years after such boards had been established in medicine, surgery, cardiology, obstetrics and gynecology, ophthalmology, and other specialties. It required three years of residency training and two years of practice for eligibility to take the examination. Harvard University, Yale University, Columbia University, the University of Michigan and the University of Iowa had residency programs in psychiatric institutes, as did some of the large private mental hospitals and a number of state hospitals, but there was very little research going on. Of the 1,889 members in the American Psychiatric Association in 1936, only 157 were psychoanalysts. In 1937, there was only one staff member at the Johns Hopkins University who had taken and passed the board examination. By World War II, there could not have been more than 3,000 psychiatrists (by 1967 there were almost 16,000, largely the result of the NIMH's financial support).
5. Kolb left the NIMH to join Braceland at the Mayo Clinic and from there went to Columbia University to head the Psychiatry Department.
6. Their work, *The Mental Hospital*, was published in 1954. It received much acclaim and led to Stanton's subsequent appointments as Medical Director of the McLean Hospital and Professor of Psychiatry at Harvard University, and Schwartz's appointment as Professor of Sociology at Brandeis University.
7. John Eberhart once said that part of his first job in the extramural program was to persuade universities to set up training programs in clinical psychology, using as an inducement the possibility of training grants and training stipends. There were few such programs at the time, and although most were eager for PHS subsidies, there was a good deal of reluctance in academic departments to begin giving Ph.D.s in such a relatively undeveloped subfield.
8. We at the NIH were not to engage in private practice. The University of Chicago at the time Mabel and I graduated was, I believe, the only full-time medical school in the country. After Eberhart and I left, Frederick Goodwin was able to obtain official permission for private practice.

9. Director of the NINDB.

10. A Civil Service ranking.

11. Axelrod agreed to come if he could be promised a professional appointment. The appointment Axelrod had at the NHI was essentially that of a technician in pharmacology while he was getting his Ph.D. at George Washington University. Axelrod's appointment was Evarts's doing, and it turned out to be a marvelous appointment.

12. One of the early projects initiated by Kety was a critical review of papers which purported to explain the development of schizophrenia. Among these was one by the Canadian psychiatrists Hoffer, Osmond, and Smythies which proposed that the illness was caused by the abnormal metabolism of adrenaline to form adrenochrome. Not only was Axelrod unable to confirm the presence of adrenochrome, but he noted that there was no reliable information about the metabolism of adrenalin. In a series of brilliant experiments that led to his Nobel Prize in 1970, he discovered the enzyme catechol-o-methyl transferase and elucidated the mechanisms that regulate the storage, release, and inactivation of noradrenaline.

13. One of Elkes's qualities that impressed me when we first met was that on a sabbatical he had spent a very considerable period at the Norwich State Hospital (Connecticut) to observe our conventional work with psychotic patients. He did not limit his interest to the work at leading universities.

14. Professor of Neurophysiology at the University of Michigan's Mental Health Research Institute.

15. Chief, Pharmacology Research Service Center, NIMH.

16. Director, LaFayette Clinic, Detroit, Michigan.

17. This achievement was the one selected by the clinical directors for the Kennedy program.

18. 56, no. 6 (1962): 960-87.

19. 61, no. 6 (1964): 1144-61.

20. 65, no. 2 (1966): 347-62.

21. The joint laboratory chiefs would attend such meetings separately throughout Kety's and Livingston's tenure. Although Kety and I had a good social relationship, he never invited me to meet with any of the laboratory chiefs in the basic research program, and I never invited him to come to our clinical branch chief meetings. And the same thing was true when Kety left and Livingston took over as scientific director. We had a cordial enough social relationship but never talked about the clinical and basic research programs together. It was not until 1960, when John Eberhart became scientific director, that we combined the basic and clinical meetings.

22. In contrast to the early days when I was looking without success for the laboratory chiefs, in subsequent years we observed with pleasure the steady growth and productivity of the men and women who came to work in the program. When Eberhart and I retired, we counted almost 30 who came as Clinical and/or Research Associates and had gone on to professorships in leading universities from coast to coast, after substantial achievements at the NIH.

Mind, Brain, Body, and Behavior
I. G. Farreras, C. Hannaway and V. A. Harden (Eds.)
IOS Press, 2004

Psychopharmacology: Finding One's Way*

Joel Elkes

On Beginning in Psychopharmacology: Activities in England and the USA

The dialectic between molecules and mind began when I was a medical student. My entry into psychopharmacology was far from direct; it happened in the mid 1940s through a fortunate play of synchronicities. I imagined the life of the mind as a molecular process but found that I knew nothing about either. I was profoundly interested in psychiatry but found little comfort in my reading on any biological correlates of mental events. Equally, my knowledge of molecules and particularly their ability to carry information was very thin to say the least. It so happened that my medical school (St. Mary's Hospital, London, where Fleming 10 years later discovered penicillin) was very strong in immunology. I began reading avidly Paul Ehrlich's writings. His concepts of receptors, accompanied by his famous lock and key diagrams, implied recognition and stereo chemical fit. I had a consuming curiosity about the molecular basis of immunological memory. Ehrlich also envisioned the fashioning (in our day we would say "engineering") of drugs that would selectively attach themselves to specific receptors. Nature could learn, and rational chemotherapy with him was an elaborate imitation of nature.

While in medical school, I was also profoundly attracted to physics. I had no mathematical gifts, but spent my first prize money on accounts of the new physics. To this day, I recall the awe with which I viewed the cloud chamber photographs that rendered visible a mysterious geometry

---

*This revised version of this article has been reprinted with the kind permission of Elsevier Science from *Neuropsychopharmacology* 12 (1995): 93-111.

of particle paths in collision. I could not go beyond first principles, and yet, as I read myself into the field, I tried to grasp the curious transformations, jumps, symmetries and asymmetries operating in particle physics, I kept on imagining the life of the mind as a molecular process, linking it in some way to particle physics. It was, of course, a fatuous exercise; yet it gave me strange satisfaction to engage in such molecular games. It was at this same time that I began to read Charles Scott Sherrington's *Integrative Action of the Nervous System*,[1] an influence which has persisted to this day. Later, I attended, by invitation, and hiding safely in the dark of a back seat, a meeting of the august British Physiological Society, in which Edgar D. Adrian (later Lord Adrian) demonstrated the firing of neurons. The loudspeaker crackled as he touched a cat's single vibrissa. It remained silent as he touched another. This strange brew of physics, immunology, and neurophysiology got me started on my interest in "drugs and the mind."

I had to wait my turn to get within reach of the brew. My chief, Alastair Frazer, to whom I owe the very foundations of my career, proposed that I put my interest in physical chemistry to use. His field was not the nervous system but fat absorption, and he suggested that I work on the structure of the surface lipoprotein of the chylomicron, a physiologically present fatty particle that floods the circulation from the thoracic duct after a fatty meal. The envelope was a lipoprotein, carrying a pH-sensitive ionic charge. I developed a microelectophoretic cell and various flocculation techniques as a means of characterizing the nature of this lipoprotein coating.[2]

I suppose what intrigued me then, and still intrigues me, was guessing the properties of a macromolecular structure from physical chemical measurements, building up a mental picture on the basis of collateral evidence. This wish to visualize, to have a map (mostly a wrong map) has stayed with me all my life. Playing with molecular configurations became quite a hobby for me and my friends. In any event, with the study of this lipoprotein envelope, my quest into the interface between physical chemistry and biology began. I started to read widely, pulled, I suppose, by a wish to penetrate the fundamental building blocks of life. I ventured into surface chemistry (or colloid chemistry) and the study of monomolecular films. It was, of course, the pursuit of an illusion. But, even then, the sense of pattern, of configuration and the effect of subtle variation of an arrangement and charge distribution became a visual game that whiled away some idle hours in medical school.

In 1941, Alastair Frazer invited me to join him in starting a Department of Pharmacology in Birmingham, England. Birmingham, even then, had the makings of the great university that it has since become. It had a splendid campus, all compact. Within five minutes' walk of the medical school there were the basic science departments: there were giants in physics (Rudolf Peierls and Mark Oliphant), chemistry (Norman Haworth), statistics (Lancelot Hogben), genetics and zoology (Peter Medawar), and science policy (Solly Zuckerman). Conversation at lunch was propitious and soon turned to the structure of the biological membranes and, of course, lipoproteins. The structure of liquid crystals—the nature of forces, polar, nonpolar, and steric—the bonding that made for their ordered cohesion, continued to excite. I found myself visualizing the architecture of membranes, streaming through special pores like a sodium ion, negotiating various channels and portals, with chains collapsing spring-like as these tiny compartments opened and closed. And then, one day, I realized that the nervous system was full of lipoproteins and that myelin was a highly ordered lipoprotein liquid crystal structure.

I came upon the papers of Francis Schmitt, who was then at St. Louis.[3] I wrote to him and got back a handsome collection of reprints describing his work on the structure of the myelin sheath. I was fascinated by his diagrams. Here was a highly ordered, aesthetically beautiful arrangement, which fitted the facts and which made it possible to envision how bimolecular leaflets were built into a highly specialized structure. Myelin, I thought, could provide a model for understanding the structure of a membrane that was ion sensitive and electrochemically responsive. My friend Alastair Frazer concurred, but I found it hard to convince others. However, one fine thing happened: Bryan Finean walked into my Laboratory as my first Ph.D. student.

Bryan Finean had obtained his degree in chemistry doing crystallography of the traditional kind. Looking at the Schmitt diagrams, we posed an obvious question. Schmitt had worked on dried nerve. Could low-angle X-ray diffraction be made to work on a nerve that was irrigated and alive? Within three months or so, we were looking at the first X-ray diffraction photograph of living sciatic nerve; I still remember the thrill of seeing that film. To me there was also a profound personal and psychological element in this engagement. I was moving from somebody else's field, fat absorption, and entering the field that mysteriously pulled me, the nervous system, albeit by creeping up the myelin sheath!

Our studies gave us a picture, a sort of basic scaffolding, into which specialized receptors could fit. Cholesterol and phospholipids were accommodated in these diagrams. We also examined the effects of temperature, moisture, alcohol, and ether on myelin structure.[4] Gradually, we developed a model of myelin for the study of the structure of biological membranes. There was much personal satisfaction. I was in the nervous system, yet, as is apparent, still edging safely at the periphery, a long way from behavior, and the mode of action of psychoactive drugs.

Pharmacology and Experimental Psychiatry in Birmingham, England

Immediately below the Department of Pharmacology there was a small subdepartment of two rooms administered from the Dean's office, called "Mental Diseases Research." In charge of it was a gifted neuropathologist, F. A. Pickworth, who held the view that mental disease was a capillary disease, and that all disorders were reflected in an abnormal cerebral vascular bed.[5] He had developed beautiful benzidine staining techniques for demonstrating the small cerebral vessels, and the laboratory was filled with innumerable slices and slides of the brain in all manner of pathological states, stained by his methods.

Pickworth retired, and again serendipity took me by the hand. The laboratory reverted to the Department of Pharmacology, and I became administratively responsible for its program. When we arrived in Birmingham in 1942 there were two people but the department grew by leaps and bounds. It seemed to me that there were five areas that had to be attended to if one were to understand the function of drugs on the brain: one, functional neuroanatomy; two, neurochemistry (A. Todrick and A. Baker); three, electrophysiology, particularly in the conscious animal when you could observe electrical activity and behavior at the same time (Phillip B. Bradley); four, animal behavior (M. Piercy); and five, the controlled clinical trial (my former wife Charmian and I). When I left, in 1950, there were 42 members in the department.

When the war ended, our military intelligence gave us insights into the secret German chemical warfare work, and particularly the anti-cholinesterases and their tremendous specificity for certain enzymes in the brain. We started mapping the cholinesterases in various areas of the brain, inhibiting the "true" and "pseudo" enzymes from birth, and observing the effect of such inhibition on the emergence of various in-born reflexes.[6] It was a long, long way from fat absorption, and some way from lipoproteins. But, at long last, it was the brain, it was drugs; and I was even beginning to "smell" the mysterious entity called behavior.

In retrospect, it becomes apparent to me that I was once again approaching my central interest, gingerly and carefully, as if I were de-fusing a bomb. For it is plain that what attracted me to research in psy-chiatry was an urge to leave the bench and get to people and what made me circumambulate this purpose was my feeling of safety with things. Somehow, mental disease research, or "experimental psychiatry" (as I was beginning to call it in my mind), presented a sort of compromise. It led inevitably to human work, but it did so by way of experiment and control. This double bookkeeping worked for a time, for an astonishingly long time; it took a further five years to break through the barrier.

As we were feeling our way through the distribution of cholinesterases, I began to read on the psychoactive drugs. I came across descriptions of the somatic and psychologic accompaniments of catatonic stupor, and saw some patients exhibiting this syndrome in the local mental hospital. We embarked on a study of the effects of drugs on catatonic stupor. We began to work at the Winson Green Mental Hospital (The Birmingham City Mental Hospital, now All Saints Hospital). Its superintendent, J. J. O'Reilly, put a small research room at our disposal and allowed us to choose patients using our criteria; he also gave us nursing help. My former wife Charmian (who was in general practice at the time) carried out the clinical trial magnificently. She examined the effects of Amytal, amphetamine, and mephenesin on catatonic schizophrenic stupor. Amytal, administered in full hypnotic doses intravenously, led to a paradoxical awakening of patients in catatonic stupor, a relaxation of muscle tone, and rise in foot temperature. The effect of amphetamine was equally paradoxical; it led to a deepening of the stupor, increase in muscle rigidity, and deepening cyanosis. Mephenesin, a muscle relaxant, produced marked muscle relaxation but little effect on psychomotor response or peripheral temperature. We also studied the ability of patients to draw—for ten minutes, without prompting—while under the influence of drugs. Amytal markedly increased this ability, and amphetamine inhibited it. The experiments thus suggested *selectivity* in the actions of drugs on catatonic stupor, and raised questions of the unexpected relation of hyperarousal to catatonic withdrawal. Most important, however, these experiments established the need of working in parallel. The laboratory and the ward became ends of a *continuum* of related activities.

It was then, I suppose, that I decided that experimental psychiatry was clinical or that it was nothing; that it depended on the continuous intentional active interaction between the laboratory and the clinic. Let it draw on the bench sciences, let it look for neural correlates of behavior in the animal model, let it delve deeply into processes governing the chemically mediated organ of information that we carry in our skull; but unless this yield from the bench is clearly and continuously related to the uniquely human events that are the business of psychiatry and of neuropsychology, the implications of such knowledge must, of necessity, remain conjectural. All this is pretty obvious nowadays. In those days, however, the late 1940s and early 1950s, in the Department of Pharmacology in Birmingham, it became part of a plan. I felt instinctively that the drugs we were working with, and the drugs still to come, could be tools of great precision and power, depending (if one was lucky) on one or two overriding properties. It is this kind of precision pharmacology of the central nervous system that made me hopeful, and made me take up my stance in the face of raised eyebrows, which I encountered not only in the Physiological Society but also in psychiatric circles, where I was regarded as a maverick, a newcomer, and a curiosity.

In 1951, I was invited to found and rename the department to the new Department of Experimental Psychiatry. I believe it was the first department of its kind anywhere. I chose the name deliberately to emphasize the research objectives of our enterprise. As indicated, the laboratory facilities were already available and had grown out of our previous work. But, as mentioned earlier, psychiatry, even experimental psychiatry, is clinical or it is nothing. Thus, quite early, we decided on the need for a clinical arm. The neurophysiology and neurochemistry laboratories were situated in the School of Medicine and in a small new building provided by the hospital board (we were already working at the City Mental Hospital). What was needed was an Early Treatment Center, comprising inpatient and outpatient facilities. Again, we were fortunate. Through the intervention of J. J. O'Reilly, a mansion that had previously been the home of the Cadbury chocolate family became available. The name of the house was "Uffculme" and the name of our Clinic thus became the "Uffculme Clinic." Standing in its own lovely grounds, it comprised 42 beds, a day hospital, and an outpatient clinic.[7]

At that time, then, there were two anchoring points for our work in the mental disease field: neurochemistry, at the bench level, and human behavior, as influenced by drugs. There was nothing in between, no indicator that could relate the effects of drugs on the brain in the conscious animal to behavior, nor any correlation between behavior and chemistry of the brain. I began to hunt again and began to read avidly into EEG studies coming from various sources. The data available were sparse, however.

Then Phillip Bradley, a trained zoologist who had carried out micro-electrode studies in insects, joined us. He spent some time with Grey Walter learning EEG techniques and then set up his own laboratory in the second of the two rooms of "Mental Diseases Research." In 1949, Bradley was developing his pioneering technique for recording the electrical activity in the conscious animal,[8] a procedure that in those days (the days of *sulfonamide*–not penicillin), was quite a trick. The work proceeded well and quickly established reference points for a pharmacology of the brain, inasmuch as it relates to behavior. We came to the conclusion that there were *families* of naturally occurring neuroactive compounds with regional distribution in the brain. Acetylcholine, norepinephrine, serotonin, and histamine were apparently compounds of this grouping, the receptors for them existed in the brain, and the drugs interacted with these receptors. The concept of families of compounds, derived and evolved from respective common chemical roots, governing the physiology of the brain (and, by implication, the chemistry of awareness, perception, affect, and memory), was a confusing idea at the time, and I must say was not very well received by the pharmacological fraternity. However, it has persisted. We went on talking particularly about the effects of drugs interfering with the turnover and interaction of these substances in the brain and gradually the idea came through and then the whole term "regional neurochemistry" began to circulate.

It is into this Department of Experimental Psychiatry that, one day, there walked W. R. Thrower, Clinical Director of May and Baker, a company in England. He showed me, in English translation, the findings of Jean Delay and Pierre Deniker concerning chlorpromazine,[9] findings that have been so admirably reviewed by Frank Ayd.[10] Thrower told me that May and Baker had acquired the British rights for chlorpromazine. They had a 500 grams supply and could make up the necessary chlorpromazine and placebo tablets if we performed a double blind-controlled trial. Being very impressed by Delay and Deniker's reports, I said we certainly would and suggested that we could do so at Winson Green Mental Hospital.

Charmian assumed full responsibility for the management of what was to prove, I think, a rather important step in clinical psychopharmacology. For, as I think back on it, all the difficulties, all the opportunities, all the unpredictable qualities of conducting a trial in a "chronic" mental hospital ward were to show up clearly, and to be dealt with clearly, in that early trial. I still remember the morning when we all trooped into the board room of the hospital, spread the data on the large oak table, and broke the code after the ratings and side effects had been tabulated. The trial involved 27 patients chosen for gross agitation, overactivity, and psychotic behavior: 11 were affective, 13 schizophrenic, and 3 senile. The design was blind and self-controlled, the drug and placebo being alternated three times at approximately six-week intervals. The dose was relatively low (350 to 300 mg per day).

We kept the criteria of improvement conservative yet there was no doubt of the results: 7 patients showed marked improvement; 11 slight improvement; there was no effect in 9 patients. Side effects were observed in 10 patients. Our short paper, which conclusively proved the value of chlorpromazine, and was the subject of an editorial in the *British Medical Journal*, was on a blind self-controlled trial.[11] But it was more; for it was a statement of the opportunities offered by a mental hospital for work of this kind, the difficulties one was likely to encounter, and the rules that one had to observe to obtain results.

Neuropharmacology and Psychopharmacology in Washington, D.C., and at the John Hopkins University, Baltimore

I had spent a year (1950 to 1951) in the United States, having had the good fortune, through the offices of Theodore Wallace of Smith, Kline, and French (SKF), to be awarded the first SKF Traveling Fellowship in England and to get a Fulbright Award. I had a stimulating time at the late Samuel Wortis' Institute at New York University, also visiting Fritz Redlich's Institute at Yale University, and also worked very productively at the Pratt (New England) Diagnostic Center at Boston with John Nemiah, later editor-in-chief of the *American Journal of Psychiatry*, who taught me much. Once again, the mental hospital exerted its pull. When I met with Redlich, I asked him whether it would not be advisable for me to get to know an American state hospital at first hand. It was duly arranged that I should spend five months at Norwich State Hospital, Connecticut.

Before returning from the United States to England, I asked my friends at SKF to arrange a visit with Seymour S. Kety, whose fundamental work on cerebral circulation I had admired from a distance for some years. This was duly done, and one morning in the summer of 1951 I was in his Laboratory at the University of Pennsylvania. We started talking and went on talking through a four-hour lunch of the possibilities of biological research in psychiatry and the exciting methods for *in vivo* work in man, which was just emerging. Kety told me that he had just been appointed scientific director of the intramural basic research program at the National Institute of Mental Health (NIMH) and the National Institute of Neurological Diseases and Blindness (NINDB), and I shared with him that I was going back to England to occupy the newly created chair of experimental psychiatry in the University of Birmingham.

When, in 1957, I received an invitation from Kety and Robert A. Cohen to create the Clinical Neuropharmacology Research Center at the NIMH,[12] we all felt that biological research would gain by being in a realistic mental hospital setting. The hospital under consideration was St. Elizabeths in Washington, D.C. Winfred Overholser, the superintendent, was duly approached and was very receptive. With Robert Felix's strong and continuous support and with Cohen's and Kety's exceptional understanding and enthusiasm, we established the Center at the William A. White building of the hospital. I will not hide the fact that it was hard going at first. We started, in 1957, with a secretary (Mrs. Anne Gibson) and myself in a large, dark, "Continued Care" building accommodating some 300 patients. However, time, energy, persistence, and support prevailed, and it became a research institute within two years. Again, the plan was the same: laboratories below, clinic above, and patients all around. The facilities grew and grew. Colleagues joined: Floyd Bloom, R. Byck, Richard Chase, R. Gjessing, R. Gumnit, Max Hamilton, Eliot Hearst, Tony Hordern, Sheppard Kellam, Donald Lipsitt, John Lofft, Richard Michael, Herbert Posner, Gian Carlo Salmoiraghi, Stephen Szara, R. von Baumgarten, Neil Waldrop, Hans Weil-Malherbe, Harold Weiner, Paul Wender, R. Whalen, and many others. In 1961, Fritz Freyhan arrived as the Center's director of clinical studies.

Again, some of the same themes (in variation) reappeared, though I cannot mention them all: microelectrophysiology, which, in Gian Carlo Salmoiraghi's hands mapped the pharmacology of respiratory neurons[13] and later with Floyd Bloom, became a pioneering technique for the study of the pharmacology of individual neurons in the central nervous system;[14] amine metabolism, under Hans Weil-Malherbe,[15] which also initiated a collaboration with Julius Axelrod,[16] the metabolism of psycho-dysleptic tryptamine derivates, under Szara;[17] animal behavioral studies, combining Skinnerian avoidance training with metabolic experiments under Eliot Hearst;[18] the effect of locally and isotopically labeled implanted hormones on behavior, under Richard Michael;[19] human behavior analysis studies under Harold Weiner;[20] the methodology of clinical drug trials under Hordern and Lofft;[21] the quantification of social interaction in a psychiatric ward under Shepherd Kellam;[22] Max Hamilton, a visiting fellow, gave seminars on the methodology of clinical research, and the conceptualization of comprehensive mental health care in a given community by Fritz Freyhan;[23] and studies on dependency, depression, and hospitalization by Donald Lipsitt.[24] Later, with Overholser's help, the Behavioral and Clinical Studies Center of St. Elizabeths was created as a complementary entity, under the direction of Neil Waldrop.

In 1963, I was invited to assume the chairmanship of the Department of Psychiatry at the Johns Hopkins University, vacated the previous year by my friend Seymour S. Kety. Here again, fate was kind. The university provided us with some new laboratories, and the old Phipps Clinic, still standing since Adolf Meyer opened it in 1913, provided room for some 80 patients and an outpatient clinic. I count myself most fortunate in the colleagues who were with us, in the residency and fellowship programs, and in major staff positions.

Footings of a New Science: Neurochemistry, Electrophysiology, Animal Behavior and the Clinical Trial

Looking back, with large national and international organizations in psychopharmacology spanning the globe, and vast industrial undertakings engaged in research, development, and manufacture, it is a little hard to visualize the sparse and intimate nature of our field some 40 years ago. As I noted earlier, neurochemistry as we know it, did not really exist. And when I began, acetylcholine was still regarded as the principal chemical mediator in the central nervous system. Regional "elective affinities" of drugs for receptors remained in Henry Maudsley's memorable phrase, still to be "shadowed out" in the brain,[25] and Paul Ehrlich's "receptors" still an analogy. I remember sitting in Heinrich Waelsch's study overlooking the Hudson in August 1951, just before returning to England to take up my newly-created post. "What is experimental psychiatry?" asked Heinrich Waelsch, giving me that whimsical penetrating look of his. The newly named professor did not rightly know. "I suppose," I said, hesitatingly, "it is the application of the experimental research method to clinical psychiatry; I suppose, in my own case, it is the application of chemistry to an analysis and understanding of behavior. I will tell you when I have done it for a while."

Later, back in England, I got in touch with Derek Richter and Geoffrey Harris; Heinrich Waelsch met with Seymour S. Kety, Jordi Folch-Pi, and Louis Flexner. Our joint hope, which we had shared at a previous small meeting, was to organize an International Neurochemical Symposium, the first of its kind. As the theme of the symposium, we significantly chose "The Biochemistry of the Developing Nervous System." As a place to hold it, we chose Magdalen College, Oxford. I was charged with being organizing secretary, but could not have done it without the devoted help of my British colleagues. Sixty-nine colleagues from nine countries participated. It may be that it was at this symposium that the term "neurochemistry" was used officially for the first time.[26]

Our small group continued to do science by correspondence; I still remember the illegible notes, often on blue airmail letters (no fax in those days!), which brought the latest news. Those were heady days, to be sure. The process felt in some way like the collective painting of a mural; it all looked a bit weird at first, but month by month, and certainly year by year, it was beginning to make increasing sense: some pieces remained blurred, but others looked quite beautiful.

The Emergence of Organizations

In the meantime, other important events were stirring. The Macy Symposia on Neuropharmacology, initiated by Harold Abramson in 1954,[27] brought a number of us together and in 1956, under the joint chairmanship of Jonathan Cole and Ralph Gerard, a milestone Conference on Psychopharmacology was held under the aegis of the National Research Council, the National Academy of Sciences, and the American Psychiatric Association,[28] during which year also Cole's Psychopharmacology Service Center was created, a step of enormous consequence for the future development of the field all over the world.

In 1957, the World Health Organization invited me to serve as consultant and convened a small study group on the subject of Ataractic and Hallucinogenic Drugs in Psychiatry. The following participated: Ludwig von Bertalanffy, U.S.A. (Systems Theory), U. S. von Euler, Sweden (Pharmacology), E. Jacobsen, Denmark (Pharmacology), Morton Kramer, U.S.A. (Epidemiology), T. A. Lambo, Nigeria (Transcultural Psychiatry), E. Lindemann, U.S.A. (Psychiatry), P. Pichot, France (Psychology), David McKenzie Rioch, U.S.A. (Neurosciences), R. A. Sandison, England (Psychiatry), P. B. Schneider, Switzerland (Clinical Pharmacology), Joel Elkes, England (Rapporteur).

At about the same time, national groups in psychopharmacology began to form, at first loosely and informally, and later in more definitive ways. That most important international body, the Collegium Internationale Neuro-Psychopharmacologicum was born in 1956, and, as mentioned earlier–reflecting E. Rothlin's and Abraham Wikler's energy and devotion–our own journal of *Psychopharmacologia*, representing our new science, saw the light of day in 1959, and has continued as a yardstick of excellence since.

Closing

There are many memories that flood the mind, but clearly these reminiscences have gone on much too long, and I must come to a close. When, through the initiatives of Ted Rothman, Paul Hoch, Jonathan Cole, and others, as I have recorded elsewhere,[29] the American College of Neuropsychopharmacology was constituted in Washington in 1960, and did me the immense honor of electing me its first president, I could not help remembering that this had happened only 15 years after I played with macromolecular models and the X-ray diffraction of myelin in my laboratory in Birmingham, and only 10 years after we had created a Department of Experimental Psychiatry in Birmingham. I could not help reflecting on the unique power of our field to act not only as a catalyst, but as a binder; a catalyst bringing into being whole new areas of science, but also as a binder and a relater of these sciences to each other. For we had not only to create fields of investigation and measuring devices in many disciplines, but also a degree of understanding and interaction between disciplines which is very rare. Speaking at a dinner that took place in October 1961, I said:

> It is not uncommon for any one of us to be told that Psychopharmacology is not a science, and that it would do well to emulate the precision of older and more established disciplines. Such statements betray a lack of understanding for the special demands made by Psychopharmacology upon the fields which compound it. For my own part, I draw comfort and firm conviction from the history of our subject and the history of our group. For I know of no other branch of science which, like a good plough on a spring day has tilled as many areas of Neurobiology. To have, in a mere decade, questioned the concepts of synaptic transmission in the central nervous system; to have emphasized

compartmentalization and regionalization of chemical process in the unit cell and in the brain; to have given us tools for the study of the chemical basis of learning and temporary connection formation; to have emphasized the dependence of pharmacological response on its situational and social setting; to have compelled a hard look at the semantics of psychiatric diagnosis, description and communication; to have resuscitated the oldest of old remedies, the placebo response for careful scrutiny; to have provided potential methods for the study of language in relation to the functional state of the brain; and to have encouraged the Biochemist, Physiologist, Psychologist, Clinician, the Mathematician and Communication Engineer to join forces at bench levels; is no mean achievement for a young science. That a chemical test should carry the imprint of experience, and partake in its growth, in no way invalidates the study of symbols, and the rules among symbols, which keep us going, changing, evolving and human. Thus, though moving cautiously, psychopharmacology is still protesting; yet, in so doing, it is for the first time, compelling the physical and chemical sciences to look behaviour in the face, and thus enriching both these sciences and behavior. If there be discomfiture in this encounter, it is hardly surprising; for it is in this discomfiture that there may well lie the germ of a new science.[30]

In our branch of science, it would seem we are attracted to soma as to symbol; we are as interested in overt behavior as we are aware of the subtleties of subjective experience. There is here no conflict between understanding the way things are and the way people are, between the pursuit of science and the giving of service. It is this rare comprehensiveness which is psychopharmacology's unique gift to medicine and to psychiatry. The pharmacology without will slowly lead to the pharmacology within, an understanding of the nature of healing and self-healing, putting psychiatry as the science of man and mind at the very heart of medicine, where it rightfully belongs.

Appendix

In 1955, I was invited by Cohen and Kety to assume the directorship of the NIMH Branch known at the time as the Psychosomatic Medicine Branch. Because of the generosity and support I had encountered in England from the University of Birmingham and the Medical Research Council I decided to stay in England.

In 1957, Cohen and Kety renewed their offer. My acceptance resulted in the creation of the Clinical Neuropharmacology Research Center at the William A. White Building of St. Elizabeths Hospital in Washington, D.C. The Center was later renamed the Division of Special Mental Health Programs of the NIMH and continued under the successive, dynamic leadership of Drs. Gian Carlo Salmoiraghi, Floyd Bloom, Ermino Costa, and Richard Wyatt, all of whom, in their subsequent, remarkable careers, made deep and lasting contributions to the neurosciences and psychopharmacology. At the closing of the Center, with the return of its activities to the intramural program in Bethesda, Maryland, I wrote the following letter to Dr. Wyatt[31]:

October 19, 1999
Dear Friends,

I am sorry I cannot be with you this evening; but my greetings and good wishes go to our beloved Richard Wyatt and to you from a full and grateful heart. I treasure my good fortune to have known some of you in person and others by their writings; and ask myself "How lucky can a person be?" How often does life bestow such riches of memories or joyous celebration of shared common work? Moments and faces spring to life as I write. I remember one such moment.

It was a fragrant crisp spring morning in, I believe, April of 1957. I had driven to Bethesda passing the cherry blossoms and suddenly found myself standing in front of the imposing facade of the William A. White building at St. Elizabeths. This was to be our new Center. Seymour Kety had sent me the plans of the building to England and sitting in my office in Birmingham, I had roughed out the general layout: Animal laboratories in the Basement; Human laboratories and offices on the fifth floor, and patients in between and all around us. But, the core question that morning was not the layout or even (in those halcyon days) the budget. It was simply this: "How do we do justice in this building to the unique qualities, the uniquely transdisciplinary nature of our field?" How do we further conversation between lab and lab and lab and clinic. How do we enhance team work? and how, in the fullness of time, do we put a team into a single head? I readily admit to a little anxiety at the time. However, the past forty years have proved profoundly reassuring.

As I said, moments and faces spring to life as I recall our efforts to develop a *continuum* of activities between neurochemistry, electrophysiology, animal behavior and clinical investigation in our dear old building, still carrying the dank, sweet smell of chronic care. I remember Nino Salmoiraghi leading me into the secrets of reciprocal discharge of respiratory neurons as we talked about the strange calming effects of deep breathing in man; I recall the excitement I felt when he and Floyd Bloom showed me the pulling of the five barrel micro pipette with which they mapped the uneven chemical susceptibilities of neurons in the hippocampus. I recall Hans Weil-Malherbe's discussions with Julie Axelrod and Steve Brody's visit to our labs. I recall Steve Szara's collaboration with Elliot Hearst on the effects of DMT derivatives on operant conditioning, making a Skinner Box a Metabolic Cage. I recall Sheppard Kellam developing a Social Interaction Matrix to study the effects of major tranquilizers in the ward; and I remember Fritz Freyman bringing me one of the first issues of his "Comprehensive Psychiatry". There was also the procession of Visiting Fellows: Von Baumgarten, Rolf Gjessing and Max Hamilton, among others. The residents were terrified of Max Hamilton. They called him "Mac the Knife".

How much more has happened since? How far have new approaches and new methods carried us under the successive leadership of Nino, Floyd, Mimo, Richard, Dan and their illustrious colleagues? How well have we grasped psychopharmacology's unique ability to *connect* disparate fields and to make dreams literally visible. Fifty years ago– before Koelle's histochemistry and the advent of the Swedish fluorescent techniques–"Regional Neurochemistry" was a game of the imagination; and the term was–shall we say–in very limited circulation. Now there are the beautiful illuminated images emerging from your laboratory. I ask you, what does the heart do with such moments of awe and gratitude? Especially now, when we stand at yet another mighty beginning. Molecular Genetics, Neuropsychoimmunology, the Human Genome and Microchip sensors beckon to create new connections and new hybrids, Psychopharmacology will expand to include even these, and will never be the same again.

When in years to come we celebrate our half century, and when new generations of drugs of extraordinary specificity and power hit the market, huge new questions will loom and will not go away. Society will ask us to face our ethical dilemma and to be accountable; and we had better be prepared. There is no better safeguard against the excesses of our own inventiveness than an informed public. In our zeal to Do you must not forget to Listen. We must Listen as we Do and train Doers who will also Listen. For ours is a peculiarly personal biology; and we will always encounter our humanity in the deepest recesses of our molecular search.

It is this rare comprehending comprehensiveness which is Psycho-pharmacology's unique gift to Medicine and Psychiatry. The Pharmacology with*out* will slowly lead to the pharmacy with*in*–to an understanding of the nature of Healing and Self-Healing, putting Psychiatry and the Sciences of the Mind at the very heart of Medicine where they rightfully belong.

So, if I thank you from a full and greatful heart, do you wonder? As we celebrate our common past we join in sending our fondest good wishes for a speedy recovery to our dear Richard and to Kay. Let us meet again from time to time. Let us go on doing what our field does so supremely well. Let us continue to *connect*.

Fondly,
Joel Elkes

Notes

1. Charles S. Sherrington, *The Integrative Action of the Nervous System* (New Haven: Yale University Press, 1911).
2. Joel Elkes, Alastair C. Frazer, and Harold C. Stewart, "The Composition of Particles Seen in Normal Human Blood Under Dark Ground Illumination," *Journal of Physiology* 95 (1939): 68.
3. Francis O. Schmitt, "X-Ray Diffraction Studies on Nerve," *Radiology* 25 (1935): 131; Francis O. Schmitt, "X-Ray Diffraction Studies on Structure of Nerve Myelin Sheath," *Journal of Cell Physiology* 18 (1941): 31.
4. Joel Elkes and J. Bryan Finean, "The Effect of Drying Upon the Structure of Myelin in the Sciatic Nerve of the Frog," in *Discussion of the Faraday Society (Lipoproteins)* (London, 1949), 134; Joel Elkes and J. Bryan Finean (1953a): "X-Ray Diffraction Studies on the Effects of Temperature on the Structure of Myelin in the Sciatic Nerve of the Frog," *Experimental Cell Research* 4 (1953a): 69; Joel Elkes and J. Bryan Finean, "Effects of Solvents on the Structure of Myelin in the Sciatic Nerve of the Frog," *Experimental Cell Research* 4 (1953b): 82.
5. F. A. Pickworth, "Occurrence and Significance of Small Vascular Lesions in Brain," *Journal of Mental Science* 87 (1941): 50-76.

6. Joel Elkes, J. T. Eayrs, and Archibald Todrick, "On the Effect and the Lack of Effect of Some Drugs on Postnatal Development in the Rat," in *Biochemistry of the Developing Nervous System*, ed. H. Waelsch (New York: Academic Press, 1955), 409.

7. William Mayer-Gross joined us as Principal Clinical Associate in 1954, and John Harrington became Director of the Clinic in 1957. There were also biochemical laboratories and an ethology laboratory to accommodate the work of M. R. A. Chance. I believe it was the first animal ethology laboratory in a psychiatric clinic. After my departure for the United States in 1957, our department was divided into a Department of Experimental Neuropharmacology, under Professor Phillip Bradley, and a Clinical Department of Psychiatry, under Professor William (now Sir William) Trethowan, later Dean of the Medical Faculty. I am glad to say that until recently Uffculme Clinic was functioning very well as a postgraduate teaching center of the Birmingham Regional Hospital.

8. Phillip B. Bradley, "A Technique for Recording the Electrical Activity of the Brain in the Conscious Animal," *Electroencephalography and Clinical Neurophysiology* 5 (1953): 451.

9. Jean Delay and Pierre Deniker, "Les Neuroplégiques en Thérapeutique Psychiatrique," *Thérapie* 8 (1953): 347.

10. Frank J. Ayd, "The Early History of Modern Psychopharmacology," *Neuropsychopharmacology* 5 (1991): 71-85.

11. Joel Elkes and Charmian Elkes, "Effects of Chlorpromazine on the Behaviour of Chronically Overactive Psychotic Patients," *British Medical Journal* 2 (1954): 560.

12. Later the Division of Special Mental Health Programs of the NIMH.

13. Gian C. Salmoiraghi, "Pharmacology of Respiratory Neurons," in *Proceedings of the First International Pharmacology Meetings* (Oxford: Pergamon Press, 1962), 217-29.

14. Gian C. Salmoiraghi and Floyd E. Bloom, "Pharmacology of Individual Neurons," *Science* 144 (1964): 493-9.

15. Hans Weil-Malherbe and E. R. B. Smith, "Metabolites of Catecholamines in Urine and Tissues," *Journal of Neuropsychiatry* (1962): 113-8.

16. Julius Axelrod, Hans Weil-Malherbe, R. Tomchik, "The Physiological Dispositions of H(3) Epinephrine and Its Metabolite Metanephrine," *Journal of Pharmacology and Experimental Therapeutics* 127 (1959): 251-6.

17. Stephen Szara, Eliot Hearst, F. Putney, "Metabolism and Behavioral Action of Psychotropic Tryptamine Homologues," *International Journal of Neuropharmacology* 1 (1962): 111.

18. Stephen Szara and Eliot Hearst, "The 6-hydroxylation of Tryptamine Derivatives: A Way of Producing Psychoactive Metabolites," *Annals of the New York Academy of Sciences* 96 (1962): 134-41.

19. Richard P. Michael, "An Investigation of the Sensitivity of Circumscribed Neurological Areas to Hormonal Stimulation by Means of the Application of Oestrogens Directly to the Brain of the Cat," in *Regional Neurochemistry, Proceedings of the Fourth International Symposium on Neurochemistry*, eds. Seymour S. Kety and Joel Elkes (Oxford: Pergamon Press, 1961), 465-80.

20. Harold Weiner, "Some Effects of Response Cost Upon Human Operant Behavior," *Journal of the Experimental Analysis of Behavior* 5 (1962): 201.

21. A. Hordern, M. Hamilton, F. N. Waldrop, and J. C. Lofft, "A Controlled Trial on the Value of Prochlorperazine and Trifluoperazine and Intensive Group Treatment," *British Journal of Psychiatry* 109 (1963): 510-22.

22. Shepherd G. Kellam, "A Method for Assessing Social Contacts: Its Application During a Rehabilitation Program on a Psychiatric Ward," *Journal of Nervous and Mental Diseases* 132 (1961): 277-88.

23. Fritz Freyhan and J. A. Mayo, "Concept of a Model Psychiatric Clinic," *American Journal of Psychiatry* 120 (1963): 222-7.

24. Donald R. Lipsitt, "Dependency, Depression, and Hospitalization: Towards an Understanding of a Conspiracy," *Psychiatric Quarterly* 30 (1962): 537-54.

25. Henry Maudsley, *The Physiology and Pathology of the Mind*, 3rd ed., Part 2 (New York: Appleton, 1882), 195.

26. Three subsequent symposia reflected the momentum that was developing at this historic first meeting. The second one was held in Aarhus, Denmark, in 1956 (Proceedings: Derek Richter, ed., *Metabolism of the Nervous System* (New York: Pergamon Press, 1957). The third one followed in Strasbourg, France, in 1958 (Proceedings: Jordi Folch-Pi, ed., *The Chemical Pathology of the Nervous System* (New York: Pergamon Press, 1961). The Fourth International Symposium was held in Varenna, Italy, in 1960 (Proceedings: Seymour S. Kety and Joel Elkes, eds., *Regional Neurochemistry* (New York: Pergamon Press, 1961).

27. Harold A. Abramson, ed., *Neuropharmacology* (New York: Josiah Macy, Jr., Foundation, 1954).

28. Jonathan Cole and Ralph W. Gerard, eds., *Psychopharmacology: Problems in Evaluation* (Washington, D.C.: National Academy of Sciences and National Research Council, 1959).

29. Joel Elkes, "The American College of Neuropsychopharmacology: A Note on Its History and Hopes For the Future," *American College of Neuropsychopharmacology Bulletin* 1 (1963): 2-3.

30. Ibid.

31. Unedited letter.

Mind, Brain, Body, and Behavior
I. G. Farreras, C. Hannaway and V. A. Harden (Eds.)
IOS Press, 2004

My Experiences as a Research Associate in Neurophysiology at the NIH (1958-1960)[1]

Sid Gilman

Why would a young man from Los Angeles come to the NIH in 1958? The answer was that there was a physician draft. The Korean War lasted for about three years, from 1950 to 1953, and there was a draft for physicians at the time. In 1954, Frank Berry became Assistant Secretary of Defense, and soon after his appointment, he devised the Berry plan. This was a system whereby physicians could put their names into a lottery, and if their number came up, they would be deferred from military service for the full extent of their residency training. If the number did not come up, however, they were subject to the draft.

I graduated from the University of California-Los Angeles (UCLA) Medical School in 1957, and during my internship at the UCLA Hospital, I learned that my number did not come up and that I was vulnerable to the draft while a house officer. I went to see Augustus Rose, who was my mentor and the chairman of the neurology department at UCLA at the time. He said, "Why don't you go to the National Institutes of Health (NIH)?" And I said, "The N-I- what?" He explained what this meant and suggested that I talk to Robert B. Livingston. Livingston had been an assistant professor in anatomy at the UCLA Medical School, and he had joined the NIH as scientific director of the National Institute of Mental Health (NIMH) and the National Institute of Neurological Diseases and Blindness (NINDB[2]) intramural basic research program. While I was still an intern, Livingston happened to visit the UCLA Medical Center and, at Rose's urging, I went to see him and asked him about going to the

NIH. He told me, "Fine, but first you have to join the Public Health Service (PHS). You have to go through a competitive examination for admission, and then you have to apply to the NIH. If you get in, we'll be glad to see you there, although I cannot take responsibility for you."

I was a very busy intern on an inpatient service, serving on-call every other night and usually staying up all night most of the nights that I was on call, but I applied to the PHS and after taking an examination, I received notification that I was accepted. The notification included a missive stating that I might be sent to an Indian reservation or a PHS station elsewhere and that I would just have to stay tuned. A few months later, I received a communication stating that I was accepted to the NIH and that I would be appointed a Senior Assistant Surgeon, which I thought was an extraordinary title. I was an intern in internal medicine and had no interest in surgery, but I accepted my fate.

On July 1, 1958, I left Los Angeles for Bethesda, Maryland, and entered the NIH Research Associates Training Program, which was marvelous. It involved special courses in some of the basic sciences that were important for physicians who had not had any research training, as was my case. The program also included a laboratory assignment with a mentor. I was one of seven physicians in the entire NIH Research Associates Program at the time.[3] The Research Associates Program spanned the entire NIH intramural program and was not confined to the NINDB and the NIMH.

I was assigned to Livingston's laboratory, and to my good fortune, Bo Ernest Gernandt was working there as a visiting scientist. Gernandt was a vestibular neurophysiologist from Sweden who had developed a technique for placing an electrode on the peripheral branches of the vestibular nerves in the inner ear of the cat, applying electrical stimulation, and then studying the downstream effects of vestibular stimulation. At that time, except for a few laboratories in the world—including the laboratory of Karl Frank and Phillip Nelson, who were studying motor neurons in the spinal cord of the cat—electrophysiology had not yet evolved widely into either cell culture or single-cell examinations. So we worked steadily, sometimes conducting two experiments in a single day, studying interactions of descending vestibular activities with neck proprioceptors and other important influences from descending pathways, including those arising in the cerebellum, the corticospinal pathway and extrapyramidal systems.[4]

The research environment was rich, with wonderful and interesting people in the adjacent laboratories whom I came to know to some extent. Karl Frank, chief of the Laboratory of Neurophysiology's Section on Spinal Cord Physiology, and Phillip Nelson were carrying out microelectrode studies of anterior horn cells. Those two investigators, plus Sir John Eccles in Canberra, Australia, were doing seminal work on motor neuron function with intracellular recordings. Walter Freygang, Jr. (Laboratory of Neurophysiology), Wade H. Marshall (chief of the Laboratory of Neurophysiology), and Edward V. Evarts (chief of the Laboratory of Clinical Science Section on Physiology) were nearby. At that time, Evarts was studying evoked potentials in the auditory system with microelectric techniques. He would later go on to classical studies of the functions of single corticospinal neurons in the cerebral cortex of the awake behaving animal. Ichiji Tasaki headed the Section on Special Senses (within the Laboratory of Neurophysiology) down the hall. Eric Kandel and William Alden Spencer were also there, working in Marshall's Laboratory of Neurophysiology. Kandel and I have remained friends since meeting at the NIH, and I participated in recruiting him to Columbia University when I was on its faculty some years back. Roscoe O. Brady headed the Section on Lipid Chemistry near me and we have remained friends throughout the years. Paul MacLean (chief of the Laboratory of Neurophysiology's Section on Limbic Integration and Behavior), William F. Windle (chief of the Laboratory of Neuroanatomical Sciences), and Lloyd Guth (within the Laboratory of Neuroanatomical Sciences) were also in the vicinity.[5] Grant L. Rasmussen (chief of the Laboratory of Neuroanatomical Sciences's Section on Functional Neuroanatomy) and Richard Gacek were working on the auditory system. Gacek later became an otolaryngologist.

I also came to know several scientists in related fields, including Mortimer Mishkin (in the Laboratory of Psychology's Section on Animal Behavior), Allan F. Mirsky (in the Laboratory of Psychology's Section on Animal Behavior), Felix Strumwasser (in the Laboratory of Neurophysiology), and Richard Coggeshall (in the Laboratory of Neurophysiology). Eugene Streicher (within the Laboratory of Psychology's Section on Aging) was there, along with Larry Embree (in the Laboratory of Neurochemistry) and Detlev Ploog (in the Laboratory of Neurophysiology's Section on Limbic Integration and Behavior). Many years after my two years as a Research Associate at the NIH, I became a member of the NINDS Advisory Council, and on my first day, Streicher came up to me and said, "Sid, welcome home." I had the good fortune to see Ploog at a meeting in Tübingen some years later as well.

During the last two years of the 1950s, the NIH had not only interesting work in many laboratories that I learned about in seminars as well as in casual conversations, but also an interesting clinical environment. G. Milton Shy was the NINDB intramural clinical director and chief of the Medical Neurology Branch at that time. Shy had grand rounds on Tuesdays and Saturdays, and as I was occupied in the laboratory on Tuesdays, I went to his extremely stimulating rounds on Saturdays. He was a challenging teacher, usually putting people on the spot and grilling them, mostly about anatomy but often about clinical disorders as well. I remember many interesting Saturday afternoons, going home, consulting anatomy books, and meeting the intellectual challenges Shy had presented.

Cosimo Ajmone-Marsan headed the Electroencephalography Branch and Maitland Baldwin and John Van Buren were neurosurgeons who headed the Surgical Neurology Branch. Trainees in the Medical Neurology Branch included Donald Silberberg, Andrew Engel, W. King Engel, and Guy McKhann.

In addition to the special courses offered to the Research Associates, there were also lectures on the nervous system that Wally Nauta gave at the Walter Reed Army Medical Center. Frank gave a series of lectures in basic electronics, and there were multiple guest lecturers and symposia offered by the NINDB, the NIMH, and other NIH Institutes.

As it is completely transformed now, let me describe Bethesda in the late 1950s. It was a small town with only one good restaurant, O'Donnell's, and nothing more than a few beer parlors. Most people would have to go into Washington for a decent dinner. Because I was a member of the PHS, however, I could go to the restaurant across the street at the National Naval Medical Research Center.

I lived with various other young physicians, including George Bray, who was a fellow Research Associate, Charles Buckner, who became a neurosurgeon, James Marsh, who went into practice in Maine, Robert Krooth, who became a professor of genetics at the University of Michigan, and was later chairman of the Department of Genetics at Columbia University, and Harold Gelboin, who remains an intramural scientist at the NIH. We initially lived in Bethesda and later in Chevy Chase.

Mishkin somehow heard that I lived in a large house with several other people and that we had plenty of room. We did; we lived in a large, rambling house on Leland Street in Chevy Chase. Mishkin said that a visiting scientist from Poland named Stefan Brutkowski would be working with him for six months and asked whether he could live with us. We could easily accommodate Brutkowski, so he moved in. He was a lovely person, and he did wonderful work with Mishkin which I heard about during many of our evenings together. Brutkowski must have thought that we were very messy, because he would put on an apron and go around the house with a broom to sweep up after the rest of us. I would like to describe the events that took place while Stefan was living with us as I recall them, and then modify them based on information that Mishkin and Mirsky have given me.

Brutkowski told us that he had an acquaintance who was coming from Bulgaria to spend some months working at the NIH. This scientist had developed a plethysmograph. Brutkowski asked me whether the visitor might stay with us for a weekend. We had a large house so we welcomed him and thus Stefan Figar came to stay with us. Unfortunately, even though his host, Mirsky, had heard otherwise, Figar was not able to sign a loyalty oath–because he belonged to the Communist Party–so he was not even able to set foot on the NIH campus at the time.

My housemates and I spent many Saturday evenings in the laboratory because although there were many interesting men at the NIH, there were almost no women, and we found ourselves with a limited social life. One of my housemates thought that we had to get acquainted with people in the "embassy circuit," and that way we would meet some eligible women. With Figar coming to stay with us, my housemate said, "Why don't we see if we can get into the Bulgarian Embassy? That'll be a way to become known in embassy row." So we asked Figar if he could arrange for us to be invited to the Bulgarian Embassy. We received an invitation and went to the Bulgarian Embassy on a Saturday evening, but the event proved to be a dreadful experience. There were perhaps two dozen of us who arrived at the embassy, and after we were in the reception area, our hosts turned off the lights and showed an awful film of young women waving red flags and doing gymnastics in Bulgaria. When the film ended, the lights came on and we were offered vodka and fried chicken that was about a week old. The food was very bad and there were no women, absolutely none. It was a bust.

On Monday, my chief, Livingston, called me into his office and said, "Sid, do you have a political agenda here? I heard you were at the Bulgarian Embassy on Saturday night." I said, "Well, no. We were there hoping to meet some interesting women." He replied, "In the Bulgarian Embassy?" Nothing further happened, but I thought at the time that the FBI must have been at or outside of the embassy on the Saturday night. I have given thought to asking for my FBI file under the Freedom of Information Act, but have never done so. I have since learned from Mirsky that Figar actually came from what was then Czechoslovakia and that we had gone to the Czechoslovakian Embassy, but the rest of the story is as I have related it.

The two years I spent at the NIH were a wonderful experience for me. When I arrived, I had not decided what I wanted to do in life, apart from working as a physician. I had not even decided on being a neurologist, although Horace (Ted) Magoun was one of my teachers in medical school, and I greatly enjoyed learning neuroanatomy, which many classmates thought was bizarre. I found the research at the NIH to be both interesting and rewarding, and I thought then that neurologically oriented research would be a wonderful way to spend one's career. When I left the NIH, I went to the Neurological Unit of the Boston City Hospital to serve a neurology residency with Derek Denny-Brown, followed by a fellowship with him in basic research. My interest in the vestibular system and cerebellum, developed at the NIH, proved to be a lifelong interest.

I remained at the Boston City Hospital and on the Harvard University Medical School faculty until Denny-Brown retired in 1967. A year later, I went to Columbia University, where Richard L. Masland, director of the NINDB after Pearce Bailey, became department chair. In 1977, I went to the University of Michigan as chairman of the Department of Neurology and have been there ever since. I have been fortunate to receive continuous training and research funding from the NIH and, in turn, I have served on multiple study sections and as a member of the NINDS Advisory Council.

It seems odd at first glance, but I have maintained closer ties with the NIH than I have with my alma mater for my undergraduate education, medical school and internship, UCLA, and other medical schools–Harvard and Columbia University–where I have been a faculty member. I have been a department chair at the University of Michigan for 25 years now and have very close ties with this institution, but when the NIH comes calling and asks me to perform a task, I will do it if I possibly can. I owe such a debt of gratitude to the NIH. I had a wonderful two years on the campus and I have had marvelous interactions with the administrators and the intramural and extramural scientists whom I have met in various contexts. So thank you, NIH; it has been a wonderful run.

Notes

1. I want to thank Dr. Ingrid G. Farreras for her help, and also Drs. Mortimer Mishkin and Allan F. Mirsky for finding the name of Stefan Figar for me.
2. Today the National Institute of Neurological Disorders and Stroke (NINDS).
3. Bauman later went into industry. Huttenlocher became a pediatric neurologist who spent many years at the University of Chicago. Cohen dropped out of the program during the first year. Smiley became an arthritis specialist at the University of Texas-Dallas. Bray is an internationally known expert in obesity, now partially retired, but still has NIH grant support. He lives in San Francisco but commutes to an institute in Louisiana. Small became a microbiologist at the University of Florida.
4. We published a series of papers based on this work, the first of which appeared in the first volume of the journal, *Experimental Neurology*, which William Windle–chief of the NINDB Laboratory of Neuroanatomical Sciences– had founded while he was at the NIH. Our second paper concerned vestibular interactions with various segmental levels of the spinal cord and was published in the *Journal of Neurophysiology*. The third article focused upon

vestibular and cortically evoked descending activity and was also published in the *Journal of Neurophysiology*. The fourth article was published in
Experimental Neurology after I left the NIH.

5. The first volume of the journal *Experimental Neurology* was published in 1959.
   Windle, the founding editor, was followed by me, then Carmen Clemente
   and then John Sladek. I became editor-in-chief in January of 2003.

Mind, Brain, Body, and Behavior
I. G. Farreras, C. Hannaway and V. A. Harden (Eds.)
IOS Press, 2004

Reflections from the Pool of Bethesda[1]

Lloyd Guth

Journey to the NIH

I was born in 1929, in the very month of the monumental stock market crash. Although I was too young to be seriously aware of the "Great Depression" that followed, I was not oblivious to it. How could it be otherwise, when there were so many motion pictures and books (such as *You Can't Take It With You*, *Modern Times*, and *The Grapes of Wrath*) which carried the message that the human spirit can triumph over degradation and misery. And in the years that followed, the successful conclusion of World War II, the establishment of the United Nations, and the initiation of the Marshall Plan seemed a confirmation of this faith in the triumph of good over evil.

By this time, I had matriculated in college as a premedical student at the University Heights campus of New York University (NYU) and was beginning to consider my future. Although biology had been the science subject of greatest interest to me in high school, the biology curriculum in college was disappointingly trivial in subject matter and dull in presentation. The course began with a series of lectures on the history of biology. These lectures included the names of significant biologists of the past, the dates of their major discoveries, and the titles of their principal monographs. All of this information had to be committed to memory for the purpose of examination. I was required to memorize information about Leeuwenhoek, Pasteur, Linnaeus, and Schleiden and Schwann, even though nothing had as yet been taught about microscopy, microbiology, taxonomy, or the structure and organization of cells. A later course on comparative anatomy was more interesting because it gave an opportunity to dissect and observe comparable organs in higher and lower vertebrates. However, no attempt was made to explain the functional purpose of such phylogenetic specializations as pronephric, mesonephric or metanephric kidneys. Many years were to pass before I realized how exciting the study of comparative anatomy could have been had the teacher only explained the relationships between structure and function in these and other organs.

Here indeed was the paradox: despite my interest in animal life, the subject of biology was unexciting. Perhaps it was fortunate that I was kept so busy memorizing trivial details that little time was left for me to question whether such a biological catechism was the best way to teach the subject. In my final year came a course in embryology, which was taught in much the same fashion—this time requiring rote memorization of facts contained in our remarkably uninspiring textbook of descriptive embryology. Not even mentioned in the book or the lectures were the remarkable experimental embryological studies for which Hans Spemann had recently won the Nobel Prize.[2] Quite by chance, in the midst of this course, I happened upon a book by Paul Weiss titled *Principles of Development*.[3] This magnificently written and scholarly textbook of experimental embryology revealed biological science as a subject in which hypotheses were tested experimentally. It conveyed the sense of excitement at the questions being studied by experimental embryologists, and it inspired me to participate in the world of experimental science. In short, the book was for me an epiphany, and from that day forward, I studied Weiss's research publications in the hope that I might some day undertake graduate studies in embryology under his direction.

But this was not to be, and after graduating from college in 1949, I matriculated at the NYU School of Medicine. I enjoyed especially the laboratory components of the courses in physiology, pharmacology, and microbiology and was especially pleased to find that students were encouraged to participate in biomedical research. I also had the good fortune to be accepted to the summer student programs of the Jackson Memorial Laboratory in Maine where, during the summers of 1949 to 1951, I worked under the supervision of Eugene Roberts, who had recently discovered the unique presence of gamma-aminobutyric acid in central nervous system (CNS) tissues. This work led to an invitation from

Pinckney Harman to continue these investigations during the academic year in the anatomy department at NYU. I accepted and for two years I spent my free time in his laboratory where we studied the neuroanatomical localization of gamma-aminobutyric acid and its behavior during neural degeneration and regeneration. By the middle of my third year at medical school, with the encouragement of Roberts and Harman, I had decided on a career in medical research. My immediate goal was to do postdoctoral research with Roger Sperry (whose research on the chemo-affinity theory of nerve regeneration intrigued me and whom I had met through the kind intervention of another professor, Hans Teuber).

When Roberts accepted a position in the Laboratory of Neurochemistry at the National Institute of Neurological Diseases and Blindness (NINDB), he promised to recommend me to Sperry, who had just been appointed to the basic research program of the NINDB laboratory. These plans fell by the wayside when both Roberts and Sperry resigned their NIH appointments in favor of positions at the City of Hope (Roberts), and the California Institute of Technology (Sperry). The lost opportunity to work with Sperry was a great disappointment, but Roberts kept his promise by recommending me instead to William F. Windle,[4] who had been appointed chief of the Laboratory of Neuroanatomical Sciences. Following an interview with Windle, I was accepted into his laboratory, commissioned as Senior Assistant Surgeon in the U.S. Public Health Service (PHS),[5] and assigned to work directly under Windle in his ancillary capacity as chief of his Laboratory's Section on Development and Regeneration. As a result, on July 1, 1954, shortly after the NINDB had been founded, I arrived in Bethesda without any idea of what the future would hold and certainly without any clue that I was about to begin an exciting, happy, and productive 21-year tenure at the NIH.

The Structure of the NINDB

It is noteworthy that during my entire career at the NIH (1954-1975) I heard little to nothing about the institute's "mission." To most basic scientists, the term "mission" was an anathema, because this quasi-military, quasi-religious term carried overtones of a structured goal with a beginning and an end. Since basic research (unlike applied research) is an endeavor in which the outcome cannot be predicted, the concept of a "mission" was considered inappropriate. As viewed by junior and senior scientists alike, we had a "responsibility" to do good research by adhering to the principles of scientific investigation, and the only goal was to increase our understanding of the anatomy, physiology, and biochemistry of the nervous system.

At that time, a fundamental tenet of the institute directors was that clinical advances depended on basic research. This view seems to be widely proclaimed today, but one caveat has unfortunately been added, viz., that basic research must justify its existence by leading to clinical advances. The founders of the NINDB, on the other hand, recognized that basic science was essential because our understanding of basic neuroscience was insufficient to guide us to more effective treatments for neurological disorders. Since clinical advances are dependent on a fuller understanding of nervous system structure and function, it is self-destructive to require basic science to validate its existence in terms of future clinical applications.[6]

Organization

When the NINDB was initiated, there were few precedents for such a government-funded biomedical research institute. Since most of the senior appointees had previously held university positions in academic departments, it is not surprising that Pearce Bailey (the NINDB's first director) and Seymour S. Kety (the first scientific director for the joint NIMH-NINDB intramural basic research program) utilized the academic prototype in structuring the intramural program.

They established a basic research division that focused on neuroanatomy, neurophysiology, neuropathology, and neurochemistry, and clinical research divisions centered around medical, surgical, and radiological neurology. This organization reflected a structure analogous to that of a medical school, where both the teaching and research responsibilities are carried out within autonomous and independent departments. Despite this structure, however, a great deal of multidisciplinary research was done by collaboration between individual investigators (within as well as between laboratories). One might say that the independence granted to the research scientist actually facilitated interactions between scientists and promoted a great deal of "self-generated" interdisciplinary research.[6] This freedom to work together also had a salutatory effect of helping reduce competition among scientists. In view of the strong administrative support for investigative freedom and the absence of competition for research funding, it is not surprising that significant "animosities" were rare.

The present-day structure of the institute's laboratories is, of course, quite different, and reflects the interdisciplinary nature of current research. But I wonder whether working on large group projects causes scientists to be fearful that open discussion of ongoing work might necessitate inappropriate discussion of the work of others in their team.

The university background of the laboratory chiefs also led them to establish procedures for ensuring the academic freedom of their scientists. In the belief that the scientists should have a voice in administrative decisions, and to provide a forum for discussion of major decisions that affected them, they established an elected Assembly of Scientists as the governmental equivalent of the university's "Faculty Council." This Assembly was designed to promote academic freedom, not restrict it; one of its major functions was to prevent the government or the NIH administration from attempting to control or micromanage intramural research. Thus, in the early days of the NINDB, the philosophy of the administration and the relationship between scientist and administration were congruent with those of academic institutions. In fact, there were pressures from some intramural scientists to expand the mission of the NIH to full university status. If my recollection is correct, Giulio Cantoni, chief of the Laboratory of Cellular Pharmacology, was a major advocate for this transformation. Although this proposal was not acted on, the NIH scientists were encouraged to participate in the teaching and research activities of the universities, and various formal collaborative arrangements with universities were established to facilitate these interactions.

In the early 1950s, new institutes such as the NINDB were just being established. Although little was known about this new research institute, university professors were beginning to accept positions at the NIH and word of this spread quickly through their institutions. For example, I learned of the NIH through those teachers who had signed on to posts at the NIH. These included Louis Sokoloff, a professor of pathology at NYU, George Jay, a geneticist at the Jackson Memorial Laboratory, and Eugene Roberts, a biochemist from Washington University in St. Louis.

Budget Process

In the 1950s, budgeting was primarily an administrative responsibility, and section chiefs and junior scientists were shielded from the intricacies of the process. Items required for the work of the laboratory were simply ordered by the scientists concerned. If, toward the end of the fiscal year, there was a shortfall in the institute's budget, a memo was sent out requesting that purchases be deferred insofar far as possible until the beginning of the next fiscal year. This simple and sensible arrangement left budget calculations in the office of the institute director, and allowed the laboratory chiefs great freedom in making the purchases necessary for their laboratory's research programs. It had the further (and not inconsequential) advantage of mitigating internecine competition for funds among the institute's laboratories. Windle once expressed appreciation that he was not held to a formal, line-item budget, and certainly the junior scientists appreciated being free of budgetary considerations; we simply ordered all inexpensive items as we needed them, and discussed more expensive purchases with our section chiefs before ordering them.

Such budgetary flexibility apparently also allowed for transfer of funds between institutes. For example, the Laboratory of Neurophysiology was funded jointly by the NIMH and the NINDB, with four sections within the NIMH and two within the NINDB. It is interesting to speculate on whether such an arrangement would now be considered an acceptable federal accounting practice.

Organization of the Laboratory of Neuroanatomical Sciences

When I arrived in Bethesda on July 1, 1954, I found only Windle and Jan Cammermeyer present, but I was told by Windle that the laboratory would soon consist of four sections: a Section on Development and Regeneration under his direction, a Section on Experimental Neuropathology under Cammermeyer, a Section on Functional Neuroanatomy under Grant L. Rasmussen, and a Section on Neurocytology under

Sanford L. Palay. Each section was to have one or two junior scientists, and I had been assigned to Windle's section because of my interest in nerve regeneration. A week or two later, I was introduced to Milton Brightman, who had been appointed to the Section on Neurocytology (and who had recently received his Ph.D. at Yale University under Palay's supervision). Soon thereafter, a third junior scientist appeared. He was R. Wayne Albers, who had the distinction of being the first and only predoctoral student of the renowned biochemist, Oliver Lowry. Albers had originally been destined for appointment to the Laboratory of Neurochemistry, but when Eugene Roberts decided against coming to the NIH, he recommended Albers to Windle. Windle's acceptance of a biochemist into his Laboratory of Neuroanatomical Sciences revealed an important aspect of his scientific philosophy. It did not matter to him whether research was done by scientists trained in biochemistry, physiology or anatomy; all that mattered was that it be good science. Indeed, Brightman recalls Windle's "pithy dictum" that "neuroanatomy is what neuroanatomists do" (a statement that helps explain why he designated his department as the Laboratory of Neuroanatomical Sciences).

Research Programs of the Section Chiefs

Windle–Spinal Cord Regeneration

In the mid-1940s, while at the University of Pennsylvania, Windle had initiated a program to identify the nerve pathways that control temperature regulation. For these experiments, he made lesions in various parts of the brain or spinal cord of animals, and he then injected a fever-inducing drug called Piromen (a bacterial lipopolysaccharide), to see whether any of these neural lesions might modify the febrile response. One of the CNS lesions that he chose to investigate was transection of the spinal cord. He injected Piromen at frequent intervals into these animals to ascertain the time course of possible changes in their febrile response to the drug. He and his colleagues observed that some of the spinal cats, after receiving the drug for several weeks, began to yowl when their tails were pinched. Careful neurohistological studies on the spinal cords of these cats revealed that the restored sensibility was accompanied by extensive growth of nerve fibers into and across the lesion. This anatomical evidence was confirmed by electrophysiological experiments showing that electrical stimulation of the cord below the lesion elicited electrical activity in the cord above the lesion. Windle continued these experiments on cats and monkeys at the NIH, and although locomotor function was never restored, his work proved that injured spinal cord nerve fibers retain their growth potential in adult animals. His research, publications, and symposia kept alive the interest in CNS regeneration for several decades and led to the present large-scale research efforts aimed at achieving functional regeneration of the injured spinal cord.

Windle–Perfusion Fixation

One of the first weekly laboratory meetings in 1954 was devoted to the problem of obtaining histological preparations that were free of artifactual changes (e.g., shrinkage, swelling, etc.). At the time, I did not understand the full significance of what was being discussed, but I do recall how impressed I was by the section chiefs' unanimous agreement that fixation by vascular perfusion was an essential step in preparing tissues for light microscopical histology. Only later did I learn that Windle and his colleagues had published in 1945 a seminal paper on the importance of perfusion fixation.[7] At that time, the concept of perfusion fixation was novel (for example, it was not even mentioned in Davenport's 1945 book on histological technique[8]). Nevertheless, its importance remained largely ignored for another two decades, and was still not considered worthy of mention in Ralph Lillie's widely-used 1965 reference book on histopathological technique.[9]

The reluctance of anatomists to accept perfusion fixation was not based on tradition so much as on scientific skepticism. For 50 years, both basic scientists and clinical pathologists had been fixing their tissues by simply dropping the specimens into a fixative solution, and most of them, being satisfied with the quality of preservation, felt no need for a change. Of course the continued testing of alternatives and additives to 10 percent formaldehyde during this time (e.g., Heidenhain's "susa" which added mercuric chloride, Bouin's fluid which added picric acid, and Zenker's solution which added chromic acid) should have provided a warning that achieving adequate tissue preservation was no simple matter. Nevertheless, the full significance of this issue was not recognized and accepted until Cammermeyer, Palay, and many others demonstrated convincingly by both light and electron microscopy, the importance of Windle's principles of perfusion fixation. Thanks in large measure to the pioneering research in the Laboratory of Neuroanatomical Sciences, perfusion fixation became the accepted standard of tissue preservation for both light and electron microscopy.

Palay

At the time of Palay's arrival, most electron microscopists fixed their specimens by immersion in osmium tetroxide solution. Because of the poor penetration of osmium tetroxide, this procedure fixed only the external surface of the specimens and left the bulk of the specimen unusable. Many years earlier, while a postdoctoral fellow in Ernst Scharrer's laboratory at Case Western Reserve University School of Medicine, Palay had learned about the importance of perfusion fixation for light microscopy from Scharrer. Now, with further encouragement from Windle, Palay set about developing a method of perfusion fixation for the electron microscopical examination of nervous tissue. His first success came when he adopted a modification of Windle's two-step procedure: he perfused the vascular system with a balanced salt solution to remove all traces of blood and followed this by perfusion with a solution of osmium tetroxide to fix the tissue. Although this procedure was a vast improvement over immersion fixation with osmium tetroxide, the fixative was very costly and, being highly volatile and caustic, required special precautions to avoid damaging the investigator's cornea and respiratory passages. The success of Palay's studies led numerous scientists world-wide to attempt further modifications that might obviate these problems. A procedure involving three successive steps was developed that soon became standard: (1) removal of blood by perfusion with an isotonic salt solution; (2) fixation of the tissues by perfusion with an aldehyde fixative (such as acrolein or a reagent grade formaldehyde that was freshly prepared from paraformaldehyde); and (3) post-fixation by immersion of the specimen in osmium tetroxide.

These improved methods of tissue fixation enabled Palay to perform his pioneering ultrastructural investigations of neurons and neuroglia. His papers on the ultrastructure of the synapse[10] delineated for the first time the synaptic cleft, synaptic vesicles, and the various presynaptic and post-synaptic membrane specializations. This description of the ultrastructure of the synapse provided the first unequivocal proof of cellular discontinuity at the synapse, the concept which was a cornerstone of the "neuron doctrine" for which Santiago Ramón y Cajal had received the Nobel Prize some 50 years earlier. In other papers, Palay played a leading role in resolving the controversy over the ultrastructural identification of astrocytes and oligodendrocytes.[11] These findings provided baseline information essential for many subsequent biochemical and physiological investigations on neurons and neuroglia.

Cammermeyer

Cammermeyer was an experimental neuropathologist and a very astute microscopist. He spent much of his first decade at the NIH investigating the effects of various fixatives (administered by immersion or perfusion) on brain volume in an effort to eliminate the swelling or shrinkage that occurs during histological procedures for preparing tissues for light microscopy. For this purpose, he made painstaking measurements of swelling and shrinkage at each stage of the fixing, dehydrating, embedding, sectioning and staining steps. These studies required expert microscopical analysis. Cammermeyer's scientific expertise and helpful attitude made him an important resource for other scientists in the laboratory. As an example, he called me into his laboratory one day and showed me an autoradiograph made with tritiated thymidine which clearly revealed silver grains over the nucleus of a large neuron. I was dumbfounded to see this evidence of a dividing adult neuron. Before I could say anything that might betray my ignorance, he told me to focus up and down with the fine adjustment. All at once it became apparent that the silver grains were not over the neuron's nucleus but over that of a glial cell located beneath the neuron. I learned that day why his motto was "one must always be cautious," and how much pleasure can be derived from teaching others to enjoy the art, craft, and science of histology and histopathology.

Rasmussen

During the 1940s, Rasmussen had discovered the olivocochlear bundle, an efferent pathway within the auditory system. For a long while the very existence of this pathway was disputed, but during his years at the NIH the issue was resolved in his favor. Its function was eventually elucidated by neurophysiological studies which showed: (a) that this pathway provided the feedback mechanism that is essential for the regulation of audition; and (b) that such feedback regulates activity in most neural circuits. Two now eminent scientists who received their early postdoctoral scientific experience in Rasmussen's section are D. Kent Morest, professor of neuroscience and director of the High Technology Center for Neuroscience at the University of Connecticut Health Center, and Thomas Reese, chief of the NINDB's Laboratory of Neurobiology's Section on Structural Biology.

Scientific Environment of the Laboratory of Neuroanatomical Sciences

Standards of Propriety

Early in my career, in 1955, Windle called me to his office to tell me that the editors of *Physiological Review* had invited him to write a review on regeneration in the central and peripheral nervous systems. He said that they were agreeable to his suggestion that so vast and unwieldy a subject would benefit by being published as two consecutive articles, one on CNS regeneration and the other on PNS regeneration. He said that he would write the review on CNS regeneration, and he invited me to be co-author with him on the PNS regeneration review article.[12] I was delighted by the opportunity and by the confidence he showed in me, especially since I had been in his laboratory only one year and had not yet published any papers. I spent the better part of the next six months working in the library where I tracked down and abstracted all (some 434) articles written from 1929 through 1955, and I then prepared a draft of the manuscript for his inspection. Knowing that Windle would have much to add to the manuscript, I presented it to him with a title page indicating the authorship as "Windle and Guth." In my presence, he took up a red pencil and began to correct the manuscript as he read it. I was spellbound at his quickness; the pencil simply flew over the page, as if unguided by human hand, marking up every sentence without any hesitation whatever. After about ten minutes he stopped and said that he would finish his task that evening.

The following day he returned to me a manuscript in which each page was filled with corrections and annotations–every correction was just and every annotation was correct. And on the title page, the name of William F. Windle was struck through, leaving that of Lloyd Guth as sole author. On that day in 1955, I learned the single most important lesson of my life about one's responsibility as scientist and teacher: it is one's duty to help advance science by suggesting research directions to one's students, and it is one's responsibility to assist them in their efforts, but it is undignified to accept the payment of authorship for these activities. To the best of my knowledge, these standards were accepted by all section chiefs in the Laboratory of Neuroanatomical Sciences, and I know of no occasion when a section chief attached his name to a junior scientist's paper unless he had participated actively in the project.

The standards of behavior regarding authorship have changed over the years since 1955, and one's *pro-bono* responsibilities now seem to be defined more in legal terms than in an ethical context. My earliest awareness of this change came in 1969 when I prepared a review of a symposium on trophic nerve function in which I cited two important experiments by Jane Overton.[13] I sent my manuscript to all of the participants for their approval, and one of them responded by informing me that Overton's experiments were done while she was a graduate student working under his supervision in his laboratory. He suggested that I make this explicit in my article because he "saw no reason for keeping this fact from the readers." Apparently, the standards of scientific propriety that were extant in the 1950s, when Overton had been granted sole authorship of these articles, had begun to change by 1969.

Standards of Scientific Investigation

Equally important to the early development of the NINDB research programs was the clear distinction between the roles of basic and clinical research. Although Windle, (who held a Ph.D.) was studying a subject that had clear-cut clinical implications (spinal cord regeneration), his goal was to understand why axonal injury was followed by continuous growth in the PNS and abortive growth in the CNS. Likewise, the research of Palay (who held an M.D.), was motivated solely by a desire to understand more fully the fundamental structure of the nervous tissues rather than by any clinical advances that might result from these findings. From the example of these men and their precepts, the junior scientists learned that to demand practical relevance as a justification for basic research is both wrong and detrimental to scientific progress.

Responsibilities of Senior and Junior Scientists

As can be seen from the foregoing, the junior scientists in the Laboratory of Neuroanatomical Sciences were encouraged to develop independent scientific careers. In this respect, they were granted consideration similar to that now given to tenure-track assistant professors at medical schools. The laboratory chief and the section chiefs did not give research assignments to the junior faculty; instead they encouraged them to develop their scientific creativity and independence. This attitude, undoubtedly a reflection of their prior academic experience, can best be illustrated by a few personal examples:

- Windle actively encouraged my incipient research programs. When I became interested in "trophic" functions of neurons, he sent me to Northwestern University to consult with Leslie Arey (a famous embryologist and author of a classical textbook *Developmental Anatomy*), who had studied mechanisms by which nerves maintain the structure of taste buds. He also arranged for me to meet W. Le Gros Clarke at Oxford University, who had studied neurotrophic interactions in the olfactory system, and Fernando de Castro, who had succeeded Ramón y Cajal and J. Francisco Tello as Director of the Cajal Institute in Madrid and who had done pioneering work on the physiological consequences of cross-reinnervation of autonomic ganglia. Windle knew how inspiring it was for a young scientist to be given the opportunity to discuss issues of scientific interest with such accomplished scientists.

- Even more important to my scientific development were the numerous discussions I had with various senior scientists who were very kind to me. Most important to my scientific maturation was the helpful friendship of Karl Frank, Chief of the Section on Spinal Cord Physiology of the Laboratory of Neurophysiology. He was a brilliant electrophysiologist, a pioneer in the then-emerging field of intracellular recording and, most important of all, a generous person who gave freely of his time to help others. When I was completing my first independent experiment, in which I had reinnervated the superior cervical sympathetic ganglion with the vagus nerve, I sought his help in interpreting my findings. He invited me to his office, spoke to me at length, and, assuring me that I was not imposing on his time, invited me to return whenever I wished. I took advantage of his kindness and spent many hours listening to him and learning from him. Little did I realize how much more I was to gain from this friendship. Two years later, I completed an experiment in which I had reinnervated the muscle of the diaphragm with the vagus nerve. I discussed the results with Frank who pointed out that the interpretation would be clarified greatly by making electrophysiological recordings of the nervous activity in the vagus nerve and its recurrent laryngeal branch. He invited me into his laboratory to observe while he performed the recordings on animals that I had prepared for him. When the resultant manuscript was ready for publication, I showed it to Windle who told me that he would like to publish it in a new journal that he had just founded. I am proud to this day that this paper, by Lloyd Guth and Karl Frank, appeared as Volume 1, Number 1, Page 1, of *Experimental Neurology*.[14]

• I want to offer one last anecdote, because it illustrates that generous helpfulness can have remarkably long-lasting effects. One day in about 1958, Frank introduced me to a visitor, Paul O. Chatfield, and mentioned that Chatfield was author of a recently published treatise on neurophysiology.[15] I purchased the book and of all its chapters I found myself most intrigued by one dealing with the crossed phrenic phenomenon. My curiosity was piqued because, despite numerous experimental investigations, the basis for this unusual phenomenon had remained elusive for more than 60 years. Furthermore, try as I might, I could not formulate an experimentally-testable hypothesis to explain it. Consequently, for the next 15 years, I put the subject out of mind while I worked on unrelated subjects. But the enigma of the crossed phrenic phenomenon must have remained within my subconscious because, in 1974, a testable hypothesis abruptly came to me. The idea did not occur as a sudden burst of inspiration nor as a result of careful re-examination of the subject. It just seemed to emerge despite my not having given serious thought to the subject for many years. At that time, Harry Goshgarian had just joined the laboratory and, when I told him of my new thoughts on this phenomenon, he initiated a comprehensive investigation into the crossed phrenic phenomenon. His investigations (which are still ongoing some 30 years later) have revealed the anatomical basis for neuronal plasticity in the respiratory pathway and have led to clinical trials of a novel treatment for patients with respiratory paralysis. In summary, Frank's kindness to an inexperienced investigator in the 1950s led directly to the notable scientific research achievements of Goshgarian many years later.

Epilogue: Dreams and Memories

It is no surprise that the National Institute of Neurological Disorders and Stroke today is vastly different from the NINDB of the 1950s, but the important premises on which the institute was founded remain valid today–as William Faulkner wrote, "The past is never dead–it is not even past." First, basic research programs must be given the freedom to investigate fundamental biological issues without consideration of practical application. Second, senior scientists have a responsibility to provide an environment in which young scientists can develop into mature, creative, and independent investigators. Third, senior scientists are also role models for junior colleagues; by their actions they should endeavor to impart respect for honor and integrity in scientific research.

It has been said that aging is a process in which dreams are transformed to memories. In this essay, I have tried to share memories of my youthful dreams and of a life in science made meaningful by the friendship and inspiration of colleagues. I hope that the present generation of young scientists will have equally rewarding experiences during their careers and equally satisfying memories to reflect upon during their retirement.

Notes

1. "Now there is at Jerusalem by the sheep market a pool, which is called in the Hebrew tongue Bethesda, having five porches….In these lay a great multitude of impotent folk, of blind, halt, withered, waiting for the moving of the water….For an angel went down at a certain season into the pool, and troubled the water: whosoever then first after the troubling of the water stepped in was made whole of whatsoever disease he had." [John: 5: 2-4].

2. Hans Spemann, *Embryonic Development and Induction* (New Haven, Connecticut: Yale University Press, 1938).

3. Paul Weiss, *Principles of Development* (New York: Henry Holt, 1939).

4. Windle had been recruited by Kety. Since both of them had been at the University of Pennsylvania, Kety was undoubtedly familiar with Windle's very distinguished scientific reputation. Windle had been honored for his work on spinal cord regeneration by an invitation, in 1945, to lecture before the Harvey Society in New York City.

5. The Commissioned Corps was especially attractive to those who held M.D.s, in part because enlistment in the PHS fulfilled requirements for service in the physician's draft. Enlistment in the Commissioned Corps was also attractive to some Ph.D.s (especially those who had served in the armed forces during the Second World War), because retirement and promotion credits earned in military service were transferable to the Commissioned Corps.

6. My later research on muscle fiber plasticity overlapped to some degree with a program on muscle fiber histochemistry in the NIH's Medical Neurology Branch. I always considered this as beneficial rather than wasteful: when two scientists work independently on a similar question, science benefits from the divergent results obtained by use of different techniques, different experimental approaches, and different interpretations.

7. H. Koenig, R. A. Groat, and William F. Windle, "A Physiological Approach to Perfusion-Fixation of Tissues With Formalin," *Stain Technology* 20 (1945): 13-22.

8. Harold A. Davenport, *Histological and Histochemical Technics* (Philadelphia: W. B. Saunders, 1945).

9. Ralph D. Lillie, *Histopathological Technique and Practical Histochemistry,* 3rd ed. (New York: McGraw Hill, 1965).

10. Sanford L. Palay, "Synapses in the Central Nervous System," *Journal of Biophysical and Biochemical Cytology* Suppl. no. 2 (1956): 193-201 and Sanford L. Palay, "The Morphology of Synapses in the Central Nervous System," *Experimental Cell Research* Suppl. no. 5 (1958): 275-93.

11. Alan Peters, Sanford L. Palay and Henry Webster, *The Fine Structure of the Nervous System,* 1st ed. (New York: Harper & Row, 1970).

12. Lloyd Guth, "Regeneration in the Mammalian Peripheral Nervous System," *Physiological Review* 36 (1956): 441-78.

13. Jane Overton, "Mitotic Stimulation of Amphibian Epidermis by Underlying Grafts of Central Nervous Tissue," *Journal of Experimental Biology* 155 (1950): 521-59 and Jane Overton, "Mitotic Responses in Amphibian Epidermis to Feeding and Grafting," *Journal of Experimental Zoology* 130 (1955): 433-83.

14. Lloyd Guth and Karl Frank, "Restoration of Diaphragmatic Function Following Vagophrenic Anastomosis in the Rat," *Experimental Neurology* 1 (1959): 1-12.

15. Paul O. Chatfield, *Fundamentals of Clinical Neurophysiology* (Springfield, Illinois: Charles C. Thomas, 1957).

Mind, Brain, Body, and Behavior
I. G. Farreras, C. Hannaway and V. A. Harden (Eds.)
IOS Press, 2004

Adult Psychiatry Research at the NIMH in the 1950s

David A. Hamburg

The review of research at the NIMH and the NINDS in the 1950s provides insight into a crucially formative phase of biomedical research, not only with respect to the nervous system and behavior, but more broadly than that. The 1950s in the National Institutes of Health (NIH) intramural program, most broadly conceived, were extremely significant. What an extraordinary group of scientists was gathered there.

How lucky we were to be at the NIH in the 1950s. The facilities and equipment were superb. It hurt me when I read in the newspapers in recent years about the so-called decrepit NIH Clinical Center. My template is the brand new, magnificent Clinical Center of the 1950s. Not only was it a wonderful facility and wonderfully supported, but the planners also wisely provided for physical proximity between basic scientists and clinical investigators, and I always thought that was one of our greatest advantages. And the NIH leadership foresaw that. Since the clinical investigators and the basic scientists were nearby, there was a great deal of incidental, informal contact, from which I learned an enormous amount, and I think the same was true for many others. We had a dynamic interplay between clinical and basic scientists. We learned so much from each other in a very hopeful atmosphere in which everything seemed possible, an open-minded atmosphere of intellectual curiosity and social responsibility. These are some of the reasons for the extraordinarily seminal influence of the NIH in that era.

No one contributed more to that atmosphere than Robert A. Cohen. He had an M.D. and a Ph.D. at a time when hardly anybody had such a broad background. He had very wide-ranging interests, was utterly open- and fair-minded, and had a facilitative personality which brought out the best in all who dealt with him.

There were other leaders of course, who were extremely helpful. All of us deeply respected Seymour S. Kety in this context. So, too, Joel Elkes. David Shakow and John Clausen were wonderful leaders in this group. Moreover, we had Louis Sokoloff, the great Julius Axelrod, Melvin Kohn, Allan F. Mirsky, Mortimer Mishkin, Marian Yarrow, Lyman Wynne, Robert H. Felix, Irving Kopin, Sheppard Kellam, Morris B. Parloff, William Pollin, Eric Kandel, and others. I am not only noting those who worked directly with me but, rather, those in other laboratories from whom I learned a great deal. We had a strong mutual aid ethic among the various laboratories. Several of the factors then that contributed to the generative and creative research of that era were: (1) visionary leadership; (2) superb facilities and support; (3) the close proximity of basic and clinical research; (4) brilliant young people; and (5) a mutual aid ethic.

I recall vividly how much we taught each other. I emphasize especially the leaders who brought extraordinary intellectual, technical, and organizational strength to bear on important and difficult problems that we wanted to address. It was all done in a great spirit of encouragement and cooperation. It is no wonder that we all feel the deepest appreciation to the people of the intramural program in the 1950s.

For psychiatry, it is not too much to say that the various research units of the NIMH intramural program laid the foundation for modern research on psychiatric problems, not only through the studies conducted at the NIH, but by the many brilliant young people who went on to positions of leadership in psychiatry and related fields of biobehavioral science.

Let me offer a few examples from my own experience as chief of the Adult Psychiatry Branch in the hope of illustrating some of the zest, vitality, and promise as well as the ongoing, long-term vision of the work at NIMH in that truly seminal era. No doubt other and better examples could be provided, but these are the ones I happen to know best. And even within these it is overly selective, but it has to be.

First, the area of stress and hormones was very new at that time and has gone on to be one of the major arenas of psychiatric research in the intervening decades. Research on stress in humans has developed a large body of evidence showing that anticipation of personal injury may lead to important changes not only in thought, feeling, and action, but also in endocrine and autonomic processes and, hence, in a wide variety of visceral functions. We established research on these problems at the NIH in 1958, following up on some earlier work that I had done elsewhere. We were fortunate to attract superb collaborators, including William Bunney, James Maas, Joseph Handlon, Francis Board, Ralph Wadeson, John Davis, and Fredric Solomon, about whom I will describe more later in this essay.

We also had a strong collaboration with the Division of Neuropsychiatry at the Walter Reed Army Institute of Research, headed by an extraordinary person, David McKenzie Rioch. In the Walter Reed Neuroendocrine Laboratory that I had helped David Rioch establish during the Korean War in the early 1950s, we had wonderful collaborations with John Mason, Edward Sachar, and Robert Rose, among others. They were major collaborators and went on to do very important work in the field afterwards.

Much work in this field has centered on adrenocortical function in association with emotional distress. Investigators have generally found the adrenal gland to be stimulated by the pituitary and, in turn, by the brain under environmental conditions perceived as threatening to a person. It has been possible to correlate systematically the extent of emotional distress with the adrenal hormone levels in blood and urine, each assessed independently.

Work in this field profited greatly from the development of precise, reliable biochemical methods for measuring hormones and related compounds. They were new at the time. When I started out in the late 1940s and early 1950s, we had to get by with bioassays, which were helpful, but not nearly as good as the various biochemical methods that were more precise and reliable; they came along later.

Since then, many hundreds of persons have been studied in various laboratories all over the world under conditions of moderately intense or severe distress. The results are consistent, showing a significant elevation of adrenocortical hormones in blood and urine compared with the levels recorded under non-distress conditions. Moreover, many of the people in the stress groups have been studied on repeated occasions, and the elevated adrenocortical hormone levels have been found to be persistent when the stress remains unabated. But with relief of the distress, substantial declines in these steroids have been observed. Similar studies have been done for adrenaline and noradrenaline under conditions of emotional distress.

Thus it is clear that distress is associated with elevated blood and urinary levels of several adrenal hormones in both the cortex and the medulla, and these elevated levels reflect not only increased secretory activity by the gland, but increased activity of the sympathetic nervous system.

So an important set of brain regulatory functions acts upon the adrenal gland, particularly through the hypothalamus and also the limbic system. Initially, this relationship was considered quite far fetched. One of my best mentors and a really good friend urged me not to go into this field because he did not see any way that the hypothalamus could influence the anterior pituitary. There were just a few nerve fibrils connecting them; there was no rich nerve connection that could do the job. We did not realize that the job was done by chemical messengers. That came along later with Geoffrey Harris in England. But it was quite counterintuitive for lots of good scientists in a variety of fields that there would be powerful brain regulatory influences on the adrenal through the pituitary—let alone hypothalamus-pituitary influences on the entire endocrine system and, hence, on every cell and tissue in the body.

Elevations in both plasma and urinary adrenal compounds are regularly observed under very difficult circumstances, perceived by the individual as threatening. Different people perceive different circumstances as threatening. It is that perception of threat that matters most, not the standardization of the external event, although some events are so terrible that they affect everybody to some degree in a stressful way.

There is a positive correlation between the degree of distress and the tendency toward hormone elevation. Consistent individual patterns have been observed both in the range within which each person's adrenal hormone levels fluctuate under ordinary circumstances and in the extent of adrenal response to difficult experiences. Those consistent individual differences particularly fascinated me, and, for reasons that there is no need to go into, had something ultimately to do with my moving from the NIH to Stanford University in order to try to pursue a behavioral-endocrine-genetic approach to stress problems.

Many of the people involved in the NIMH-Walter Reed group on stress and hormones went on to make important contributions at other institutions in later years. They and other investigators in other countries have elucidated the importance and much of the nature of the hypothalamic-pituitary-adrenal axis in depressive disorders particularly. Jack Barchas, who, for almost a decade, edited the *Archives of Psychiatry*, has told me that there probably has not been anything more important in psychiatric research in the past decade than the great elaboration—and much greater depth, of course, than we had—of that work on the hypothalamic-pituitary-adrenal axis, particularly in depressive and bipolar disorders. These findings in depressed patients were counterintuitive. When we made the initial discoveries, we were actually quite apprehensive that we must be wrong because it was assumed at the time that a person sitting quietly, not communicating, and rather withdrawn and despondent would not have physiological or biochemical alarm responses, but that turned out not to be the case. Indeed, that work on depression has turned out to be extremely interesting in many contexts.

The findings of consistent individual differences in adrenal cortical response to environmental conditions touch on the important problem of differential susceptibility to psychological stress. Clinicians have long observed the precipitation and exacerbation of a variety of illnesses in association with emotional crisis, not only psychiatric disorders, but also clinical problems coming to the attention of other disciplines. Most of the specialties of internal medicine, in one way or another, see that phenomenon of stress-induced disorders or exacerbation.

Yet it is abundantly clear that many individuals undergo the common stressful experiences of living without developing clinical disorders. A number of genetic and environmental factors must contribute to these individual differences in stress response and, hence, to the differential susceptibility to illness.

One promising line of inquiry on this topic, which we began in a rudimentary way, was based on human biochemical genetics, relating genetically determined differences in metabolism of hormones to behavior under stress. In pursuit of such questions, I formulated a behavioral-endocrine-genetic approach to stress problems that I think still offers, much more so now than then with recent advances in genetics, a promising opportunity for mental health research. We pursued that at Stanford University, particularly with the excellent work of Barchas and Roland Ciaranello.

There was in the 1950s an interesting possibility that abnormal concentrations of steroids might affect brain function adversely under highly stressful conditions, particularly if there were genetically determined abnormalities in steroid hormone synthesis, transport, or disposal. There is considerable evidence that a variety of fat-soluble steroids have access to the brain and many produce neurophysiological, pharmacological, and behavioral effects. This line of inquiry has been fruitfully pursued in Bruce McEwen's laboratory at Rockefeller University in the past couple of decades.

Another aspect of this problem area is stress-related coping and adaptation. Psychological responses to stressful experiences are central to the work of most psychiatrists. Hence, the psychiatric literature has provided abundant documentation of the ways in which many common experiences can be traumatic. Some of these are inherent components of the life cycle; others are major features of urbanized, industrialized societies. Many kinds of difficult experiences have been described in psychiatric clinical practice that have adverse effects.

What do humans typically do in the face of painful elements of experience? The psychiatric literature and that of closely related fields in the 1950s mainly gave the impression that what we did was to avoid the painful elements at all costs, reject them as part of ourselves, even if this required extensive self-deception. The classical mechanisms of defense functioned largely in this way, being centrally concerned with minimizing recognition of potentially distressing aspects of personal experience. They relied heavily upon avoidance and reduction of information. That seemed strange to me, coming from a background in evolutionary biology. It was hard for me to see how human adaptation could be based essentially on the reduction of information and particularly the avoidance of information that was more or less life-threatening in character. I could see how that might be true sometimes under some circumstances, but I could not see how that could characterize human behavior as the general way in which we responded to stressful experience.

So we asked whether there might be other ways in which the human organism coped with stressful experiences and began to investigate coping, interpersonal problem solving, and adaptive behavior. In the early 1950s, initially during the Korean War, at Brooke Army Hospital in Texas, particularly in collaboration with my wife, Beatrix Hamburg, we started this work with severely burned patients. A series of studies over the next two decades explored the ways in which individuals drawn from a broad range of the general population coped with difficult circumstances. Some of these studies dealt with situations of life-threatening illness and injury, such as severe burns; then severe poliomyelitis in the days before the vaccine; and studies of childhood leukemia patients and their parents at the NIH Clinical Center. There were also studies involving psychosocial transitions that were not life-threatening in character, like going away to college for youth who had not been away from home much before, stressful but not intrinsically life-threatening. Much of this research was done in the intramural program and in various field locations derived from the intramural program.

These studies of coping behavior described how people actually seek and utilize information under stressful conditions. We found that under difficult circumstances, the human organism tends to seek information about several questions: How can the distress be relieved? How can a sense of personal worth be maintained? How can a rewarding continuity of human relationships be maintained? How can the requirements of the stressful task be met or the opportunities utilized?

Psychological preparation centers on the availability of time to answer those questions prior to a threatening event. Then the blow, if it must come, can be absorbed in the prospect of substitute, alternative sources of self-esteem and rewarding interpersonal relationships. On the other hand, if a threatening event occurs without warning, as in the situation of sudden illness or injury, then the time for "preparation" is likely to be bought by temporary self-deception, and here is where we get back into the classical mechanisms of defense. In this way, by not recognizing right away the gravity of the situation, the recognition of threatening elements is made gradual and manageable. A time scale of weeks or a few months for preparation, as in chronic diseases of slow onset, appears to have considerable utility, and where there is a time scale of many months or a few years, as in the transitions of youth, then there are exceedingly gradual, usually thorough, multifaceted preparations that occur.

The threatened person seeks to answer personal questions in many ways and from many sources. Strategies for obtaining and utilizing such information are formed at all levels of awareness and may be employed over long periods of time. Strategies that were established earlier in a person's psychological repertoire and that have served similar functions in earlier stress are likely to be employed first, but distress of high intensity and/or long duration is a powerful impetus to the formation of new strategies that are effective and are likely to become available for use in a future crisis. So individuals tend to build a behavioral repertoire that through adolescent and young adult development can broaden the individual's problem solving capacity. To a certain extent, that continues through the entire life span. Even at my age, I delude myself by thinking that now and then I learn something useful in adaptation that I did not know before. In any case, we studied stress in the framework of human adaptation. We stimulated research at the NIMH and elsewhere on the development of competence, of interpersonal problem solving, and coping behavior.

This is another frontier on which psychiatrists are joining with other behavioral scientists in interdisciplinary efforts to clarify important problems. The work has had wide-ranging impact on clinical practice in many ways. There were important contributors to the NIMH program in the 1950s: George Coelho, Earle Silber, Roger Shapiro, Elizabeth Murphey, Morris Rosenberg, Leonard Pearlin, Stanford Friedman, and Fredric Solomon, with whom I later had five fruitful years of collaboration when I was president of the Institute of Medicine of the National Academy of Sciences and he was chief of the Division of Mental Health and Behavioral Medicine. This effort was highly interdisciplinary; there were psychiatrists, psychologists of different breeds, sociologists, a pediatrician, and endocrinologists. We were relating stress-hormone responses to various coping variables over a wide range of situations.

Such studies across several decades have now illuminated successful and unsuccessful coping patterns and some of the conditions that favor success, and that opens up possibilities for disease prevention that have been pursued in recent years. For example, there are toxic and non-toxic ways of trying to cope with the stress of early adolescence. The toxic ones include heavy smoking, high intake of alcohol or other drugs, wild driving, unprotected sexual activity, and a preference for violent pseudo-solutions. Early adolescence is a crucial phase of human development that had been scientifically neglected until the 1950s. My wife, Beatrix Hamburg, a child psychiatrist with pediatric training, played a crucial role in clarifying early adolescence, delineating it as a distinctive phase of adolescence, a distinctive phase of the life cycle in which crucial choices are made in the face of high-risk behaviors.

The high-risk behaviors are typically undertaken on an exploratory basis. By understanding the developmental tasks and coping strategies, preventive measures may be taken before these exploratory patterns get cast in concrete, before health-damaging patterns are firmly established. There is currently much interest in discovering ways to help people improve their coping strategies, and further utilization of basic learning principles in this field is a line of inquiry well worth pursuing.

In years to come, a deeper understanding of human coping behavior can be useful in devising reasonable therapeutic and preventive interventions. The promise of such interventions is clearest in mental health; but they also have direct relevance to general health, because health-damaging coping efforts, such as smoking, alcohol use, and risky driving weigh heavily in the burden of illness. Epidemiologists roughly estimate that about half the burden of illness of the American population is behavior related, so how we cope matters in a lot of ways.

Let me write a word about sleep and its disorders. It was my privilege to establish a sleep laboratory at the NIMH headed by Frederick Snyder, with Irwin Feinberg as a major contributor in that effort. Since the mid-1950s, psychiatrists have joined with scientists of various disciplines, and we have awakened—no pun intended—to the fact that we spend one third of our lives in a state about which very little was then known. In the intervening years, the problems of sleep have become a major frontier of science through the efforts of such pioneers as William Dement, with whom I had the privilege of working for many years at Stanford. These scientists' studies of brain waves, heart rate, breathing, movement, attention, and sleep loss have illuminated a variety of sleep disorders and symptoms of mental illness. During that period, the very important discoveries about the differences between REM sleep and non-REM sleep became clear. That was a really stunning discovery–that for about a quarter of a night's sleep the brain is in some ways very active. And when you awaken people during that time, they are usually dreaming, far more dreaming than anybody had anticipated.

I had high hopes that the biological and psychological significance of dreaming would be clarified by these discoveries of REM and non-REM sleep, and to some extent that has happened, but much remains to be done. In recent years, one hope of mine has been fulfilled–the entry of geneticists into this field, for instance in Dement's laboratory.

Dreams were one of the principal building blocks of psychoanalysis, which was dominant in the late 1940s and the 1950s in academic psychiatry as well as in the practice of psychiatry. Yet the meaning of dreams remains much more of a mystery than I would wish.

One of the interesting findings about REM sleep is the compensatory rebound. If you deprive people of REM sleep by waking them consistently, when they go into REM, they make it up at the first chance they get, as if there were some quota of REM sleep that the brain requires. When *total* sleep time is sharply restricted for days on end, severe disturbances are likely to occur: sensory disorders, lapses of attention, micro-sleep intervals, and a tendency to withdraw. So sleep deprivation has a widespread importance as a clinical and social problem, especially for, but not limited to, adolescents. Adolescents, as a group in our society, are sleep deprived, and it affects their academic performance, as well as their involvement in serious accidents.

In recent decades, narcolepsy, a disorder characterized by frequent lapses into sleep during the day, began to be clarified, particularly its genetic basis. Psychiatric research concentrated especially on sleep disorders in depression and schizophrenia. The work at the NIH Clinical Center in the 1950s and ever since has been very important–particularly in depressed patients who show striking sleep abnormalities, most prominently in psychotic depression. In general, the more severe the depression, the greater is the tendency toward sleep abnormalities, and the NIMH laboratory has had a very stimulating effect in this field, in its own work and its effect throughout the world. And there is today a distinct field of sleep medicine, thanks to such pioneers as Dement, Snyder, and Feinberg. One of the great opportunities in the first decade of the twenty-first century lies in the integration of sleep medicine into primary health care. Another is the education of the general public about the serious risks of major sleep deprivation (e.g., truck accidents). The American Sleep Foundation is pursuing this opportunity.

I want to close with a brief word about interdisciplinary collaboration and progress in psychiatric research. Many scientists and clinicians have noted the value of the interdisciplinary climate that we had at the NIH in the 1950s, and this valuable climate has continued in a powerful way to the present time.

One of the main thrusts, not only in the Adult Psychiatry Branch but in the entire NIMH intramural program, was to promote contact, lively exchange, and mutual assistance among the various scientists concerned with psychiatric problems. Certainly Kety and Cohen, as the two administrative leaders who also were scientific leaders, encouraged that kind of interplay. Psychiatry's scientific position is at the interface between biological and behavioral sciences. No sharp line of separation may be drawn. Psychiatrists have learned from poignant experience that the human problems they face are too complex to be understood in any narrow, doctrinaire way. By and large, we have emerged from that phase of the field's history. The tools of no single discipline will suffice. The present mood of the field is one that searches for new opportunities, welcomes diversity, and turns away from dogmatism. I believe that much of this spirit arose in the 1950s, particularly in the NIMH intramural program, and has had stimulating effects throughout the nation and beyond.

This work continues to link behavioral inquiry with the neurosciences, and there are now far-reaching ramifications in both basic science and clinical investigation. The field of stress research illustrates how advances in neurobiology stimulate the scientific study of behavior in its own right, an urgently needed enterprise in the modern world. Consider, for example, the stress-related field of aggression and violence in which I have been so deeply involved in the past two decades.

The extraordinary success of basic research in the neurosciences, and also in genetics, provides a continuing flow of illuminating glimpses into the most wondrous of machines, the human brain. The promise for socially useful applications in health and disease is undeniable. By the same token, exposure to clinical or social problems can be exceedingly stimulating for basic sciences, as has so vividly been the case in genetics and also in neurosciences.

Just a short time ago, the great geneticist, James Watson, made a public confession that is illuminating for our field. In their classic paper, Watson and Crick did not mention the classic Avery, McLeod, and McCarty paper of 1944 on the pneumococcus transformation experiments, which came about a decade earlier, showing that DNA was the genetic material–a profound discovery. Of course they stood on the shoulders of Avery, McLeod and McCarty. What is especially interesting about their fundamental work is that they were clinicians trying to understand pneumonia. This was the pre-antibiotic era. They wanted to understand the pneumococcus organism in order to do something about treatment and perhaps immunization vis-à-vis pneumonia, and they discovered the deeply important fact that DNA is the genetic material.

As Axelrod has clearly pointed out, there has been a similarly stimulating effect of stress problems and clinical disorders on basic neuroscience. There is a dynamic interplay between basic and clinical research which has been fostered over decades, probably better in the intramural NIH than anywhere else. Yet the full promise of this approach will probably require even higher levels of cooperation because we have now entered an era of exploring the extent to which the methods of the sciences can be brought to bear on the entire range of factors that determine the health of the public and to delineate well-tested interventions for diagnosis, therapy, and prevention. This is especially important for psychiatric progress. It requires excellent basic science at every level of biological organization; it requires a dynamic interplay between basic and applied science; it requires a widening of horizons to include new or neglected lines of inquiry; and it requires an enduring commitment to the scientific study of behavior.

Mind, Brain, Body, and Behavior
I. G. Farreras, C. Hannaway and V. A. Harden (Eds.)
IOS Press, 2004

Reflections on the Intramural Research Program of the NIMH in the 1950s

Melvin L. Kohn

The perspective that I bring to bear on the National Institute of Mental Health (NIMH) in the 1950s is that of a newly minted Ph.D. coming to an intramural research program so recently established that it had only two laboratories and, to the best of my recollection, was not even a distinct organizational entity. I joined the NIMH in June, 1952, as a Commissioned Officer in the United States Public Health Service (PHS), then part of the Navy, having signed up one step ahead of the draft board's assigning me to the infantry. I did not have the slightest compunction about serving in the armed forces of the United States, which I saw as the savior of civilization, having defeated the Nazis, but I was extremely reluctant to waste two years of my life in dreary non-research activity while my research skills deteriorated. I intended to spend my two years of compulsory military service doing research, with every expectation of then moving on to some university. But I remained at the National Institutes of Health for 33 exciting years, until driven out of the intramural research program and the government by the animus to social research of the Reagan Administration and the consonant practices of a like-minded scientific director, Frederick Goodwin.

In my description, I will only give a bare minimum about my own early research, of which I remain very proud, and instead address three general issues. The first is my impression of the NIMH, the intramural research program, and the Laboratory of Socio-Environmental Studies, both when I came to Bethesda and as the intramural research program developed during its first decade. Then I shall discuss the research program of that particular laboratory, and my sense as a very junior member of the intramural research program at that time of the research program of the intramural research program more generally as it developed under the leadership of Robert A. Cohen and Seymour S. Kety. I shall discuss only briefly the relationship between the basic and clinical portions of our laboratory and of the intramural research program more generally. Finally, I shall examine something that did not seem at all noteworthy at the time, but which would be extraordinary today: the inclusion of social science in a predominantly biological intramural research program.

The Intramural Research Program and the Laboratory of Socio-Environmental Studies in the 1950s

When I arrived in Bethesda, the Laboratory of Socio-Environmental Studies—"the Lab," as its members called it then and ever after, knowing full well that we were not the only laboratory in the NIMH, but signifying that it was our intellectual and emotional home—was squeezed into a minuscule few square feet of a building aptly named T-6, the "T" standing for temporary. Building T-6 was not only temporary but ramshackle, and this was before air conditioning, so it was also beastly hot. There was almost no room to work, and certainly no place on campus to conduct research in this pre-Clinical Center era.

What we lacked in physical amenities was partially recompensed by the excitement of being part of a wonderful social experiment: we were going to make this part of the government an ideal research institution. Even in that very first decade we succeeded, in large part because of the inspired leadership of Cohen and Kety. I would also like to add that never, not in that decade or later, were the resources adequate for research. Certainly, it was never easy for the investigators to secure even the minimum of needed resources, but the freedom to do unfettered inquiry, and the spirit of inquiry and of cooperation that pervaded the intramural research program, more than compensated for the lean resources.

At the beginning, when there was no place on campus for us to conduct our research, we worked off-campus, doing surveys in Washington, D.C., doing studies of the social structure of St. Elizabeths Hospital in Washington, D.C., and in my case, being shipped off to Hagerstown, Maryland. My experience provides a glimpse of the *ad hoc* way that the NIMH operated in those early days. The founding director of the institute, Robert H. Felix, was put on the griddle at a meeting of the Appropriations Committee (or some subcommittee thereof) of the House of Representatives, for having closed a research clinic in Phoenix, Arizona. It had been a huge success as a clinic, for which one of the appropriators praised it whole-heartedly, but a failure in terms of doing any research. Felix, no scientist but a skilled administrator and politician, assuaged the Committee by telling them that the NIMH was about to open a research field station in Hagerstown, a city well known to the Committee as the site of past PHS triumphs, and that the NIMH had already hired an expert in community studies to set up that field station.

That purported expert was *me*–a 23-year old who had done participant-observation research on race and ethnic relations in the Jewish community and what was then called the Negro community of Elmira, New York, as a Cornell graduate-student research assistant and as part of his Ph.D. thesis. That experience was of no possible relevance to a community study of mental disorder, even assuming that a community study was appropriate to the study of mental disorder. Dispatching me to Hagerstown served Felix's political purposes, and it turned out to serve my research purposes as well.

I was assigned, as my office, the storeroom of an existing PHS unit. After I swept out the coal soot deposited by three nearby railroads, I realized that the records of Antonio Ciocco's morbidity studies of Washington County's school children, which filled the many filing cabinets in that storeroom, were a gold mine. From those records, I was able to design a comparison-group study, in which I matched everyone from Washington County who had been hospitalized for schizophrenia in any public or private hospital in the state of Maryland during a 13-year period with a former classmate of the same age and gender, who had lived in the same neighborhood and whose parents had similar socio-economic status, long before the patient's hospitalization. It was a fluke that Felix's political gambit had scientific payoff, but we had to use what opportunities presented themselves. It took all the political ingenuity at Felix's command, and all the research ingenuity at his staff's command, to get research underway before we had appropriate facilities, an administrative structure, and a modicum of resources.

Gradually, other laboratories and branches were founded at the NIMH, and a remarkable group of laboratory chiefs and investigators was hired. I was not privy to the deliberations of the directors and their laboratory chiefs in those years. For my first couple of years, I was not even living in the vicinity, but in Hagerstown, then a two-hour drive from Bethesda. I visited the NIH once every week or two to meet with the Laboratory of Socio-Environmental Studies chief, John A. Clausen; to purchase tax-free bourbon at the Navy store; and, often, to give a seminar on my research, for there was a huge demand in the institute for research seminars and, as yet, scant research to report. By the time I had completed my fieldwork in Hagerstown, the NIH Clinical Center had been built and there was a real locus of research.

Although there were complaints about insufficient opportunity to learn about each other's research, we at the NIMH actually had vastly more opportunity to learn about our colleagues' research than universities provide. As a telling example, I may hold the world record among sociologists for attending seminar presentations about catecholamines and for being able to spot where any particular biochemical agent stood in the seemingly inevitable course from being *the* hypothesized cause of schizophrenia, to becoming *a* hypothesized genetic marker for schizophrenia, to perhaps being the cause of what was then termed manic-depressive psychosis, to perhaps being a genetic marker for that disorder. I was not forced to attend such seminars. It happened that I really was interested, because I very much wanted a genetic marker for schizophrenia for research I wanted to do (and still want to do) on the interaction of genetic and social factors in the etiology of schizophrenia. The serious point is that mutual interest and cross-disciplinary discussion prevailed.

What was true of the intramural research program in general was even more dramatically true of the Laboratory of Socio-Environmental Studies. The laboratory was a disparate group of people from several disciplines and of diverse orientations, who learned from each other in spirited, ongoing discussions. John Clausen was a gambler in his hiring practices, which is rather surprising to me in retrospect, because he was also an anxious man, not at all a gambler in his administrative practices.

He hired a wide range of talented people, many of whom might not have done as well in securing university employment–including women in that sexist age (a notable example being Marian Yarrow), young men subject to the draft (such as me), and an occasional oddball who was either a genius or a wild man. The outstanding example of the latter category was Erving Goffman, who was to become one of the most prominent sociologists of the latter half of the twentieth century. Clausen hired sociologists, developmental and clinical psychologists, anthropologists, a couple of social workers, even a population geneticist. We honed our research and analytical skills from intensive, continuing discussion. I would add that I especially honed my skills in research design from discussions with Clausen himself.

Research Programs of the Laboratory of Socio-Environmental Studies

The very term, research programs, brings to mind an image of experienced elders laying out a program of research for their juniors to implement. If Seymour S. Kety and Robert A. Cohen had any such vision in mind, they kept it well hidden from me and the other young scientists at the NIMH. Their expressed philosophy, which they exemplified in their every action, was to recruit the best scientists they could find in any and every scientific discipline that might contribute to our understanding of human behavior, and to give them all the encouragement and support that they could. By their choice of laboratory chiefs, they, of course, had considerable influence on the directions that research in the several laboratories and branches would take, but their choices seemed to be influenced more by the quality of the research their appointees had done and were likely to support in their laboratories than by a particular research agenda.

Within particular laboratories and branches, of course, it could be and often was quite another matter. Some chiefs seemed to think they owned their laboratory or branch, and that all the scientists in that unit worked for them; others seemed to think their scientists autonomous. The difference showed, even then, in numerous ways: first, in whether the chiefs claimed co-authorship on all of the papers written in their laboratory or branch; second, in how they exercised their power and responsibility for "clearing" manuscripts for publication; and third, in how much freedom their scientists had to choose their own research projects. Since I am far from knowledgeable about the actual practices in other laboratories and branches at that time, I shall only describe the one I know best, Socio-Environmental Studies.

Clausen's policies changed decisively during the decade of the 1950s. At first, he was, or so it seemed to his scientific staff, preoccupied with proving the value of social science to the NIMH and to the PHS. Mainly, this meant that research conducted in the laboratory had to be addressed to questions close to the heart of the NIMH's concern with mental disorder, unless it was even closer to the heart of the PHS's mission, as in the case of one rather mundane study of who had participated in a large-scale trial of a polio vaccine. Mainly, though, we worked on studies of mental disorder—even though the very name of the National Institute of Mental *Health* gave us license to study normal human functioning as well. The first study undertaken in the laboratory, one in which Clausen himself was involved in a major way, was a study of the families of men hospitalized for schizophrenia. Several other members of the laboratory did studies of the structure and functioning of mental hospitals—initially, and to some extent continuing even after the construction of the NIH Clinical Center, studies of St. Elizabeths Hospital; later, also studies of some of the psychiatric wards in the Clinical Center. I did research on social factors in the etiology of schizophrenia.

Most of these studies were first-rate, methodologically and substantively. They were particularly valuable in clearing away myths. Clausen, Yarrow, and their collaborators dispelled sociological myths about the processes by which people were legally committed to mental hospitals— in those days, most often involuntarily—and cast deserved doubt on a then-prominent theory that mental disorder results primarily from societal reactions to, and labeling of, deviant behavior. Erving Goffman, in a work that became famous, not only within sociology and psychiatry but even to the lay public, reconceptualized how mental hospitals resocialize their inmates. In his study, St. Elizabeths was the prototype of what he called "the mental hospital as a total institution." Leonard Pearlin, Erwin Linn, and other members of the laboratory did valuable studies of the institutional dynamics of mental hospitals, particularly as such hospitals were affected by the introduction of psychotropic drugs. Clausen and I dispatched a myth beloved by our sociological brethren that social isolation causes schizophrenia. We also recast psychiatric understanding of the possible role of parent-child relationships in the etiology of schizophrenia, by showing that families whose offspring became schizophrenic were not so different from normal families of their socioeconomic level as prior studies had mistakenly concluded. In fact, they were typical of families of the lower socioeconomic strata from which schizophrenics disproportionately come. These studies were valuable in clearing away misconceptions and for reconceptualizing important theoretical issues. But most of them were not, in my judgment, of fundamental importance for our understanding of human behavior.

Well before the end of the decade, however, Clausen seemed to grow confident that our work need not be limited to the study of mental disorder, but could encompass much broader and more fundamental issues of social psychology, which was what his staff wanted to do. By the end of the 1950s, the Laboratory of Socio-Environmental Studies was clearly in transition from a singular focus on the study of social factors in the etiology and treatment of mental disorder, to a far-reaching program of fundamental research on social structure, culture, and personality. To give an accurate picture of this transformation of the laboratory's program, I have to describe not only what was being done by the end of the 1950s, but also where the investigators were headed in their research. (For this part of my comments, I leave out the developmental psychologists—at that time: Roger Burton, John Campbell, and Marian Yarrow. After the decade of the 1950s, they became a laboratory of their own, under the distinguished leadership of Marian Yarrow.) William Caudill was then a new arrival, best known for his participant-observation study of a mental hospital, but he and Carmi Schooler were soon to undertake their incisive studies of culture, childhood socialization, and personality in Japan and the United States. Leonard Pearlin was at that time doing a study of the nursing staff at St. Elizabeths Hospital, with his cross-national research on the family not yet underway, and his pioneering research, with Schooler, on stress and coping not yet envisaged. Morris Rosenberg was then beginning the research on the self-concept that made him the leading figure in this field. Schooler, who in ensuing years was central to nearly all of the core studies of the laboratory, was then solely engaged in experimental studies of chronic schizophrenics at St. Elizabeths Hospital. And I was completing my small-scale, exploratory study of social class and parent-child relationships in Washington, D. C., the forerunner of what would become Carmi Schooler's and my long-term and far-reaching studies of social structure, job conditions, and personality in the United States, Poland, and Japan. The research that would define the laboratory for decades to come was only just getting underway, and the evidence of its quality was not yet firmly in place, but the investigators were all on board and thirsting to do fundamental research.

How did the directors of the intramural research program react to this radical shift of emphasis? So far as I was able to tell, they responded positively to every research project that anyone in the laboratory ever undertook, provided only that it was high-quality research, as it generally was. It was not Kety and Cohen who dictated that we had to limit our research to mental disorder, or who thought that every ward in the Clinical Center needed to have a social scientist as resident participant-observer. When I argued, as a typical example, that to understand the role of the family in the etiology of schizophrenia, I had to move beyond comparisons of families that produced schizophrenic offspring with families of similar socioeconomic status that did not, to research on social class and family relationships in the population generally, they properly questioned the rationale of my research design, but not the appropriateness of my studying the normal population.

This may be as appropriate a place as any to describe the division of the laboratory into its basic and clinical components. From my vantage point, which in this regard was very limited, the division was merely a convenient administrative and fiscal device, and in no way a constraint on our research activities. I do not remember just when it was that the laboratory first had sections, some of which were designated "basic" and others "clinical." Whenever it was, the studies of the mental hospital were called clinical. Studies done outside of any hospital setting, even studies of former patients living in the community, were called basic. So far as I know, no one in the laboratory was ever prevented from doing research because he or she was in the wrong component of the laboratory. I was in what formally was Kety's "basic" jurisdiction and not in Cohen's "clinical" jurisdiction, but I always thought of these two men as working together. What mattered more to me, as a first-level investigator with only modest administrative responsibility, was that I knew that both of them were interested in and supportive of my research.

The Place of Sociology and of Social Science in the Intramural Research Program

It may have been happenstance that a social science laboratory was one of the first two laboratories in the intramural research program, for Clausen was already in the employ of the NIMH as an expert advisor, and Robert H. Felix, the founding director of the institute, was extremely good at spotting talent and gambling on talented people. But it was certainly not happenstance that the director of the institute thought it necessary to include social science among its core disciplines, nor that the leaders of the intramural research program sustained that decision. On the contrary, it was breadth of imagination, a non-reductionist belief on the part of some very wise men that the social sciences might well have something important to contribute to our understanding of human behavior, and should therefore be included in the program.

I want to add something about Seymour S. Kety's and Robert A. Cohen's day-to-day treatment of sociology as a discipline and of sociologists, me included, as members of their staffs. Kety is reputed to have said that when he came to the NIMH he knew nothing about sociology and even had some prejudices against the field, but that, if sociology were to be part of his responsibilities, he would wipe that slate clean and approach the field with an open mind. Even if this story is apocryphal, Kety certainly demonstrated his open-mindedness at every turn. He proved again and again that he supported good research in every discipline, and sociology was most certainly included. For Cohen, there are no comparable stories, not even apocryphal ones. It is not that every psychoanalyst can be assumed to be favorable to social research, but that Cohen was so evidently open-mindedness incarnate that no investigator in any scientific discipline could ever doubt his interest in and support for the work of that discipline. The directors of the NIMH's intramural research program, Cohen, Kety, and for many years thereafter, John Eberhart, gave us the encouragement and provided the structural conditions to do the best work we were capable of doing.

How did social science perform under these supportive conditions? I would venture the opinion that the Laboratory of Socio-Environmental Studies, even in its formative years, performed as creditably as did any laboratory in the program. But I have already noted that the program of the laboratory changed dramatically during its first decade and was in decided transition even before the end of that decade. One must take a longer term view. Even by the end of the 1950s, the Laboratory of Socio-Environmental Studies was well on its way toward becoming one of the most productive centers of social scientific research anywhere in the world. Small though the laboratory always was, it was astonishingly productive, and it launched its members on notable careers. You need not take my word for it. The laboratory whose members Clausen had recruited and whom the intramural research program supported from their early careers into their full maturity, produced, inter alia; two presidents and a vice president of the American Sociological Association; four winners of the Association's Cooley-Mead Award for distinguished contributions to social psychology, one of them John Clausen himself; and the only person trained as a *psychologist* ever to be elected chair of the American Sociological Association's Section on Social Psychology–Carmi Schooler–who is the current chief of what is now the Section on Socio-Environmental Studies.

My point is hardly subtle, but no less true for that. Social science has made and can continue to make, important contributions to the intramural research program of the NIMH; and the program has made and can continue to make important contributions to social science.

Mind, Brain, Body, and Behavior
I. G. Farreras, C. Hannaway and V. A. Harden (Eds.)
IOS Press, 2004

Psychopharmacology Research in the 1950s

Irwin J. Kopin

I am delighted to have been asked to review the historical and critically important contributions of the NIH to neuroscience and behavioral research in the 1950s. In 1957, I arrived at the NIH after completing an internship and a residency in internal medicine at Boston City Hospital. During the end of my residency I applied to the Public Health Service and was interviewed for an appointment at the then new NIH Clinical Center. Philippe V. Cardon, Jr., hired me as a Clinical Associate beginning July 1, 1957, but after a few months, I joined the first group of physicians that began the Research Associates Training Program; Seymour S. Kety was my mentor in that program.

My initial responsibility was to select and care for relatively healthy schizophrenic patients who were admitted for a study of potential biological abnormalities that could account for their mental disorder. Because I was obtaining spinal fluid from them for diagnostic purposes, I was able to use some of the fluid to determine levels of 5-hydroxyindole acetic acid (5-HIAA), the metabolite of serotonin, in the cerebrospinal fluid (CSF). Albert Sjoerdsma's group, in the National Heart Institute, had recently discovered serotonin as the biogenic amine secreted by malignant carcinoid tumors. This amine was also present in the brain and it was reasonable to suppose that its metabolite could be found in CSF. Marian Kies, who was chief of the Section on Biochemistry in Kety's Laboratory of Clinical Science and who was working on a review of experimental allergic encephalomyelitis, gave me some space in her laboratory. I set up a relatively large desalting apparatus so that I could concentrate the spinal fluid and perform paper chromatography.

At that time, Kety had organized seminars during which there was discussion of various biological factors that might be involved in schizophrenia. Due to my interest in this area and the study that I had undertaken, Kety asked me to join the Research Associates Program. There was considerable excitement about the putative role of amines in brain function and in amine metabolism as a means for evaluating amine activity. Discussions included descriptions of the several theories that were being proposed about the biological basis of schizophrenia, all of which were being examined and ultimately disproved. Because so much effort had been expended over a number of years in the failed efforts to identify a biochemical abnormality as the basis for the psychotic symptoms, Kety referred to the study of the biological basis of schizophrenia as the graveyard of biochemists. Extraordinary findings were reported, but later it was found that the findings had a rational basis unrelated to schizophrenia. Since amino acids were the precursors of the biogenic amines, each of us tackled the hypotheses associated with compounds derived from a particular amino acid. Tryptophan, the precursor of serotonin was my area. Phenylalanine and tyrosine, the precursors of catecholamines and adrenochrome, an oxidation product of epinephrine that had been suggested by Canadian psychiatrist, Abram Hoffer, as an endogenous hallucinogen in schizophrenics, became Julius Axelrod's domain.

At that time—the end of the 1950s—there was a revolution in the approach to understanding and the treatment of mental illness, particularly of the psychoses. Up to the early 1950s, psychiatry dealt mainly with interviewing patients; shock therapy with insulin-induced hypoglycemia or electrical current was the major therapeutic intervention to attempt to treat psychotic patients. In extreme cases, frontal lobotomy was an option. By the second half of the decade, there had been a huge change in perception, a paradigm shift, based on the observations that chemicals could alter the mind, and the last lobotomy was performed in 1960.

The discovery of chlorpromazine, monoamine oxidate (MAO) inhibitors, reserpine, and psychedelic agents was taken as proof that chemicals could alter brain function. This provided a strong basis for the concept

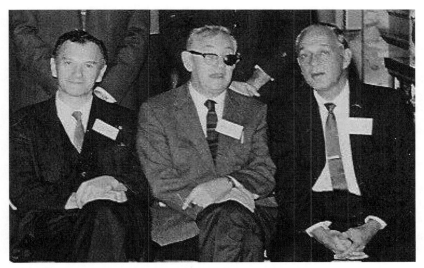

Left to right: Joel Elkes, Julius Axelrod, and Seymour S. Kety, 1969
Donated to the Office of NIH History by Dr. Irwin Kopin

that drugs could be important therapeutic agents. Chlorpromazine was accidentally discovered; it was introduced as a better antihistamine but was found to have strong sedative effects. When Henri Laborit, a military surgeon in France, tried it as a pre-anesthetic, he found that the patients developed what he described as "euphoric quietude." A fellow surgeon told his brother-in-law, Pierre Deniker, an assistant to Jean Delay, head of the Psychiatry Department at Sainte Anne Hospital in Paris, about the effect observed by Laborit. Delay and Deniker were the first to report the spectacular effects of chlorpromazine in psychotic patients and introduced the term "neuroleptic" to describe this type of drug. Patients who were unmanageable before became manageable; patients that were immobile became mobile; psychotic symptoms were alleviated. Chlorpromazine was the first breakthrough in drug treatment of schizophrenia and was approved by the Food and Drug Administration (FDA) in 1954. Although the therapeutic effects did not return all patients to a normal state, the mental hospitals began to empty and psychopharmacology was born.

Then, again by chance, MAO inhibitors were discovered. Iproniazid was first tried as a substitute for Isoniazid to search for a better treatment of tuberculosis. The patients became euphoric, had boundless energies, but their X-rays did not improve. Nathan Kline called this drug a "psychic energizer" and suggested that it be used for the treatment of depression. The results were so encouraging that by 1957 or 1958, hundreds of thousands of depressed patients were beginning to take this MAO inhibitor. Iproniazid was withdrawn from the market because of toxic side effects, but other less toxic MAO inhibitors were found and came into wide use. The efficacy of these drugs provided a strong argument for linking to amines to mental illlness.

Another link to amines resulted from the introduction of reserpine. For many centuries, the root of *Rauwolfia serpentina*, snakeroot plant, was used for treating snake bites, but it also was used for treating anxiety, insomnia, and "general insanity." In 1948, reserpine was isolated from this source and CIBA put this drug on the market. It was first used as a sedative and an antihypertensive agent, but its use declined when it was found to induce depression. When it was discovered that reserpine was a powerful means for depleting brain amines (serotonin and catecholamines), another link of amines to brain function was established.

Also, in the 1950s, psychedelic agents were popularized by the publication in 1954 of Aldous Huxley's *The Doors of Perception*. The hallucinogenic effects of agents such as mescaline or lysergic acid diethylamide (LSD) were described as "mind expanders." Mescaline was the most active of the components of peyote, a cactus plant that had been used in Mexico for centuries to induce a hallucinogenic, "mystic" state. LSD, a derivative of ergot, was accidentally discovered to be an hallucinogen in 1943 by Albert Hofmann in Switzerland, He had been working on drugs related to ergot alkaloids that might be useful for treatment of migraine headaches and had synthesized LSD. Infinitesimal amounts of this material cause hallucinations and when Hofmann inadvertently ingested or inhaled the chemical, he became sick and developed hallucinations. Because the hallucinations were recognized as similar to those experienced by schizophrenic patients, many investigators throughout the world, including at the NIH, began to study the effects of LSD.

The studies of LSD at NIH typify the results of Seymour Kety's philosophy of directing science. Seymour Kety had invented the means for measuring cerebral blood flow and brain metabolism. He started out as a physiologist but ended up as a psychiatrist, responsible for the development of the concept that schizophrenia has a genetic basis. Kety was my respected and admired mentor, as well as the mentor of many other scientists. His leadership, research and teaching led many, including me, to regard him as the father of biological psychiatry. In confirmation of this, in 1999, just six months before his death, Seymour Kety received the Albert Lasker Award for a Lifetime Special Achievement in Medical Science. Seymour Kety's approach directing research is best described in his own words, quoted from an oral interview by his colleague Philip Holzman, a professor of psychiatry at McLean Hospital in Belmont, Massachusetts: "I had confidence that the best way to direct people's interest toward mental illness was by having it directed by themselves. One could hope that this could be accomplished in a consortium of scientists working in their own field but getting together once in a while at lunch, at conferences, learning a little bit about mental illness and perhaps finding out how something they were interested in might fit into the picture."

And how successful Kety was at accomplishing this! Some of the many studies conducted at the NIH that examined different aspects of the effects of LSD listed in Table 1 are examples of the outcome of his direction. The first paper listed is one in which Louis Sokoloff, Seymour Perlin, and Conan Kornetsky collaborated with Kety in describing the effects of LSD on the cerebral circulation and brain metabolism. In the next paper, Julius Axelrod, Roscoe O. Brady, Bernhard Witkop and Edward V. Evarts described the metabolism of LSD. All four of these scientists were later elected as members of the National Academy of Sciences. Edward Evarts and Wade Marshall examined the electrophysiological effects of LSD. After World War II, because of the electronic advances, it was possible to record, without noise, signals from the brain and even from single cells. A whole room on the fourth floor of the NIH Clinical Center was devoted to the equipment required for these studies. There were no microchips at the time, and recordings required relatively large electronic tubes. As some may remember, the first computers occupied a whole building. Even this one little equivalent of a computer occupied a whole room, and so many wires went across the room, draped from the ceiling, that it was called the spaghetti room.

Table 1. NIH Studies of LSD (1955-1957)

Edward V. Evarts and Wade H. Marshall, "The Effects of Lysergic Acid Diethylamide on the Excitability Cycle of the Lateral Geniculate," *Transactions of American Neurological Association* 80 (1955): 58-60.

A. Sjoerdsma, Conan Kornetsky, and Edward V. Evarts, "Lysergic Acid Diethylamide in Patients With Excess Serotonin," *Archives of Neurological Psychiatry* 75 (1955): 488-92.

Julius Axelrod, Roscoe O. Brady, Bernhard Witkop, and Edward V. Evarts, "The Distribution and Metabolism of Lysergic Acid Diethylamide," *Annals of the New York Academy of Sciences* 66 (1957): 435-44.

Louis Sokoloff, Seymour Perlin, Conan Kornetsky, Seymour S. Kety, "The Effects of D-lysergic Acid Diethylamide on Cerebral Circulation and Overall Metabolism," *Annals of the New York Academy of Sciences* 66 (1957): 468-77.

Seymour S. Kety, "The Implications of Psychopharmacology in the Etiology and Treatment of Mental Illness," *Annals of the New York Academy of Sciences* 66 (1957): 836-40.

Marian W. Kies, D. Horst, Edward V. Evarts, and Norman P. Goldstein, "Antidiuretic Effect of Lysergic Diethylamide in Humans," *Archives of Neurological Psychiatry* 77 (1957): 267-9.

Conan Kornetsky, "Relation of Physiological and Psychological Effect of Lysergic Acid Diethylamide," *Archives of Neurological Psychiatry* 77 (1957): 657-8.

Marian Kies, Edward Evarts, Norman Goldstein, and Dale Horst, who was a normal volunteer, studied the anti-diuretic effects of LSD; Conan Kornetsky, the physiological and psychological effects. As indicated above, Albert Sjoerdsma had described serotonin, produced by malignant carcinoid tumors, as causing problems in the circulation; serotonin was also found in the brain. It was Kety who was putting all of this together in an attempt to explain mental illness in biological terms and introduce drug treatment of psychiatric patients; this heralded a new discipline that came to be called psychopharmacology.

At that time, a major laboratory research tool for separating and identifying compounds found in the urine and the tissues was paper chromatography; column chromatography with ion-exchange resins was just being introduced. The fluorescence spectrophotometer, invented by Robert Bowman in the National Heart Institute, was one of the new workhorses for quantitative assay of amines. Radioisotopes were just being introduced as a means for studying amine metabolism. Kety purchased the first liquid scintillation counter to come to the NIH. It was the third such instrument that the Packard Instrument Company built.

In order to count the disintegrations of the radioisotope, the investigator had to take a vial, put it into the "pig," a lead container inside of a freezer. First the freezer was opened, then the "pig" was opened, the sample was placed in the appropriate space, the "pig" was closed, the freezer was closed, and the researcher pressed a button to begin the count. After watching the little lights on the tubes, the number of counts indicated after the selected time (a minute or two) was recorded, and then the next sample was put in. Naturally, since then, all of this has been automated, of course. Today, with the development of newer, more sensitive techniques, the use of radioisotopes has diminished, but for several decades radioisotopic methods predominated in the studies of amine metabolism and disposition.

It was Kety's idea to use radioisotopes for such studies. He contracted with what was then a small company called the New England Nuclear Company—subsequently taken over by DuPont—to make the first radioactive epinephrine and norepinephrine. This led to some of the most important discoveries about catecholamine metabolism and inactivation by uptake into sympathetic neurons, a discovery for which Julius Axelrod was awarded the Nobel Prize. While working with Julius Axelrod, I synthesized the first ^{14}C-S-Adenosyl-methionine using ^{14}C-methionine supplied by the New England Nuclear Co. We needed that to make ^{14}C-O-methyl-metanephrine for a double-label experiment that I had designed to determine the initial metabolism of tritiated epinephrine. ^{14}C- and ^{3}H-S-Adenosyl-methionine also became important for the discovery of new methylation reactions.

Another important factor was the enthusiastic financial support given to the NIH by Congress. I do not believe there was any resistance to building up this new research enterprise at the NIH. Furthermore, there were several important new programs responsible for bringing to the NIH many physicians who subsequently became important scientists. The Research Associate and Clinical Associate Programs allowed physicians who were United States citizens to become Commissioned Officers in the United States Public Health Service (PHS), which satisfied the military service obligation. At that time, the Korean War was in progress and later on, the war in Vietnam. Many found it preferable to serve their compulsory military service at the NIH instead of going into the army.

The Visiting Scientist Program for foreign citizens also started at that time. Georg Hertting from Austria and Shiro Senoh from Japan were among the first of the Visiting Scientists. Senoh was working in Bernhard Witkop's laboratory in the National Institute of Arthritis and Metabolic Diseases (now the National Institute of Diabetes and Digestive and Kidney Diseases). When Axelrod needed the O-methylated derivative of epinephrine to prove that this compound was formed from epinephrine, Senoh was assigned the task of synthesizing the compound, called metanephrine. Three days later, Senoh delivered the required compound to Axelrod and, using paper chromatography, the compound that was enzymatically formed from S-Adenosyl-methionine and epinephrine was shown to be identical to the authentic metanephrine synthesized by Senoh.

As explained earlier, paper chromatography was one of the most important techniques used to study metabolites excreted in urine. Jay Mann and Elwood LaBrosse were using this method to examine the urinary excretion of phenolic acids, metabolites of many amines. There had been several reports of a compound found using paper chromatography of excreted urinary metabolites of schizophrenic patients that was absent in urine from normal subjects. Mann and LaBrosse examined phenolic acids excreted in the urine from the schizophrenic patients and the normal subjects housed at the NIH. I remember the initial excitement when a spot was found on the chromatograms of urine from almost all of the schizophrenics, whereas only one of the normals excreted the compound. The one schizophrenic who did not excrete that compound was younger and behaved differently from the other patients. All, except the one normal subject who excreted the compound, were Mennonite normal volunteers. The one who excreted the compound was older and also had different habits than the younger Mennonite subjects. It was soon determined that the compound in question was

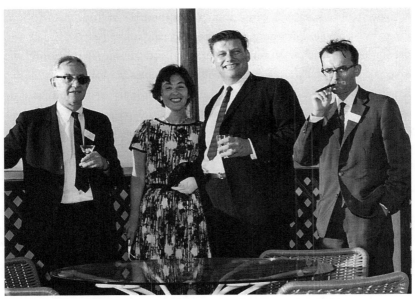

Left to right: Julius Axelrod, Rita Kopin, Irwin Kopin, and Georg Hertting, 1965
Donated to the Office of NIH History by Dr. Irwin Kopin

derived from coffee! The Mennonites did not drink coffee, whereas the single normal subject whose urine contained the compound did drink coffee. Conversely, all the schizophrenics, except this one younger patient whose urine did not contain the compound, drank coffee. There were a number of other similar reports of "spots" appearing in the chromatograms of urine from schizophrenic subjects that were not present in urine from normal subjects. These also were subsequently found to be of dietary origin.

Another example of the pitfalls encountered in psychiatric research at that time was a report that after an oral loading dose of tryptophan, schizophrenic patients failed to have the normal increase in urinary concentration of 5-HIAA. I repeated the study, but collected 24-hour urine specimens. I also found that the urinary concentrations of 5-HIAA were lower in the schizophrenic subjects, but this was the result of the enthusiasm of the nursing staff in urging schizophrenic patients to drink excessive quantities of water to ensure adequate urine flow to facilitate collection of urine specimens, whereas this was not necessary in the normal subjects. The 5-HIAA concentrations were lower in the urine of schizophrenic patients because their 24-hour urine volumes were about three-fold greater than those of the normal control subjects.

Another hypothesis about a biochemical abnormality in schizophrenia involved adrenochrome. Abram Hoffer, Humphrey Osmond, and John Smithies had published a monograph[1] based on an anecdote that during World War II, when supplies of adrenaline were running out, vials containing outdated adrenaline that had turned pink had to be used. It was rumored that when pink adrenaline was injected, some of the patients developed hallucinations. Since pink adrenaline is the result of auto-oxidation of the adrenaline to form adrenochrome, this anecdote was the basis for the hypothesis that schizophrenia resulted from adrenochrome formed by abnormal metabolism of adrenaline. Stephen Szara and Axelrod showed that adrenochrome could not be demonstrated in the blood of normal or schizophrenic patients.

Thus, some of the earliest efforts of the scientists in Kety's laboratory were directed at critically examining several hypotheses regarding biochemical abnormalities in schizophrenic patients.

At that time, studies of catecholamines were an exciting research area. Ulf von Euler had proven that norepinephrine was the transmitter released from sympathetic nerve endings and many grant applications were coming into the NIH study sections requesting funding to support research on the role of catecholamines in various diseases. However, little was known about sensitive and specific methods for measurement of catecholamines in plasma or about catecholamine metabolism. To inform the scientific community better, a symposium was held in October 1958 at the NIH Clinical Center to review what was known about catecholamines: how they could be measured, how they were formed in the body, how they produced their effects, how their actions were terminated, and what their role in brain function is. I do not think that any of the organizers anticipated that five Nobel Prizes would be awarded to the participants of this symposium on catecholamines. The symposium was published in *Pharmacological Reviews*.[2] Between the time that this symposium was originally proposed and when it was actually held, there had been a number of striking advances in the field.

Marvin D. Armstrong, Armand MacMillan and Kenneth N. F. Shaw had found that the major urinary metabolite of epinephrine and norepinephrine was a deaminated and O-methylated product, vanillylmandelic acid (VMA).[3] They had assumed that deamination occurred first and O-methylation followed. As indicated above, Axelrod found that O-methylation of the catecholamines could occur first and that this was the more important pathway for metabolism of administered catecholamines.[4] VMA could be formed by deamination of the metanephrines. Axelrod's demonstration of O-methylation of epinephrine and discovery of the enzyme, catechol-O-methyl transferase, was possible because he could obtain S-adenosylmethionine, required for all methylation reactions, from Giulio Cantoni's Laboratory of Cellular Pharmacology, which was just down the hall.

At the symposium, von Euler, who was awarded a Nobel Prize in 1970, described the method that was then being used in his laboratory for catecholamines. This method was based on the formation of a fluorescent trihydroxyindole formed by oxidizing catecholamines and became the most widely used method for many studies during the next decade. Robert Furchgott, who was awarded the Nobel Prize in 1998 for his discovery of nitric oxide as a signaling molecule, talked about the adrenergic receptors, how the drugs act at these receptors. Earl Sutherland presented for the first time his discovery of adenosine-3',5'-phosphoric acid (cyclic AMP), which was formed from ATP in the presence of epinephrine. The discovery of this crucial "second messenger" in the actions of hormones and neurotransmitters was the reason that he won the Nobel Prize in 1971.

In his presentation, George Koelle, who was one of the organizers of the symposium and was professor of pharmacology and physiology at the University of Pennsylvania, emphasized the importance of understanding how the actions of catecholamines were terminated by mechanisms that do not involve metabolic transformation. He listed five different mechanisms, which Thomas Butler had discussed, as the means of terminating the actions of norepinephrine. None of them were correct. Axelrod found the right answer, which was one of the discoveries that led to his Nobel Prize awarded in 1970.[5] As discussed above, Axelrod's first discoveries were in relation to the importance of O-methylation, and the major route of metabolism of administered epinephrine or norepinephrine. When injected into the bloodstream, O-methylation is the major means of terminating the action of these catecholamines. But at nerve endings, that is not the case. The proof that reuptake into the sympathetic nerve terminals was the major means for terminating the actions of norepinephrine released at the nerve terminals was obtained with radioactive norepinephrine. If the nerves degenerated, the norepinephrine was not taken up into the tissues. Hertting, the Visiting Scientist who was then working in Axelrod's laboratory, and I performed the experiment in which a cat's right superior cervical ganglion was removed. A week later, after the sympathetic nerves had degenerated, almost no administered radioactivity was found in the denervated tissues, indicating the importance of the nerves for accumulating the catecholamine. This, along with the known supersensitivity of denervated tissues exposed to catecholamines, indicated the physiological importance of the uptake process. This was further supported when it was demonstrated that cocaine-induced supersensitivity to catecholamines was attended by a blockade of the neuronal uptake process.

Arvid Carlsson was also at this symposium, where he first presented the observations that were the basis for his Nobel Prize in 2000. He showed that dopamine was present in the corpus striatum, that when reserpine depleted the content of dopamine in the brain, the animal appeared Parkinsonian, and that the behavioral motor deficit could be reversed by treatment with the dopamine precursor, dihydroxyphenylalanine (DOPA). The essentials for DOPA treatment of human Parkinson's disease were there, but it was not until ten years later, in 1968, that George Cotzias successfully treated patients with sufficiently high doses of DOPA to obtain therapeutic effects on the motor deficits.

Kety, in providing an overview of the symposium and the central actions of catecholamines, wrote "In biochemistry as well as pharmacology, the brain is often the last organ to be tackled and will certainly be the last to be understood."[6] This is as true today as it was then. We are still looking for answers about the biological bases for mental disease; the role of molecules in the brain is still a challenging problem. Many Nobel Prizes are awaiting the scientists who unravel these perplexing processes that regulate brain function, but I think it unlikely that there will be a symposium in which as many as five future Nobel Prize laureates will participate.[7]

Notes

1. Abram Hoffer, Humphry Osmond, and John Smythies, "Schizophrenia: A New Approach," *Journal of Mental Science* C, no. 418 (January 1954).
2. 11 (1959): 241-566.
3. Marvin D. Armstrong, Armand McMillan, Kenneth N. F. Shaw, "3-Methoxy-4-hydroxy-D-Mandelic Acid, a Major Urinary Metabolite of Norepinephrine," *Biochimica et Biophysica Acta* 25 (1957): 422-3.
4. Julius Axelrod, "O-Methylation of Catecholamines In Vitro and In Vivo," *Science* 126 (1957): 400.
5. Georg Hertting, Julius Axelrod, Irwin J. Kopin, L. G. Whitby, "Lack of Uptake of Catecholamines After Chronic Denervation of Sympathetic Nerves Nature," *Nature* 189 (1961): 66.
6. Seymour S. Kety, "Central Actions of Catecholamines," *Pharmacological Reviews* 11 (1959): 565-6.
7. I would like to acknowledge the contributions of Joel Elkes. At that time, Elkes was Kety's equivalent at St. Elizabeths Hospital, where he headed the Clinical Neuropharmacology Research Center, a branch of the NIMH, and he greatly fostered the development of biological psychiatry. We all miss Kety greatly.

Mind, Brain, Body, and Behavior
I. G. Farreras, C. Hannaway and V. A. Harden (Eds.)
IOS Press, 2004

A Forty-Year Journey

Guy McKhann

I want to describe a 40-year journey. I was a Clinical Associate at the National Institutes of Health (NIH) from 1957 to 1960, when my mentors were Richard L. Masland and Donald B. Tower, in neurochemistry. Gerald Fischbach then asked me in 2000 to return to work with him, Audrey Penn, and Story Landis as associate director for clinical research in the institute, so I have a perspective on the National Institute of Neurological Disorders and Stroke's (NINDS) intramural research program that is a little different than that of others. In my comments I would like to take the tack of discussing what the Neurology Institute actually did for neurology.

When I arrived at the NIH in the late fifties, neurology, like psychiatry, was unsure what its roots were. To some extent, it overlapped with neuropsychiatry. But that was not biological psychiatry; at the time it was Freudian psychiatry. How did that overlap with neurology? It was not an easy marriage. On the other hand, there was the question of whether neurology was simply a branch of internal medicine. Was the brain, like the liver or the heart, part of internal medicine? Why should neurology be considered a separate entity?

I think one can argue that what the NINDS brought to the table was the introduction of neuroscience to neurology. For clinicians, neuroscience should be our natural base and that is how we should link the fields. And I think that what occurred over the intervening period of time between 1960 and 2000 is very much due to what went on in the Neurology Institute in the 1950s and 1960s. As an aside, it is rather ironic that we fought so hard to separate ourselves from psychiatry 50 years ago and yet now neurology and psychiatry are very much coming back together again. We describe cognitive neuroscience as a joint field. We talk jointly about approaches to disease. We talk jointly about approaches to medications that may alter, say, epilepsy, on the one hand, or mood disorders, on the other. We have also made an interesting liaison again with internal medicine. We now have fields we call neurovirology, neuro-oncology or neurocardiology, so all of a sudden neurology is returning to internal medicine, but it is now on our own terms.

Now, what did the NINDS intramural research program in the 1950s and 1960s bring to neurology? I have already mentioned one part of it, that is, it provided a scientific basis. It was also—as in psychiatry—a breeding ground for academic clinician scientists. The people who came to the NIH did not necessarily work with people in the Neurology Institute; they may have worked with people in the Mental Health Institute. There was tremendous overlap; some people in physiology were in the NIMH and some were in the Neurology Institute. It was a very rich environment for a group of people that came here with almost no research experience. These were bright men right out of medical school or a few years of residency, and most of them had had very little research experience before they arrived. It is a tribute to colleagues like Louis Sokoloff or Tower that they would put up with someone like me during those periods of time.

The other thing that I believe began to take place in the intramural research program at that time was the ability to focus on long-term problems. If I ask myself what the intramural research program's contributions were, they were in areas that would probably have been impossible to fund within the medical school framework. One example is the field of slow viruses that began at the National Institutes of Health. It is inconceivable to me that Joseph Gibbs and Carleton Gajdusek could have carried out those research studies for the many years that they did in the usual format of a medical school's vagaries of financing.

Another example takes Roscoe O. Brady as a model. He was working in an area that I started in as a pediatric neurologist. At the time, Brady was becoming interested in metabolic disorders and he would talk about enzyme therapy and genetic manipulation. In the 1950s we had to deal with family history. We had simple genetic patterns: dominant, recessive, x-linked. But our major lead-in was the pathology, and the pathology was almost showing accumulation of some material. Brady was working on disorders of glycolipids: Tay Sachs disease, Gaucher disease, and other diseases of lipid metabolism. First, the accumulation was identified, then the enzymes involved, and later they were used for diagnosis. That was a pattern that really started at the NIH with Brady and he carried the research forward: in the mid 1970s, by bringing other techniques in enzyme therapy, and now in the 2000s, by looking at risk-factor genetics, transgenics. That is not so much looking at enzymes anymore but at what proteins are abnormal in these disorders.

If we take another disorder, like Alzheimer's disease, we go through exactly the same steps that Brady began at the NIH. When I first began in neurology, it was considered a very rare disease; it was considered a pre-senile dementia. It had about the same frequency as Creutzfeldt-Jacob disease, and if a neurologist saw one or two cases in his practice, that would be a lot. In the 1960s, we did not think the disease existed. In the 1980s, we had anti-cholinesterases and antioxidants as therapies. Now we have a whole pattern of approaches—none of them magic bullets—but at least we have a logical approach to what we are trying to do. What changed all this was the work of the group at the Albert Einstein College of Medicine who recognized that the pathology of what was called pre-senile dementia and what we were calling senility or hardening of the arteries was essentially the same. Raymond Adams, with whom I trained, made essentially the same observations. So, in the 1970s, we were looking at disease incidence and the dominant forms, but we went back to exactly the same steps that Brady had gone through with his diseases: the accumulation of a particular compound, the mechanism by which that compound was being metabolized, the enzymes involved, how they might be used for diagnosis, and how they might be used for therapy. I would argue that the genetic approach that Brady pioneered in the NINDS intramural research program is now, some 25 to 30 years later, currently being applied very effectively to another disease process.

Another field was cognitive neuroscience, because at that time we were not doing much better than Paul Broca had done in the nineteenth century. We talked about lesions in disease and postmortem, and that was our approach to the association of behavior and neurological lesions. Patients were examined, some years later they died, and then the brains were looked at.

On the other hand, at the same time, there were a lot of people in the field of theories of cognition who did not know very much about the brain at all. These fields were brought together, not by clinicians, but by people like Mortimer Mishkin, who could look at systems in primate brains and say, "These are how some systems work." The challenge to us as clinicians was, how do we get from that kind of primate physiology to human physiology? What has done it has been the advent of imaging: lesion location, functional imaging, and, it is to be hoped, functional correlations that are going to be closer to online images than are current imaging techniques.

There were no cellular therapies when we were in the NINDS intramural research program in the 1950s. If a person had gone to an NIH study section in the 1950s and said, "I think we would like to transplant some cells into the brain," not only would the application have been rejected, but the person would have been locked up as well. Cellular therapy began in the 1970s in a small way but no one paid too much attention to it. Now, of course, Richard Sidman and others are right on top of stem cells, using genetic vectors as cellular therapies, and so on.

I want to move to the present. The 1950s were a golden era. We have learnt about this from a number of people. The NIH was a great place for a young investigator to be, whether in psychiatry, neurology or neurosurgery. What about now in 2000? Having spent a year working with Landis and others on aspects of clinical research, I would argue that the NINDS and the NIMH intramural research programs are still very special places. They allow people to do research that would be very difficult to do in the medical school environment. First of all, at the NIH there is a unique inpatient facility, the Clinical Center, which makes it possible for a researcher to bring in people–at very little expense to families–and keep them for much longer than can be done in any other hospital environment that I am aware of. Second, there are excellent imaging facilities at the NIH that are absolutely crucial to asking a lot of the questions a researcher would like to ask. Finally, specific cohorts of patients can be attracted and studied over long periods of time, another thing that is very difficult to do in the current medical school environment.

However, I do have some suggestions for change. Anyone who has run a neurology department is aware of the fact that you cannot do everything. You have to focus and identify what the strengths of your department are going to be. I believe that the NIH has to do the same thing. When I was here in the 1950s, the NIH was unique. The NINDB was a spin off, in a sense, of the Montreal Neurological Institute. Thus, it very much focused on epilepsy, and there were not many other epilepsy-oriented programs then. But, over time, epilepsy programs sprang up all over the country, so one could now argue whether the NIH has a unique role to play in epilepsy or not. If it does, one ought to rethink how it would be different from the programs for which it was essentially a model.

The problem of maintaining flexibility with scientific staff is not unique to the NIH. Every medical school faces this problem—aging faculty, tenure problems—yet still wants this atmosphere of bright young people. Forty years ago, we were all in our late twenties or early thirties. That was what made this a really great place. It is very important that that group of young people be established and maintained. It is hard to do.

Many people who came to the NIH in the 1950s did not know what the NIH was. They did not know much about research, and they did not know much about what their laboratories were doing. I would argue that, sadly, to some extent, this is still a problem and that one of the NIH's challenges is to get out and tell the young people what a great opportunity it can offer.

My last comment has to do with a problem of insularity. This, again, is in no way unique to the NIH, but I think it is very important that, as the NIH develops, ways are found to work outside the NIH with other institutions. This is not easy because of all of the problems with the data, the relationship with who is on the study section and who is not, but these can be solved.

I would like to conclude by noting that I am one of many people, both in neurology and psychiatry, who essentially owes his career to the NIH. I, like Sid Gilman, have had grant funds from the NIH ever since I was here in the 1950s. As a child, an adolescent—I will not say an old man—a maturing man in the field of neurology, all stages in my career have been supported by the NIH, so I owe the institution an enormous debt.

Mind, Brain, Body, and Behavior
I. G. Farreras, C. Hannaway and V. A. Harden (Eds.)
IOS Press, 2004

The Onset of Developmental Neuroscience in Mammals[1]

Richard L. Sidman

I was one of the lucky ones–a young physician pulled out of residency training at the Massachusetts General Hospital, Boston, and assigned to the National Institutes of Health (NIH) for the required two years of military service. I stayed on for an extra six months, so my service at the NIH spanned from July 1, 1956 through December 1958. My assignment was to William F. Windle's Laboratory of Neuroanatomical Sciences in the National Institute of Neurological Diseases and Blindness (NINDB[2]).

A little of my personal background history is useful to set this phase of my professional life in perspective. Most of the physician-soldiers assigned to the NIH were gaining their first research experience. When I came to the NIH, I was a neurologist still at an early stage in my residency training but well into my laboratory research career, with eleven published papers between 1950 and 1956 and first authorship on five of them. My research interests had come to focus on developmental neuroscience, although such a term for this field had not yet evolved. We have celebrated, in 2003, the 50th anniversary of the landmark Watson and Crick paper on the structure of DNA,[3] but looking back, it is curious how little impact that momentous publication had on most of us, whether senior or junior scientists, in the late 1950s. Genetics had been only a very minor subject in my formal education at Harvard College and Harvard Medical School and had made little impact as yet on thinking or practice in developmental biology or neurological research.

The Laboratory of Neuroanatomical Sciences was based in a little, one story structure, Building 9, near the massive Clinical Center. What excited me most as I became familiar with the NIH research scene was, first of all, the dynamic, experimental work of my next door neighbor, Lloyd Guth. Guth taught me, through his example, the importance of designing an experiment thoroughly in advance, and refining it as needed when the results begin to come in.[4]

The second influence was the remarkable progress of Sanford L. Palay (chief of the Laboratory of Neuroanatomical Sciences's Section on Neurocytology) and his colleagues in mapping new territory in the central nervous system by electron microscopy and developing new functional concepts from their extraordinary pictures.[5]

Palay's section was one flight downstairs, in the basement. A great many good things in science move forward in basements and in attics. For example, I became acquainted in those years with David Hubel's early work across town at the Walter Reed Army Medical Center in Silver Spring. Hubel also toiled away in a basement, painstakingly working out how to fashion extracellular electrodes that would come to allow him to make prolonged recordings from the visual system in living animals.[6]

My own work was to be centered on use of organ-culture techniques to investigate the actions of peripheral nerves on target organs, a technique I had learned from Dame Honor Fell at the Strangeways Laboratory in Cambridge, England, during a research year abroad in 1954-55, between internship in medicine and assistant residency in neurology. The Strangeways, on the outskirts of Cambridge, was typical of the best in British science, a dedicated group of unassuming individuals quietly pursuing very new ideas. The immediate attraction for me was Fell's own work on the direct effects of defined agents such as vitamin A on developing organs. However, other Strangeways research projects had subliminal influences that affected my subsequent NIH and Harvard research directions, particularly Aaron Moscona's use of trypsin to dissociate tissues into single cell suspensions which he could then reassemble *in vitro* into organotypic patterns; Alfred Glücksman's demonstration of reproducible patterns of programmed cell death during development; Audrey Glauert's formulation of epoxy resins for embedding and sectioning tissue specimens for electron microscopy; and above all, Stephen R. Pelc's pioneering autoradiographic studies on the timing of DNA synthesis in relation to cell division.

Windle, my new chief at the NIH, had no personal interest in the organ culture line of research. He had done distinguished work on trajectories of the earliest axons to form during fetal development of the mammalian brain and spinal cord, and was mainly preoccupied in those formative years of the recently launched institute with axonal regeneration in injured spinal cord and in development of an NIH-operated, free-ranging rhesus monkey colony in Puerto Rico.[7] He generously gave me full freedom to pursue any research direction I chose, a remarkable difference from today's pattern in which most junior investigators become cogs in some senior person's research machine.

Soon after my arrival in the summer of 1956, I ran into the NIH's biggest intramural problem, a problem that, in an odd twist of fate, became my salvation. The NIH at that time was already a marvelous place for scientific work, permeated by a creative spirit, wonderfully equipped, covering an enormous range of biomedical fields. However, it was also hostage to the government's employment system—designed to assure that nobody was treated unfairly, but a system in which many non-professional workers found a sure road to a long, quiet life by taking on an attitude that any job assignment is better done tomorrow than today.

Windle submitted all the proper requisitions calling for a small half-room to be converted for me from office space into a tissue-culture cubicle. It then took the NIH's Building and Maintenance bureaucracy more than a year and a half of my required two-year stint to install a sink and a sliding door. Since I could not do the intended organ-culture work, I had lots of time to spend in the elaborate library in the Clinical Center, where I was able to delve deeply and uninterruptedly into the scientific literature, and even obtain free translations of articles in foreign languages.

Research that caught my attention was the initial work of Walter L. Hughes and his colleagues at the Brookhaven National Laboratory with a new radioactive reagent developed in 1956 at Brookhaven, called tritiated thymidine, and tested in adult normal and irradiated mice.[8] Thymidine was already known to be capable of serving as an exogenous precursor of DNA, and Hughes' plan was to use a radioactive version of it to radiate and kill dividing cancer cells. This, like most later mitosis-targeted drugs, failed as a cancer therapy, but the 1957 studies from

Brookhaven showed that in the days after a single injection of this agent into human subjects, radioactive white blood cells began to appear in the circulating blood. Clearly the tritium had been incorporated into dividing cells in the bone marrow, and those cells then matured and entered the circulation. After passage of more days, the radioactivity per blood cell decreased progressively because their precursors in the bone marrow (stem cells, in today's terminology) were diluting the radioactivity that had been incorporated into DNA about 50 percent with each new cell division that was taking place in the absence of further radioactive precursor.

Here, then, was a visualizable reagent that could target specifically on dividing cells or be rapidly degraded and the tritium excreted as tritiated water. It occurred to me that most cells in the developing nervous system, unlike those in the bone marrow, ceased dividing early and permanently, and therefore should not go on synthesizing new DNA. The radioactivity would be expected to remain indefinitely in those brain cells undergoing their final or penultimate round of cell division, and since tritium has a 12.5-year half-life, should serve to trace where and when cells are dividing in a fetal mammal's brain, where they will reside in the adult brain, and what those cells are destined to become.

Making arrangements at the science level, as opposed to the building-renovation level, was marvelously efficient at the NIH. We found a newly established commercial source of tritiated thymidine—the New England Nuclear Company—and chose the mouse as the experimental animal, not because of some clairvoyant recognition that the mouse would be the animal of central importance in the medical research world of the future, but simply because it was small and would need less of the expensive reagent than a larger animal. We obtained permission to do our experiment across the NIH campus in Building 14, a site that had been designated as the only place on campus where radioactive compounds could be injected into experimental animals. There were three of us working together at the laboratory bench: Ned Feder, a medical school classmate, Irene Miale, a postdoctoral fellow, and me. Miale's mentor, Mac Edds, had sent her from Brown University to his friend, Windle, because Miale's husband was just being assigned to duty in Washington, D.C., in the U.S. Diplomatic Corps. Windle then assigned Irene to me.

There was a lot for us to learn, some with help from other scientists at the NIH and some on our own. I contacted Clifford Grobstein, the outstanding developmental biologist of his era and a tower of strength at that time in the National Cancer Institute, because of our mutual interest in organ culture. He taught me about the existence of inbred strains of mice, and showed me how to breed mice and how to recognize the first day of gestation so that the pregnancies could be timed.[9]

In addition to all that we learned from others, we also taught each other from descriptions of methods on journal pages. One example was mastering how to work in complete darkness to make autoradiograms by dipping microscope slides into liquid photographic emulsion and then hanging them with clothespins onto a wire suspended above the laboratory bench to dry, a technique based on the newly published method of the distinguished Canadian histologist, Charles P. LeBlond.[10]

A bit of luck always helped, and we were fortunate in choosing mice at the eleventh day of gestation for the first trial injections of tritiated thymidine. Younger embryos, as we learned later, do not receive enough of the radioactive compound after its injection into the mother because the placental circulation connecting mother and embryo is not yet well enough developed. The patterns of radioactive cells in older fetuses might have been too complex for us to analyze and understand at that initial phase of our venture into uncharted territory. No one before us had used tritiated thymidine to look at the nervous system or indeed, at any tissues in mammalian embryos.

We killed the first four injected pregnant mice at 1, 6, 24, and 48 hours after injection. The embryos were fixed for histological and autoradiographic workup. Beta rays from the tritium produce a latent image in the photographic emulsion layer just as light does with the film in a camera. The difference from the camera is that for autoradiography, exposure time of the film to tritium is measured in weeks or months, not in fractions of a second. However, at the end of the exposure time, the slides with the emulsion are developed in the darkroom with the standard chemicals used for photographic development, and the cells with sufficient radioactivity in their nuclei are then seen to be overlaid with reduced (black) silver grains in the emulsion.

When we came to examine those slides from the first experiment, we were gratified to see with the microscope that there was indeed a pattern of labeled cells and that the pattern in the embryonic brain was different at each of the three time points.[11] In the brain sampled at one hour after injection, most of the radioactive cell nuclei were oval-shaped with their long axis radial to the brain surfaces, and were located at a distance from the inner surface of the brain, while in the six-hour specimen, most labeled nuclei were near the inner surface (that is, the ventricular surface), and all cells that were actually dividing at the moment of fixation were radioactive.

It took some time to figure out what this meant, but the two keys were already in the published literature. First, I found a trio of very obscure, largely forgotten papers from the mid-1930s by a Midwestern embryology professor named Frederick Sauer, in which he showed that many so-called "multi-layered" epithelia were actually composed of pseudo-stratified, elongated cells with their nuclei at different distances from the surface.[12] The nuclei of these cells, he inferred correctly, dynamically moved toward the inner surface as the cells prepared to divide, and cell division actually took place at that surface. It seemed that in our specimens, those cell nuclei which lay at a distance from the surface were the ones to become radioactive, as seen at one hour after injection of tritiated thymidine, and that those same nuclei must then move toward the inner surface of the brain, taking about six hours to get there, and divide at that surface.

The other key publication was a more recent and timely one–a brief, conceptually vital paper by the Strangeways Laboratory investigator, Stephen Pelc, which established that cells replicate their DNA prior to cell division, not during cell division.[13] Pelc was responsible for the nomenclature everyone has come to use: S for the DNA synthesis phase, M for the mitosis phase, G1 for the gap phase between mitosis and synthesis, and G2 for the later gap phase between synthesis and mitosis.[14]

In one of those rare flashes of insight that make the labor of scientific work unmatchably rewarding,[15] the conclusion seemed to me unavoidable that in the developing brain, cells in S phase have their nuclei at a distance from the ventricular surface, and that those nuclei translocate toward the surface during G2, go through mitosis, M, at the surface and then withdraw again from the ventricular surface during G1. Examination of our 24-hour specimen indicated that some of the heavily labeled cells already had entirely left the germinal zone near the ventricular surface. Most of these were destined never to divide again. That is, they would differentiate and retain their full complement of radioactive DNA for the life of the mouse, while other cells remained in the germinal zone and returned to synthesis activity, diluting their radioactivity in half with each subsequent division. The cells that had ceased dividing migrated outward in patterns that had been only dimly guessed at before, to make a cerebral cortex,[16] a cerebellar cortex,[17] a retina,[18] and so on.

This, then, was the beginning of our precise and semi-quantitative understanding of the genesis of form in the mammalian brain. The work underscored the fundamental new idea, now accepted as commonplace, that cell migration is a major event in neurogenesis. These studies also led to the concept that a large repertory of new cell interactions, made possible by the migration patterns, plays a dominant role in formation of the incredibly complex nervous system. Understanding the molecular genetic control of these migrations and interactions occupies world-wide attention today as the central challenge in basic and clinical developmental neuroscience. It all began so simply at the NIH.

Notes

1. I would like to express my thanks to Drs. Ingrid G. Farreras and Victoria A. Harden, who organized the symposium and publication, for the invitation to participate.
2. Today the National Institute of Neurological Disorders and Stroke (NINDS).
3. James D. Watson & Francis H. C. Crick, "A Structure for Deoxyribonucleic Acid," *Nature* 171 (1953), 737-8.
4. Lloyd Guth, "Functional Recovery Following Vagosympathetic Anastomosis in the Cat," *American Journal of Physiology* 185 (1956): 205-8.
5. Sanford L. Palay, "The Morphology of Synapses in the Central Nervous System," *Experimental Cell Research 14, Suppl. 5 (1958):* 275-93.
6. David H. Hubel, "Cortical Unit Responses to Visual Stimuli in Nonanesthetized Cats," *American Journal of Ophthalmology* 46 (1958), 110-21.
7. William F. Windle, J. L. Littrell, J. O. Smart, and J. Joralemon, "Regeneration in the Cord of Spinal Monkeys," *Neurology* 6 (1956), 420-8.
8. W. L. Hughes, V. P. Bond, G. Brecher, E. P. Cronkite, R. B. Painter, H. Quastler, and F. G. Sherman, "Cellular Proliferation in the Mouse as Revealed by Autoradiography With Tritiated Thymidine," *Proceedings of the National Academy of Sciences* 44 (1958), 476-83.

9. Grobstein, like so many NIH scientists of that era, later went out to create modern medical academia. He went first to Stanford University, and a few years later to the University of California–San Diego, where, as dean and then as vice chancellor, he was central to the creation of its innovative new medical school.

10. B. Messier and Charles P. LeBlond, "Preparation of Coated Radioautographs by Dipping Sections in Fluid Emulsion," *Proceedings of the Society for Experimental Biology and Medicine* 96 (1957), 7-10.

11. Richard L. Sidman, I. L. Miale, and N. Feder, "Cell Proliferation and Migration in the Primitive Ependymal Zone: An Autoradiographic Study of Histogenesis in the Nervous System," *Experimental Neurology* 1 (1959): 322-33.

12. F. C. Sauer, "Mitosis in the Neural Tube," *Journal of Comparative Neurology* 62 (1935): 377-405.

13. Stephen R. Pelc, "Quantitative Aspects of Autoradiography," *Experimental Cell Research* 13, Suppl. 4 (1957): 231-7.

14. L. F. La Cour, and Stephen R. Pelc, "Effect of Colchicine on the Utilization of Labelled Thymidine During Chromosomal Reproduction," *Nature* 23 (1958): 506-8.

15. See A. Lightman, "A Sense of the Mysterious," *Daedalus* 132, no. 4 (2003), 5-21, for a vivid discussion of this phenomenon.

16. J. B. Angevine, Jr., and R. L. Sidman, "Autoradiographic Study of Cell Migration During Histogenesis of Cerebral Cortex in the Mouse," *Nature* 192 (1961): 766-8.

17. I. L. Miale, and Richard L. Sidman, "An Autoradiographic Analysis of Histogenesis in the Mouse Cerebellum," *Experimental Neurology* 4 (1961): 277-96.

18. Richard L. Sidman, "Histogenesis of Mouse Retina Studied with Thymidine-H3," in *The Structure of the Eye*, ed. G. K. Smelser (New York: Academic Press, 1961), 487-506.

Mind, Brain, Body, and Behavior
I. G. Farreras, C. Hannaway and V. A. Harden (Eds.)
IOS Press, 2004

The 1950s Clinical Program at the NINDB[1]

Donald B. Tower, M.D., Ph.D.

We have had 50 good years of research since April of 1953 when G. Milton Shy and Maitland Baldwin arrived at the National Institutes of Health (NIH) to start the clinical program at the National Institute of Neurological Diseases and Blindness (NINDB, today the National Institute of Neurological Disorders and Stroke). The points of emphasis that I would like to make are four or five. First of all, the original contingent to the NINDB's clinical program came primarily from the Montreal Neurological Institute (MNI). It was the largest single group of Montrealers in training that went anywhere. Wilder Penfield established the Montreal Neurological Institute at McGill University in 1934, and he operated a very successful institute during and after World War II.

The NINDB began mostly as part of the NIH intramural program, as authorized congressionally in 1951. Neurology in the United States, Canada, Mexico, and Europe was at a nadir at that time. Training in neurology was restricted to a handful of places. There was an argument, very active especially in government, as to whether programs should be in neuropsychiatry or in neurology and psychiatry separately. Pearce Bailey was head of the Navy neurology program in Philadelphia and after the war he was chosen to head the neurology program in the United States Veterans Administration (VA). This gave him an opportunity to begin, in a very small way at the VA hospitals around the country, the resurrection of neurological training and neurological services. To start a program at the NIH in the new Clinical Center, he turned to Montreal and invited Shy and Baldwin to come. They, in turn, invited those of us who comprised the initial contingent.

There were nine people from the MNI to head up the various units. Milton Shy (from Denver (via Montreal) was clinical director and head of neurology. Maitland Baldwin (also from Denver (via Montreal) was head of neurosurgery. Choh-luh Li was a microelectrode neurophysiologist and neurosurgeon, originally from Canton and Shanghai in China. John Van Buren rounded out the neurosurgeons with emphasis on neuroanatomy. Cosimo Ajmone-Marsan was head of EEG and clinical neurophysiology; he came originally from Torino (Turin), Italy, also via Montreal. Two were originally from Poland: Igor Klatzo (in neuropathology) via the Vogt's Institute at Freiburg-im-Breisgau and then Montreal; and Anatole Dekaban (in pediatric neurology) from Poland via Montreal. I was part of the group; I came in the summer of 1953 to set up a clinical neurochemistry laboratory. In addition, Shirley Lewis was an operating room nurse at Montreal and came to be Baldwin's surgical nurse; later they married. Lastly was John Lord, from Maine and Montreal, who was in private practice as a neurosurgeon but also a consultant to the NINDB program.

These nine people represented the nucleus from which the program grew. These were the people who made the "golden age" of the 1950s golden. Programs were established in neuromuscular disorders, epilepsy, and lots of different approaches to problems of spinal cord regeneration, voltage-clamp techniques, etc. Training was offered for those who wanted to come and learn from the experts.

We had a dual personnel system at that point: partly Civil Service and partly Public Health Service Commissioned Corps. The latter was a uniformed service. It was a time when the physician's draft was in effect. If you were acceptable otherwise, you could come to the NIH, get a commission in the Public Health Service, and join whatever program you and the program leaders agreed upon to satisfy your draft obligation. I was one of those. I left the U.S. Navy base at Subic Bay (Philippines) when they said: "You're finished. Thank you and goodbye." That was in 1946. In 1953, while I was in Montreal, they said: "You owe us 18 months more service." And I was obliged to come back, so research at the NIH provided a means to satisfy this obligation.

But I think that that system was invaluable not only to the people who were in the program but to the program as a whole. I do not think we could have started on such a high note, such a golden-age approach, if we had not had this opportunity to bring top-flight people to Bethesda. To the Montreal contingent should be added: Giovanni DiChiro (neuroradiology), Paul O. Chatfield (neurophysiology), and Laurence L. Frost (neuropsychology).

In addition, we should not overlook the basic neuroscientists who regularly interacted with their clinical colleagues: Kenneth S. Cole (Laboratory of Biophysics), Wade H. Marshall (NIMH Laboratory of Neurophysiology), Karl Frank (Section on Spinal Cord Physiology, within Marshall's Laboratory of Neurophysiology), William F. Windle (Laboratory of Neuroanatomical Sciences), Jan Cammermeyer (Section on Experimental Neuropathology within Windle's Laboratory of Neuroanatomical Sciences), and Roscoe O. Brady (Section on Lipid Chemistry, within the Laboratory of Neurochemistry).[2]

There is a tendency to distinguish between clinical research and basic research. I think that is wrong. In looking back over our programs, it seems to me that there was a constant undulation in which at one point you were in a clinical phase and at the next point in a research phase. It would not have worked to get the answers that we sought and some of which we got if we had not done it that way. I think of Brady's program as a prime example.

Brady started out looking at lipid storage diseases (lipodystrophies). He spent a long time with a good many people in his laboratory to define the fact that these diseases were due to genetic absence or genetic attenuation of various key degradative enzymes. And he went on to study Tay-Sachs disease, Gaucher disease, Niemann-Pick disease, and a number of others from the standpoint of trying to achieve enzyme replacement. So here we are starting out with a completely basic research program and no patients. Then you moved to patients who would donate tissue samples to see if you could find what was wrong in their enzymology. And then you moved to a ward of patients where you were trying to treat them by replacing the missing enzyme. And it worked. As far as I know, this is one of few programs that has worked from such historic starts to finishes. Many have tried but only a very few have succeeded.

We also had opportunities during the 1950s to learn ourselves. I remember Shy and I went down to Oak Ridge, Tennessee, to the Oak

Ridge Institute of Nuclear Studies (ORINS) in order to take their course on radioisotope techniques and thus qualify to use isotopes in our research. Today everyone takes for granted that you learn in your own institution and get certified there. We had to go to Oak Ridge to get a certificate after three weeks of training and hands-on work in order to be able to go back to Bethesda and qualify for using radioisotopes in our research.

We were able to invite consultants in as well. I stress this because a brand new program may take some time before one can reach the point of inviting consultants. We had within the first two years people like J. Godwin Greenfield (from Queen Square Hospital) in neuropathology and muscle physiology; and Henry McIlwain (from the University of London) as the leading neurochemist in Britain and Europe. I like to think of McIlwain because he worked with Choh-luh Li. Li could make beautiful microelectrodes, and McIlwain had the apparatus in which to incubate a slice of brain so that it could be stimulated. All that was necessary was to drop the microelectrode into a neuron in that slice of brain in order to see what the effect of stimulation or change in the ionic environment might be. They obtained injury potentials from neurons in these slices—the first such records obtained—and McIlwain went on to show that he could drain the cell, so to speak, of potassium and then get the cell to pump the potassium back in again. Thus began a great deal of work on brain slices that took place later on.

I think the foregoing gives you a flavor of the clinical program and its broad-ranging activities. I wish it well for the next 50 years. May I conclude with a quote from my 25th anniversary paper, about where we stood in 1950 as this enterprise began:

> Consider for a moment the 1950s state of knowledge. My examples come from areas of my interests and experiences, but they will suggest many others. At the time the NINDB was founded our knowledge of the Krebs cycle of intermediary metabolism was newly established....The concept of the mechanism of neuromuscular transmission had just changed from an electrical to a chemical one, and the

mechanisms of action of cholinesterase and the anti-cholinesterase agents were just in the process of elucidation. The electric eel and the squid were among the earliest of 'exotic' species to prove especially valuable to the neuroscientist....[A]xoplasmic flow was known, but its bidirectional transport characteristics were still unknown. The voltage clamp technique and studies of the details of axonal conduction were in their infancy...

Isotropic tracers were few and not widely used....The preparative ultracentrifuge was just coming off the drawing boards....We knew something about the macromolecular arrangement of the myelin sheath–one of the first biological membranes subjected to study by physical techniques such as X-ray crystallography. But we did not yet understand the intricacies of its structure or the role of oligodendroglia or Schwann cells in its genesis and maintenance....

We were beginning to learn about the simple peptide nature of the posterior pituitary hormones, but we had only rudimentary appreciation of the role of the hypothalamus in pituitary hormone control....We knew about inborn errors of metabolism, but we did not know about enzyme deletions or attenuations, so that the biochemical lesions responsible for phenylketonuria (PKU), galactosemia, and the like were still to be demonstrated....Neuroviruses like rabies and polio were known, but the polio vaccines were still experimental and would require the development of tissue culture for commercial production to become feasible....

In 1950 there were only three really effective anticonvulsant drugs...[O]nly neostigmine was available for myasthenia gravis; antibiotics were just beginning to make inroads into the bacterial infection of the nervous system, with some of them creating new problems because of their...toxicity...

For all [of the advances since then]...we must credit the biomedical research and research training effort spearheaded by the NIH and contemporary federal and private sector

organizations in the post-World War II era. For the neurosciences and the communicative sciences the NINDB
provided the major resources through its research grant,
training grant, and special training programs.[3]

Over 50 years much has been accomplished, but many more challenges continue to confront us. May the next anniversary enlighten us
even more.

Notes

1. The sources employed in this account were: Pearce Bailey, "National Institute
    of Neurological Diseases and Blindness: Origins, Founding, and Early
    Years (1950 to 1959)," in *The Nervous System: A Three-Volume Work
    Commemorating the 25th Anniversary of the National Institute of Neurological
    and Communicative Disorders and Stroke, Vol. 1: The Basic Neurosciences,*
    eds. Donald B. Tower and Roscoe O. Brady (New York: Raven Press, 1975),
    xxi-xxxii; Donald B. Tower, "Introduction,"Ibid., xvii-xx; Donald B. Tower,
    "The Neurosciences–Basic and Clinical," in *NIH: An Account of Research in
    its Laboratories and Clinics,* eds. DeWitt Stetten, Jr., and W. T. Carrigan
    (Orlando: Academic Press, 1984), 48-70.
2. I have not included here the Ophthalmology Branch, headed by Ludwig
    von Sallmann. It would seem more appropriate to include it in a review
    of programs of the National Eye Institute.
3. Donald B. Tower, "Introduction," in *The Nervous System,* xix-xx.

Epilogue: Bridge To The Present

The intramural program at the National Institute of Neurological Disorders and Stroke (NINDS), one of the largest basic and clinical neuroscience programs in the world, has always been highly visible. According to Lewis P. Rowland, in his history of the institute, *NINDS at 50,** five investigators from the NINDS intramural program have won Lasker Awards—one of the country's most prestigious awards in biomedical research—and one has been awarded the Nobel Prize. But even those who have not won renown for their discoveries have made major contributions to the advancement of the neurosciences by training, mentoring, and launching the careers of the next generation of biomedical scientists.

The types of programs in the NINDS intramural division have always been diverse. Some have been basic science investigations, based in laboratories on the Bethesda campus or in buildings nearby. Some have been conducted in the field, such as Nancy Wexler's investigations into the genetic origins of Huntington's disease on Lake Maracaibo in Venezuela. Clinical investigations, in the National Institutes of Health (NIH) Clinical Center or in nearby hospitals, have existed since the beginning of the institute's history.

Intramural programs at the NINDS have also been interdisciplinary from the beginning. In 1951, when Pearce Bailey arrived as the first director of the National Institute of Neurological Diseases and Blindness (NINDB), he discovered that the NIH would provide administrative funds for the fledgling institute, but no money for training and research. For the first several years, he had to depend upon the National

---

* Lewis P. Rowland, *NINDS at 50: An Incomplete History Celebrating the Fiftieth Anniversary of the National Institute of Neurological Disorders and Stroke*, October 2001, NIH Pub. 01-4161.

Institute of Mental Health (NIMH) for money, and its scientific director, Seymour S. Kety, to head the intramural program for the NINDB as well as the NIMH.

Most scientific directors would have made the NINDB research more biological, and guided the NIMH research in psychoanalytic or sociological directions, but from the start Kety chose to make psychiatry research more biological, and hired neuroscientists on the basis of their research skills, regardless of the institute with which they would be affiliated. This is how neuroscience research began at the NIH, in tandem with the behavioral sciences, in laboratories that encouraged an interdisciplinary exchange between the physiological and psychological study of the brain.

But even as the NINDS grew, split off from the NIMH, and spun off other institutes (the National Eye Institute, and the National Institute of Deafness and Other Communication Disorders), it never strayed from its mission—to reduce the burden of neurological disorders by finding ways to prevent or to treat these diseases. The intramural division has always had a steady commitment to clinical investigations. Programs for neuromuscular diseases and epilepsy were initiated when G. Milton Shy arrived in 1953 to act as the first intramural clinical director. The neuromuscular diseases section, now in its fiftieth year and its third generation of leadership, is still a pioneer in studies of muscle diseases. From 1953 to 1980, epilepsy surgery was a dominating specialty in the clinical program, and it was later joined by neurosurgery programs that made technical advances in brain tumor surgery.

In 1968, when stroke research was added to our portfolio, the NINDS began clinical programs in stroke prevention and treatment that built a strong foundation for the rapid treatment of acute stroke. Clinical research continues to identify and test promising experimental stroke therapies.

In basic research, the intramural division encompasses programs in every important area of neuroscience, investigating neuromechanisms at the molecular, cellular, and neural network levels. Neurogenetics research continues to identify single and multiple gene interactions that can cause common and rare neurological diseases. Imaging programs are developing new techniques and tactics to diagnose and measure disease in the brain. Epidemiological studies are tracking the incidence of neurological diseases within specific populations.

NINDS intramural researchers also lead the way in stem cell research. Their studies have contributed to fundamental advances in understanding embryonic and adult stem cells; to improved methods for isolation, proliferation, and specialization of stem cells; and to promising therapeutic attempts in animal models of stroke, spinal cord injury, Parkinson's disease, demyelinating diseases, brain tumors, and inherited metabolic disorders.

The NINDS intramural division will continue to be a place for basic research of uncertain outcome that may take years to complete. Our challenge is to balance research that pushes the neurosciences forward with research that pushes treatments for neurological diseases forward. Translational research encompasses the many steps needed to move from basic research insights to a therapy ready for human testing in clinical trials. It is one way of quickly moving discoveries from the laboratory to life-saving treatments. We will continue to energize our efforts to translate opportunities into practical therapies.

I am fortunate to have become director at a pivotal time in the history of the NINDS and the NIH. Before taking my present position as the NINDS Director, I was the scientific director of the institute's intramural research program, and worked with my counterparts at other neuroscience institutes to integrate our intramural research programs through a common seminar series, a shared website, shared resources, and joint recruitment of outstanding scientists.

The emergence of an inter-institute and multidisciplinary community of intramural neuroscientists has led to the development of the concept for the new National Neuroscience Research Center (NNRC) on the Bethesda campus. Scientific directors from seven intramural programs worked together to select cross cutting neuroscience research themes, and researchers whose approaches to those themes complemented one another. Laboratory space in the Center is assigned according to the potential for catalyzing scientific interactions rather than by institute affiliation. Investigators from each of the participating NIH institutes will be joining in this effort to "put the brain back together" and set the standard for collaborative research in neuroscience.

In the course of the past 53 years of neuroscience research at the NIH, we have seen the pendulum swing one way, and then another, and then back to where we began, as we consider an intramural neuroscience program without institutional boundaries. Neurologists, neurosurgeons, psychiatrists, neuroscientists, developmental neurobiologists, behavioral scientists, and other researchers with an interest in how the brain works, are now working together to advance discoveries in basic, clinical, and translational research at the NIH. The discoveries they make, and the treatments that will derive from them, are likely to revolutionize the practice of medicine in ways we can only begin to imagine.

Story C. Landis, Ph.D.
Director, NINDS

Appendices

Appendix A
Intramural Research Program Organizational Chart, 1950s

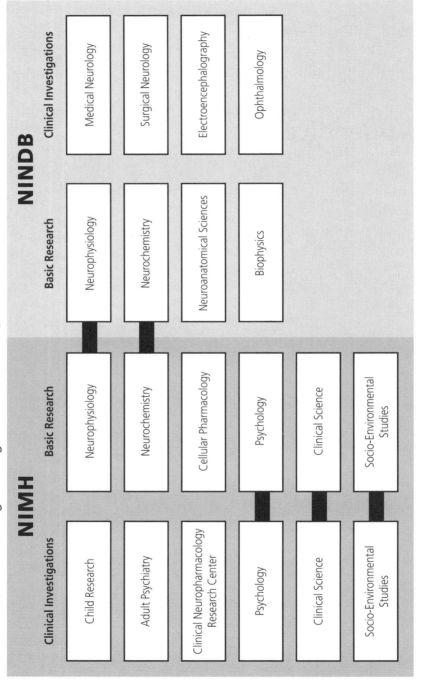

NIMH

Clinical Investigations

- Child Research
- Adult Psychiatry
- Clinical Neuropharmacology Research Center
- Psychology
- Clinical Science
- Socio-Environmental Studies

Basic Research

- Neurophysiology
- Neurochemistry
- Cellular Pharmacology
- Psychology
- Clinical Science
- Socio-Environmental Studies

NINDB

Basic Research

- Neurophysiology
- Neurochemistry
- Neuroanatomical Sciences
- Biophysics

Clinical Investigations

- Medical Neurology
- Surgical Neurology
- Electroencephalography
- Ophthalmology

Appendix B

NIMH and NINDB Laboratory and Branch Members

The *NIMH* and *NINDB Annual Reports* include Project Description Sheets for every study that the Laboratories and Branches conducted. The Principal and Other Investigators involved in each study are listed on these sheets. Not all scientists listed in the first column (i.e., Principal Investigators) of the following Appendices were official members of that Laboratory or Branch. However, they were Principal Investigators of studies listed under that Laboratory or Branch, collaborating with the official members of that Laboratory or Branch.

Adult Psychiatry Branch, NIMH

Principal Investigators	Other Investigators
Boomer, Donald S.	Alexander, Irving
Bowen, Murray	Auster, Simon
Cardon, Jr., Philippe V.	Basamania, Betty
Charlton, Arlyn	Brodey, Warren M.
Cholden, Louis S.	Bunney, William
Day, Juliana	Cabrera, Carmen
Deasy, Leila Calhoun	Campaigne, Howard H.
Dittmann, Allen T.	Coelho, George
Dysinger, Robert	Duhl, Leonard
Elkes, Charmian	Duncan, Pam
Fishman, Jacob R.	Evarts, Edward V.
Goodrich, D. Wells	Farber, Leslie H. (psychiatric consultant)
Greenberg, Harold A.	Fisher, Thais
Hamburg, David A.	Flint, Arden
Hirsch, Stanley I.	Friedman, Stanford
Jenkins, Jr., William C.	Geisser, Seymour
Perry, Stewart E.	Goffman, Erving
Pittenger, Robert E.	Greenberg, Irwin
Rioch, Margaret	Greenhouse, Samuel W.
Ryckoff, Irving M.	Hall, Edward T.
Savage, Charles	Halperin, Alexander (psychiatric consultant)

Principal Investigators	Other Investigators
Schaffer, Leslie	Handlon, Joseph H.
Scher, Jordan M.	Hirsch, Stanley I. (psychiatric social worker)
Shapiro, Roger L.	Jordan, Nehemiah
Shurley, Jay T.	Kwiatkowska, Hanna Y. (art therapist)
Silber, Earle	Lewis, Thomas
Snyder, Frederick	Loveland, Nathene
Wadeson, Ralph	Maas, James
Weinstein, E.	Marvin, Sidney
Wynne, Lyman C.	Mason, John
	Murphey, Elizabeth
	Newman, Ruth
	Parloff, Morris B
	Pearlin, Leonard I.
	Perry, Stewart
	Rosenbaum, C. Peter
	Rosenberg, Morris
	Ryckoff, Irving (psychiatric consultant)
	Sacher, Edward
	Schaffer, Leslie
	Schwartz, Charlotte G.
	Searles, Harold (psychiatric consultant)
	Shakow, David
	Singer, Margaret Thaler (consultant)
	Smith, Jr., Henry Lee
	Solomon, Fredric
	Stephansky, Anne (research assistant)
	Sweet, Blanche S.
	Toohey, Margaret (research assistant)
	Trager, George
	Usdansky, George (psychologist)
	Waldman, Marvin
	Weigert, Edith
	Wilkie, Charlotte (psychiatric social worker)
	Wolff, Carl

Laboratory of Biophysics, NINDB

Principal Investigators

Adelman, Jr., W. J.
Binstock, L.
Chandler, W. K.
Chang, J. J.
Cole, Kenneth S.
Dalton, J. C.
FitzHugh, R.
Goldman, D. E. (NMRI)
Hodgkin, A. L. (Cambridge)
Julian, F. (NMRI)
Kishimoto, U.
Moore, J. W.
Mullins, L. J. (Purdue)
Sjodin, R. A. (Purdue)
Whitcomb, E. R.

Other Investigators

Antosiewicz, H. A. (NBS)
Castillo, José del
Franck, U. F.
Friess, S. L. (NMRI)
Taylor, R. E.

Laboratory of Cellular Pharmacology, NIMH

Principal Investigators

Ames, Bruce N.
Bridgers, William F.
Cantoni, Giulio L.
Durrell, Jack
Gabriel, O.
Gelboin, H. V.
Greengard, O.
Haba, Gabriel de la
Jamieson, Graham A.
Kaufman, Seymour
Klee, Werner A.
Levenberg, Bruce
Levin, Ephraim
Luborsky, S. W.
Mann, Jay D.
Mudd, S. Harvey
Pollock, M. R.
    (Institute of Medical Research, Mill Hill, England)
Yarmolinsky, Michael

Other Investigators

Barnhard, Sidney
Blanc, Claude
Butler, Robert N.
Clancy, C. W.
Gellert, Martin (Naval Medical Center)
Goodfriend, Theodore
Hertzenberg, Leonard
Kalckar, Barbara (NHI)
Mars, Robert de (NIAID)
Morrison, Raymond A.
Richards, H.
Singer, Maxine (NIAMD)
Sokoloff, Louis
Szilard, Leo (Rockefeller Institute)
Tompkins, Gordon (NIAMD)
Weiss, Peter

Child Research Branch, NIMH

Principal Investigators

Bell, Richard Q.
Black, Florence
Bloch, Donald A.
Boomer, Donald S. (trans. to Lab of Psychology)
Dittmann, Allen T.
Goodrich, D. Wells
Gordon, Gene (resigned 7/12/56)
Guest, H.
Iflund, Boris
Jacobson, S.
Kaplan, David (resigned 9/21/56)
Kitchener, H.
Longley, H. (resigned 9/28/56)
Maxwell, Jay
Newman, Ruth
Noshpitz, Joseph
Raush, Harold L.
Redl, Fritz
Siegel, Leonard
Silber, Earle (resigned 6/29/56)
Spielman, P.
Sweet, Blanche S.
Vernick, J.

Other Investigators

Bell, Richard Q.
Berman, S.
Blank, Paul
Burkhardt, Jane (resigned 7/20/56)
Campbell, John
Citrin, E.
Crawfort, S.
Ellis, B.
Faegre, Chris
Farber, Leslie H.
Flint, Arden A.
Glaser, J.
Greenberg, H.
Handlon, Joseph H.
Littman, Richard A. (visiting scientist)
Long, N.
Lourie, R.
Maeda, E.
Pearlin, Leonard I.
Perry, H.
Perry, Stewart
Ramana, C.
Rosenberg, Morris
Ryckoff, Irving M.
Sceery, Walter
Scher, Jordan
Taylor, Thaddeus
Waldman, Marvin

Clinical Neuropharmacology Research Center, NIMH

Principal Investigators

Byck, Robert
Cambosos, Nicholas
Carlson, Virgil
Chassan, J. B. (St. Elizabeths Hospital)
Cosmides, George
Feinberg, Irwin
Fotheringham, John B.
Geller, Max
Gentry, Robert
Grossman, Robert G. (WRAIR)
Gumnit, Robert J.
Hamilton, Max
Harwood, Theresa
Hearst, Elliot S.
Hordern, Anthony
Kellam, Sheppard G.
Koresko, Richard
Lipsett, Donald R.
Lofft, John G.
McDonald, Roger
Michael, Richard P.
Posner, Herbert S.
Salmoiraghi, Gian Carlo
Schwartz, Arthur S.
Smith, E. R. B.
Snyder, Frederick
Sodd, Mary Ann
Solomon, James D.
Stewart, Allan
Stopp, P. E.
Szara, Stephen
Taylor, Wilson L.
Waldrop, Francis N.
Weil-Malherbe, Hans
Weise, Virginia
Whalen, Richard E.

Other Investigators

Axelrod, Julius
Baumgarten, R. von
Benjamin, Mary E.
Bigelow, William
Bohrer, Charles
Bowles, Grace
Chace, Marion (St. Elizabeths Hospital)
Chassan, J. B. (St. Elizabeths Hospital)
Clyde, Dean
Epps, Viola H.
Fong, Ching
Greenberg, Harold
Handlon, Joseph H.
Hertting, Georg
Hrubeck, Zdenek
Kales, Arthur
Konchegul, Leon (St. Elizabeths Hospital)
Leacock, Yvonne
Libow, Leslie
Mann, Morris G., Jr.
Mathson, Henrietta (St. Elizabeths Hospital)
McCamey, Arliene
Peacock, Bonnie J.
Pearlin, Leonard
Perlin, Seymour
Putney, Frances K.
Rockland, Lawrence H.
Rosenthal, David
Seinato, Helen K. (St. Elizabeths Hospital)
Sidman, Murray (WRAIR)
Thaxton, Lewis
Tomchick, Robert
Torovsky, Alice

Laboratory of Clinical Science, NIMH
(formerly the Clinical Biochemistry Section, Clinical Physiology Section, and Psychosomatic Medicine Branch)

Principal Investigators

Ader, Robert
Axelrod, Julius
Bihari, Bernard
Bradley, Dan F.
Brady, Roscoe O.
Brown, Donald D.
Butler, Robert N.
Cardon, Jr., Philippe V.
Cobb, Reneal C.
Cochin, Joseph
Dastur, Darab K.
Davies, David R.
Dittmann, Allen T.
Durell, Jack
Evans, Franklin T.
Evarts, Edward V.
Falsenfeld, Gary
Feinberg, Irwin
Felsenfeld, Gary
Fleming, T. Corwin
Gjessing, L. R.
Goldstein, Norman P.
Hansen, Douglas B.
Haverback, Bernard J.
Hotta, Shoichi S.
Huttenlocher, Peter
Iflund, Boris
Kellam, Sheppard G.
Kendig, Isabelle
Kety, Seymour S.
Kies, Marian W.
Kopin, Irwin J.
Kornetsky, Conan
LaBrosse, Elwood H.
Lane, Mark H.
Lassen, Niels A.
Lee, A. Russell
McDonald, Roger K.
Müller, Peter S.
Pare, C. M. B.
Parloff, Morris B.

Other Investigators

Aberle, David F.
Agranoff, Bernard W.
Albers, R. W.
Alvord, Jr., Ellsworth C.
Birren, James E.
Blank, Paul
Blow, David M.
Bowman, Robert L.
Brounstein, Sybil
Burriss, William T.
Carlson, Virgil R.
Chassan, Jacob B.
Clementi, C.
Clink, Daniel W.
Cohen, Robert A.
Cox, Robert R.
Crick, F. H. C.
Daly, J. W.
Eddy, Nathan
Fishman, J.
Freygang, Jr., Walter H.
Geisser, Mary Lee
Goldin, Samson
Goodrich, D. Wells
Gordon, Robert S.
Gordon, Spencer
Greenhouse, Samuel
Guerney, Lillian M.
Hertting, Georg
Horning, Evan
Horowitz, D.
Humphries, Ogretta
Inscoe, Joseph K.
Isselbacker, Kurt (NIAMD)
Johnson, Jean
Kalckar, H. M. (NIAMD)
Kammen, Edith
Kaufman, Seymour
Kessler, Edith K.
Kurland, Albert A.
Laatsch, Robert

Principal Investigators

Patrick, Raymond W.
Perlin, Seymour
Pollin, William
Posternak, Jean
Rich, Alexander
Rockland, Lawrence H.
Rosenthal, David
Schweig, Noel
Shakow, David
Snyder, Frederick
Sokoloff, Louis
Szara, Stephen
Vates, Thomas
Weise, Virginia K.

Other Investigators

Ladusky, Walter
Landau, William
Laroche, M-J.
MacLean, Paul D.
Mann, Jay D.
Marshall, Wade H.
Mercer, M.
Miller, Alice
Mirsky, Allan F.
Mishkin, Mortimer
Moore, Harvey C.
Morgenbesser, S.
Morrison, Donald
Murphy, Joseph B.
Orgel, Leslie
Paterson, P. Y.
Peacock, Bonnie
Petit, John M.
Putney, F.
Roboz, Elizabeth
Schaefer, Earl S.
Schaffer, Leslie
Scher, Jordan
Schmidt, Rudi
Schooler, Carmi
Silverman, Milton
Sjoerdsma, Albert
Solomon, Fredric
Taylor, W.
Tomchick, Robert
Tomkins, Gordon
Treadwell, Carleton
Wagner, Jr., Henry N.
Weil-Malherbe, Hans
Weiss, William P.
Weissbach, Herbert
Werner, Martha M.
Whitby, G. L.
Wilkie, Charlotte
Witkop, Bernhard
Wynne, Lyman C.
Wynne, Ronald

Electroencephalography Branch, NINDB

Principal Investigators

Abraham, Kristof
Ajmone-Marsan, Cosimo
Castillo, José del
Chatfield, Paul O.
Doudoumopolous, Alexander
Enomoto, Takayuki Francis
Gerin, Paul
Henry, Charles
Long, R. Gordon
Mirsky, Allan F.
Morillo, Arturo
Obrist, W. D.
Ralston, Bruce L.
Strang, Raymond
Tower, Donald B.
Tradhan, S.
Van Buren, John M.
Widen, Lennart

Other Investigators

Baldwin, Maitland
Birren, James E.
Dekaban, Anatole S.
Lewis, William
Mateos, José H.
Millichap, G.
Moore, J. W.
Primac, D. W.
Richards, Nelson G.
Stevens, J. R.
Wells, Charles E.

Medical Neurology Branch, NINDB

Principal Investigators

Altrocchi, Paul H.
Baldwin, Maitland
Berg, Leonard
Bradley, Robert
Caughey, John Egerton
Chatfield, Paul O.
Cummings, Donald J.
Curtis, William C.
Dekaban, Anatole S.
DiChiro, Giovanni
Dingman, Wesley
Drager, Glenn A.
Engel, Andrew G.
Engel, W. King
Eyerman, Edward L.
Fatt, Paul
Haase, Guenther R.
Horvath, Beni
Irwin, Richard L.

Other Investigators

Ajmone-Marsan, Cosimo
Alvord, Jr., Ellsworth C.
Bale, William (Rochester University)
Castillo, José del
Cohen, Maynard (University of Minnesota)
Drachman, Daniel
Drews, Genevieve A.
Garry, Barbara
Gasteiger, Edgar L. (Harvard Medical School)
Greenfield, J. Godwin
Hamp, Edward
Henriksson, K. G.
Huebner, Robert
Jaffe, Israeli
Kalckar, Herman (NCI)
Kenerson, Lamar
Klatzo, Igor
Li, Choh-luh
Lord, John T.

Principal Investigators

Jaffe, Israeli
Korengold, Marvin C.
Krooth, Robert
Kurland, Leonard T.
Lane, Mark
Li, Choh-luh
Magee, Kenneth R.
Matthews, William
McKhann, Guy
Meiller, Fred H.
Morel, Joseph
Norris, Jr., Forbes H. (visiting scientist)
Peters, Edmund L.
Prockop, Darwin
Rowley, Peter T.
Rubin, Martin
Shepherd, James A. (PHS)
Shy, G. Milton
Smith, Bushnell
Sokoloff, Louis
Sporn, Michael
Tower, Donald B.
Wanko, Theodor
Wells, Charles E.
Wherrett, John L. (visiting scientist)

Other Investigators

Marshall, Wade H.
McIlwain, Henry (consultant)
Miquel, J.
Mumenthaler, Marco
Norris, Ted
Payne, Charles
Phoenix, John
Pogorelskin, Milton A.
Proctor, Joseph
Resnik, Robert
Rowland, Lewis P.
Sabin, A.
Silberberg, Donald
Smith, III, Henry J.
Spar, Irving (Rochester University)
Trams, Eberhard G.
Van Buren, John M.
Wells, Jay B.
Windle, William F.

Laboratory of Neuroanatomical Sciences, NINDB

Principal Investigators

Albers, R. Wayne
Altmann, Stuart A.
Bailey, Clark J.
Bernstein, Jerald J.
Boord, Robert L.
Brightman, Milton W.
Cammermeyer, Jan H. W.
Campbell, J. B. (consultant)
Combs, C. M.
Dawes, Geoffrey S. (consultant)
Dennery, J. M.
Dorrill, Elizabeth
Feder, Ned (NIAID)
Feringa, Earl R.
Frontera, José G.
Gacek, Richard R.
Guth, Lloyd
Hack, M. H.
Jacobson, Howard N.
Joralemon, Jane
Koford, C. B.
Maiale, Irene
Malm, Mignon
Massopust, Jr., Leo C.
Morest, Donald Kent
Palay, Sanford L.
Ramirez de Arellano, Marisa I.
Ramsey, Helen
Ranck, J. B.
Rasmussen, Grant L.
Saxon, Sue V.
Sidman, Richard L.
Smart, John O.
Vollman, R. F.
Wilcox, Harry H. (by contract)
Windle, William F.
Wolf, M. Kenneth

Other Investigators

Ashburner, Roberta
Bairati, Angelo
Bassett, A. (consultant)
Brady, Roscoe O.
Chandler, K.
Comerford, John
Crigler, Catherine
Curran, Doris
Dohlman, Gosta
Embree, Larry
Frank, Karl
Gavan, J.
Glees, Paul
Gordon, Spencer
Johnston, J. G.
Koval, G.
Lloyd, John G.
Long, Samuel E.
Manuelidis, E. E.
McCrane, Edna P.
McCrosky, D. L.
McGee-Russell, S. M.
McKhann, G.
Miale, Irene
Mott, Joan C.
Pelegrina Sariego, Ivan
Pfeiffer, Carroll A.
Ramirez de Arellano, Max
Rosenbluth, Jack
Salvador, Richard
Shelley-Houton, Heather
Shy, G. Milton
Sordyl, Frank
Soutter, Lamar (Boston University)
Stiehl, W.
Thuline, C.
Tobias, Cornelius A.
Van Wagenen, Gertrude
Walther, Jost B.
Ziemnowicz, Stanislaw

Laboratory of Neurochemistry, NIMH-NINDB

NIMH

Principal Investigators

Allen, Gordon
Bernhard, Sidney A.
Botwinick, Jack
Bradley, Dan F.
Dastur, Darab K.
Davies, David R.
Duda, William L.
Dunitz, Jack D.
Eichhorn, G. L.
Felsenfeld, Gary
Gewirtz, Jacob L.
Glauser, Stanley C.
Kety, Seymour S.
Kornetsky, Conan
Rich, Alexander
Sokoloff, Louis
Weise, Virginia K.
Weiss, Alfred D.
Wolf, M. Kenneth
Youmans, E. Grant

Other Investigators

Berger, Arieh
Birren, James E.
Blum, J. J.
Chen, John
Clark, Carl
Crick, Francis H. C.
Elden, Harry
Freygang, Jr., Walter H.
George, Philip
Hansen, Douglas
Johnson, Jean M.
Katchalski, Sphraim
Kaufman, Seymour
Kendrew, J. C.
Landau, William M.
Lane, B. Mark
Lewis, Benjamin M.
Livingston, Robert
Miles, H. Todd
Perlin, Seymour
Rowland, Lewis P.
Stone, Audrey L.
Taylor, John
Tower, Donald B.
Viswanatha, T.
Watson, J.
Wells, Charles

NINDB

Agranoff, Bernard W.
Brady, Roscoe O.
Burton, Robert M.
Cole, Kenneth S.
Gernandt, Bo E.
Hecht, Eugen
Iranyi, Magdolna A.
Livingston, Robert B.
Moore, J. W.
Trams, Eberhard G.

Antosiewicz, H. A. (NBS)
Axelrod, Julius
Freygang, Jr., Walter H.
Friess, S. L. (NMRI)
Gilman, Sid
Goldin, Abraham
Hendricks, S. B.
Miller, Donald L.
Robinson, Joseph D.
Salvador, Richard (visiting scientist)
Siegelman, H. W.
Spyropoulos, Constantin S.
Stadtman, Earl R.
Tasaki, Ichiji

Laboratory of Neurophysiology, NIMH-NINDB

NIMH

Principal Investigators

Adrian, R. H.
Bak, Anthony
Brinley, Jr., F. Joseph
Coggeshall, Richard E.
Evarts, Edward V.
Fleming, T. Corwin
Freygang, Jr., Walter H.
Gernandt, Bo E.
Gorgan, John
Hansen, D.
Huttenlocher, Peter
Kandel, Eric R.
Kety, Seymour S.
Landau, William M.
Leao, A.
Lilly, John C.
MacLean, Paul D.
Marshall, Wade H.
Ploog, Detlev W.
Posternak, Jean
Renkin, B. Z.
Robinson, Bryan W.
Spencer, William Alden
Spyropoulos, Constantin S.
Strumwasser, Felix
Tasaki, Ichiji

Other Investigators

Bacon, M.
Carmichael, Martha
Cobb, Caroline
Cox, Robert R.
Ferreira, Martins
Frank, K.
Gaither, D.
Galkin, Thelma W.
Gergen, John
Gilman, Sid
Highes, John R.
Iranyi, Magdolna
Johnson, M.
Lerner, S.
Livingston, Robert B.
Magoun, H. W.
Miller, Alice M.
Peacock, Bonnie
Peek, Bobby C.
Ploog, Frauke
Rosenthal, S.
Schulman, Arnold
Sokoloff, Louis

NINDB

Principal Investigators	Other Investigators
Agranoff, B. W.	Bak, Anthony
Arvanitaki-Chalazonitis, A.	Becker, Mary
Brady, Roscoe O.	Bennett, M.
Chalazonitis, N.	Eagle, H.
Chang, J. J.	Ezzy, M. E.
Erulkar, S. D.	Gilman, Sid
Franck, U.	Hayward, G.
Frank, Karl	Hild, W.
Freygang, Jr., Walter H.	Iranyi, Magdolna
Fuortes, Michelangelo	Lane, M. D.
Gernandt, Bo E.	Livingston, Robert B.
Hagiwara, S.	Naka, K. (visiting Fellow)
Morrell, R.	Nims, L.
Nelson, Philip G.	Rall, W.
Oikawa, T. (visiting scientist)	Rioch, David McKenzie
Paton, W.	Sands, R.
Spyropoulos, Constantin S.	Siegelman, W.
Tasaki, Ichiji	Sprague, James M.
Tasaki, L. N.	Wolfe, M.
Teorelk, T.	
Terzuolo, C.	
Trams, Eberhard G.	

Ophthalmology Branch, NINDB

Principal Investigators

Alphen, Gerard van
Aronson, Samuel
Bell, Joseph A.
Bonting, Sjoerd L.
Bornschein, Hans
Caravaggio, Leo
Cohan, Bruce E.
Copenhaver, Richard M.
Curtis, Howard J.
Dodt, Eberhard
Fuortes, Michelangelo
Goodman, George
Gouras, Peter
Greenfield, J. Godwin
Grimes, Patricia
Gunkel, Ralph D.
Hart, William M.
Holland, Monte G.
Huckel, Hubert
Huebner, Robert J.
Iser, Gilbert
Jacobs, Leon (NMI)
Jones, III, Ottiwell W.
Kaufman, Herbert E.
Kuhlman, Robert E.
Lele, P. P.
Macri, Frank J.
O'Connor, G. Richard
Oglesby, Richard B.
Okun, Edward
O'Rourke, James F.
Parrott, Robert H.
Paton, David
Reid, Mary E.
Resnik, Robert A.
Rushton, W. A. H.
Ryan, Ralph W.
Sallmann, Ludwig von
Scullica, Luigi
Simon, Kenneth A.
Tanaka, Chie
Tansley, Katharine
Thomas, Louis B.
Wanko, Theodor
Wolf, M. Kenneth

Other Investigators

Black, Roger L.
Bradley, Robert
Bunim, Joseph J.
Caldwell, Lee A.
Collins, Eleanor
Culligan, John J.
Gavin, Mary Ann
Irwin, Richard
Kenton, Edith
Kolacskovszky, Edith
Papaconstantinou, John
Patton, Humphrey
Remington, Jack
Roberts, Nancy L. (orthoptic technician)
Robinette, Sarah
Sperling, Frederick W. (NIAMD)
Suggs, Frank G.
Tasaki, Kyoji
Trams, Eberhard G.
Weaver, Kirk
Wolff, Ann R.
Wyngaarden, James B. (NHI)

Laboratory of Psychology, NIMH

Principal Investigators	Other Investigators
Alexander, Franz	Aberle, David F.
Allen, Gordon	Adland, Marvin
Bayley, Nancy	Axelrod, Julius
Bell, Richard Q.	Barbehenn, Kyle R.
Bergman, Paul	Baroff, George S.
Berlyne, Daniel E.	Battig, Karl
Birren, James E.	Brown, Thomas
Blough, Donald S.	Brush, Elinor
Bondareff, William	Brutkowski, Stefan
Boomer, Donald S.	Butler, Robert
Botwinick, Jack	Butter, Charles M.
Calhoun, John B.	Cholden, Louis
Campbell, John	Cromwell, Rue L. (visiting scientist)
Cardon, Jr., Philippe V.	Day, Juliana
Carlson, Virgil R.	Deasy, Leila C.
Caron, Albert J.	Eichorn, Dorothy H. (University of California, Berkeley)
Clausen, John A.	Elkes, Charmian
Cohen, Robert A.	Evarts, Edward V.
Dittmann, Allen T.	Feinberg, Irwin
Evarts, Edward V.	Fishman, Jacob
Fiedler, Miriam	Goldberg, Ivan
Garbus, Joel	Goldstein, Norman
Gewirtz, Jacob L.	Gordon, Gilbert S.
Goffman, Erving	Gordon, R.
Goodrich, D. Wells	Greenberg, Harold A.
Handlon, Joseph H.	Hess, Eckhard H. (University of Chicago)
Hertz, Roy	Hirsch, Stanley I.
Iflund, Boris	Hoffman, Jay
Jerome, Edward A.	Honzik, Marjorie P.
Jordan, Nehemiah	Huebner, Robert J.
Kallmann, Franz J.	Jenkins, William C.
Kelman, Herbert C.	Jones, William
Kendig, Isabelle V.	Kay, Harry
Kety, Seymour S.	Kincannon, James
Kohn, Melvin L.	Kline, John
Kopin, Irwin J.	Kuypers, Henricus G. (consultant)
Kornetsky, Conan	Kwiatkowska, Hanna (art therapist)
La Brosse, Elwood H.	Lawlor, William G. (special consultant)
Mirsky, Allan F.	Lisser, Hans (University of California Medical School, San Francisco CA)
Mishkin, Mortimer	
Parloff, Morris B.	Lodge, Ann
Pearlin, Leonard	Mann, Jay D.
Perlin, Seymour	Marshall, Wade H.
Quinn, Olive Westbrooke	Moore, Harvey C.

Principal Investigators

Rheingold, Harriet L.
Robinson, Bryan W.
Rosenberg, Morris
Rosenthal, David
Rosvold, Haldor E.
Schaefer, Earl S.
Schwartz, Charlotte Green
Shakow, David
Stein, Morris
Streicher, Eugene
Szwarcbart, Maria K.
Turk, Herman
Van Buren, John M.
Waldman, Marvin
Warren, Richard M.
Weiss, Alfred D.
Will, Gwen Tudor
Wynne, Lyman
Yarrow, Marian Radke
Zahn, Theodore P.

Other Investigators

Müller, P.S.
Murphy, Harriet S.
Pollin, William
Rapaport, David
Redl, Fritz
Riegel, Klaus
Riegel, Ruth
Rosenbaum, Peter
Sank, Diane
Schaffer, Leslie
Skinner, William D.
Snyder, Frederick
Sokoloff, Louis
Steinberg, Daniel
Straight, Belinda (guest investigator)
Sweet, Blanche S.
Tassone, Eugene
Taylor, Thaddeus
Theban, John
Unger, Sanford
Waskow, Irene
Wilkie, Charlotte
Wilson, Robert
Yarrow, Leon
Youmans, E. Grant

Laboratory of Socio-Environmental Studies, NIMH

Principal Investigators	Other Investigators
Allen, Gordon	Auster, Simon
Boggs, Stephen T.	Baroff, George S.
Burton, Roger V.	Blank, Paul
Butler, Robert N.	Carroll, Eleanor
Campbell, John D.	Cholden, Louis S.
Caudill, William	Coelho, George
Clausen, John A.	Flint, Arden A.
Deasy, Leila Calhoun	Golden, Samson
Diamond, Stanley	Greenberg, Irwin
Ember, Melvin	Handlon, Joseph H.
Gillette, Thomas	Hawkins, Doris E.
Goffmann, Erving	Hoffman, Jay
Goodrich, D. Wells	Kendig, Isabelle V.
Hamburg, David A.	Landusky, Walter
Hertz, Roy	Lawlor, William G. (visiting scientist)
Jordan, Nehemiah	Lee, A. Russell
Kellmann, Franz J.	Mason, John
Kohn, Melvin L.	Murphey, Elizabeth
Lefcowitz, Myron J.	Murphy, Harriet S.
Linn, Erwin L.	Parloff, Morris B.
Lochen, Yngvar	Rockland, Lawrence
Pearlin, Leonard I.	Ross, Lucille
Perlin, Seymour	Sank, Diane
Pollin, William	Sceery, Walter
Quinn, Olive Westbrooke	Schachter, Joseph
Raush, Harold L.	Schweig, Noel
Rosenberg, Morris	Shakow, David
Schaffer, Leslie	Snyder, Frederick
Schooler, Carmi	Sweet, Blanche S.
Schwartz, Charlotte G.	Theban, John
Silber, Earle	Wadeson, Ralph
Turk, Herman	Whiting, John W. M.
Van Buren, John M.	Wynne, Lyman C.
Wallin, Paul	Yarrow, Leon
Will, Gwen Tudor	
Yarrow, Marian Radke	
Youmans, E. Grant	

Surgical Neurology Branch, NINDB

Principal Investigators

Ajmone-Marsan, Cosimo
Alvord, Jr., Ellsworth C.
Baird, Robert L.
Baldwin, Maitland
Bender, Michael (Oak Ridge Laboratory)
Blevins, Mildred L.
Chou, Shelley N.
Crowe, Joan
Dekaban, Anatole S.
Engel, W. K.
Frost, Laurence L.
Galindo, Anibal
Greenfield, J. G.
Hall, Kenneth D.
Klatzo, Igor
Landsdell, Herbert
Laskowski, Edward J.
Li, Choh-luh
Lord, John T.
Miquel, Jaime
Norris, Jr., Forbes H.
Obrist, Walter D.
Ortiz-Galvan, Armando
  (Mexico General Hospital)
Pritchard, William Lee
Ralston, Bruce L.
Seitelberger, Franz
Shy, G. Milton
Van Buren, John M.
Wells, Charles E.

Other Investigators

Adamkiewicz, Joseph
Bach, Sven A.
Barbee, Peggy
Birren, James E.
Brace, Kirkland
Bucknam, Charles A.
Caldwell, J.
Chatfield, Paul O.
Cone, T. E. (Naval Medical Center)
Cornman, T.
Edgar, Robert
Emmart, Emily
Farrier, R.
Ferris, P.
Frei, Emil
Gajdusek, D. Carleton
Garry, B. J.
Geisler, Philip H.
Geppert, L. J. (Walter Reed Army Hospital)
Gills, J.
Goldstein, Norman
Gordon, Spencer
Gouras, Peter
Haymaker, Webb
Hertz, R.
Hill, H. H. (Naval Medical Center)
Horvath, Beni
Johnston, George
Jones, S.
Kendall, Marie
Lanauze, Harold
Lewis, Shirley
Lilly, John C.
MacCubbin, D.
Mannarino, M.
Mateos, J. H.
McIlwain, Henry

Other Investigators

Merzig, John
Miller, Joseph
Millichap, J. Gordon
Mills, N.
Mirsky, Allan F.
Morrell, Roger M.
Mullins, Charles
Olhoeft, Joyce
Otenasek, Richard
Pearlman, William
Piraux, A.
Riva, H. L. (Walter Reed Army Hospital)
Roring, Martha
Rowe, A.
Rubin, Philip
Ryan, Ralph
Savard, Robert
Smith, Carolyn May
Smith, F.
Tobias, C.
Tower, Donald B.
Urbach, N.
Weissbach, J.
Whitlock, David G.
Wood, Charles D.
Zigas, V.

Appendix C
NIMH and NINDB Laboratory and Branch Selected Landmark Papers

Adult Psychiatry Branch, NIMH

Bunney, Jr., William, and David Hamburg. "Methods for Reliable Longitudinal Observation of Behavior: Development of a Method for Systematic Observation of Emotional Behavior on Psychiatric Wards." *Archives of General Psychiatry* 9 (1963): 280-94.

Coelho, George, David Hamburg, and Elizabeth Murphey. "Coping Strategies in a New Learning Environment: A Study of American College Freshmen." *Archives of General Psychiatry* 9 (1963): 433-43.

Fishman, Jacob, David Hamburg, Joseph Handlon, John Mason, and Edward Sachar. "Emotional and Adrenal Cortical Responses to a New Experience: Effect of Social Environment." *Archives of General Psychiatry* 6 (1962): 271-8.

Friedman, Stanford, P. Chodoff, John Mason, and David Hamburg. "Behavior Observations on Parents Anticipating the Death of a Child." *Pediatrics* 32 (1963): 610-25.

Friedman, Stanford, John Mason, and David Hamburg. "Urinary 17-hydroxycorticosteroid Levels in Parents of Children With Neuroplastic Disease." *Psychosomatic Medicine* 25 (1963): 364-76.

Hamburg, David, chairman. "Some Observations on Controls in Psychiatric Research." *Report no. 42.* New York: Group for the Advancement of Psychiatry, 1959.

Hamburg, David. "Recent Trends in Psychiatric Research Training. *Archives of General Psychiatry* 4 (1961): 215-24.

Hamburg, David. "The Relevance of Recent Evolutionary Changes to Human Stress Biology." In *Social Life of Early Man*, edited by S. Washburn, 278-88. Chicago: Aldine Publishing, 1962.

Hamburg, David. "Plasma and Urinary Corticosteroid Levels in Naturally Occurring Psychological Stresses." In *Ultrastructure and Metabolism of the Nervous System*, edited by S. Korey, Association for Research in Nervous and Mental Disease, vol. 40, 406-13. Baltimore: Williams and Wilkins, 1962.

Hamburg, David. "Emotions in the Perspective of Human Evolution." In *Expression of the Emotions in Man*, edited by P. Knapp, 300-17. New York: International University Press, 1963.

Handlon, Joseph, Ralph Wadeson, Jacob Fishman, Edward Sachar, David Hamburg, and John Mason. "Psychological Factors Lowering Plasma 17-hydroxycorticosteroid Concentration." *Psychosomatic Medicine* 26 (1962): 535-42.

Silber, Earle, David Hamburg, George Coelho, Elizabeth Murphey, Morris Rosenberg, and Leonard Pearlin. "Adaptive Behavior in Competent Adolescents: Coping With the Anticipation of College. *Archives of General Psychiatry* 5 (1961): 354-65.

Wadeson, Ralph, John Mason, David Hamburg, and Joseph Handlon. "Plasma and Urinary 17-OHCS Responses to Motion Pictures." *Archives of General Psychiatry* 9 (1963): 146-56.

Laboratory of Cellular Pharmacology, NIMH

Kaufman, Seymour. "A New Cofactor Required for the Enzymatic Conversion of Phenylalanine to Tyrosine." *Journal of Biological Chemistry* 230 (1958): 931-9.

Kaufman, Seymour. "Phenylalanine Hydroxylation Cofactor in Phenylketonuria." *Science* 128 (1958): 1506.

Kaufman, Seymour, and B. Levenberg. "Further Studies on the Phenylalanine Hydroxylation Cofactor." *Journal of Biological Chemistry* 234 (1959): 2683-8.

Levin, E., B. Levenberg, and Seymour Kaufman. "The Enzymatic Conversion of 3,4-dihydroxyphenylethylamine to Norepinephrine." *Journal of Biological Chemistry* 235 (1960): 2080-6.

Sokoloff, Louis, and Seymour Kaufman. "Effects of Thyroxin on Amino Acid Incorporation Into Protein." *Science* 129 (1959): 569.

Child Research Branch, NIMH

Bloch, Donald A., Earle Silber, and Stewart E. Perry. "Some Factors in the Emotional Reaction of Children to Disaster." *American Journal of Psychiatry* 113 (1956): 416-22.

Goodrich, D. Wells, and Donald S. Boomer. "Some Concepts About Therapeutic Interventions With Hyper-Aggressive Children." *Social Casework* 39 (1958): 207-13.

Goodrich, D. Wells, and Donald S. Boomer. "Some Concepts About Therapeutic Interventions With Hyper-Aggressive Children. Part II." *Social Casework* 39 (1958): 286-92.

Raush, Harold L. "Interaction Sequences." *Journal of Personality and Social Psychology* 2, no. 4 (1965): 487-99.

Raush, Harold L., Allen T. Dittmann, and Thaddeus J. Taylor. "The Interpersonal Behavior of Children in Residential Treatment." *Journal of Abnormal and Social Psychology* 58 (1959): 9-26.

Raush, Harold L., Allen T. Dittmann, and Thaddeus J. Taylor. "Person, Setting, and Change in Social Interaction." *Human Relations* 12 (1959): 361-78.

Raush, Harold L., Irwin Farbman, and Lynn G. Llewellyn. "Person, Setting, and Change in Social Interaction: II. A Normal Control Study." *Human Relations* 13 (1960): 305-32.

Raush, Harold L., and Blanche Sweet. "The Preadolescent Ego: Some Observations of Normal Children." *Journal for the Study of Interpersonal Processes* 24, no. 2 (1961): 122-32.

Redl, Fritz. "What is Normal for Children." *National Conference of Social Work, Casework Papers, 1954*, 99-109. Oxford, England: Family Service Association of America, 1956.

Redl, Fritz. "The Concept of a "Therapeutic Milieu." *American Journal of Orthopsychiatry* 29 (1959): 721-36.

Redl, Fritz. "The Life Space Interview: Workshop, 1957. I. Strategy and Techniques of the Life Space Interview." *American Journal of Orthopsychiatry* 29 (1959): 1-18.

Silber, Earle, Stewart E. Perry, and Donald A. Bloch. "Patterns of Parent-Child Interaction in a Disaster." *Psychiatry: Journal for the Study of Interpersonal Processes* 21 (1958): 159-67.

Clinical Neuropharmacology Research Center, NIMH

Axelrod, Julius, Hans Weil-Malherbe, and R. Tomchik. "The Physiological Dispositions of H(3) Epinephrine and Its Metabolite Metanephrine." *Journal of Pharmacology and Experimental Therapeutics* 127 (1959): 251-56.

Freyhan, Fritz, and J. A. Mayo. "Concept of a Model Psychiatric Clinic." *American Journal of Psychiatry* 120 (1963): 222-7.

Hordern, A., M. Hamilton, F. N. Waldrop, and J. C. Lofft. "A Controlled Trial on the Value of Prochlorperazine and Trifluoperazine and Intensive Group Treatment." *British Journal of Psychiatry* 109 (1963): 510-22.

Kellam, Sheppard G. "A Method for Assessing Social Contacts: Its Application During a Rehabilitation Program on a Psychiatric Ward." *Journal of Nervous and Mental Diseases* 132 (1961): 277-88.

Lipsitt, Donald R. "Dependency, Depression, and Hospitalization: Towards an Understanding of a Conspiracy." *Psychiatric Quarterly* 30 (1962): 537-54.

Michael, Richard P. "An Investigation of the Sensitivity of Circumscribed Neurological Areas to Hormonal Stimulation by Means of the Application of Oestrogens Directly to the Brain of the Cat." In *Regional Neurochemistry: The Regional Chemistry, Physiology, and Pharmacology of the Nervous System*, edited by Seymour S. Kety and Joel Elkes, 465-80. Oxford: Pergamon Press, 1961.

Salmoiraghi, Gian Carlo. "Pharmacology of Respiratory Neurons." In *Proceedings of the First International Pharmacology Meetings*, 217-29. Oxford: Pergamon Press, 1962.

Salmoiraghi, Gian Carlo, and Floyd E. Bloom. "Pharmacology of Individual Neurons." *Science* 144 (1964): 493.

Szara, Stephen, and Eliot Hearst. "The 6-hydroxylation of Tryptamine Derivatives: A Way of Producing Psychoactive Metabolites," *Annals of the New York Academy of Sciences* 96 (1962): 134-41.

Szara, Stephen, Eliot Hearst, and F. Putney. "Metabolism and Behavioral Action of Psychotropic Tryptamine Homologues." *International Journal of Neuropharmacology* 1 (1962): 111-7.

Weil-Malherbe, Hans, and E. R. B. Smith. "Metabolites of Catecholamines in Urine and Tissues." *Journal of Neuropsychiatry* (1962): 113-8.

Weiner, Harold. "Some Effects of Response Cost Upon Human Operant Behavior." *Journal of the Experimental Analysis of Behavior* 5 (1962): 201-8.

Laboratory of Clinical Science, NIMH

Axelrod, Julius, J. K. Inscoe, S. Senoh, and B. Witkop. "O-Methylation, the Principal Pathway for the Metabolism of Epinephrine and Norepinephrine in the Rat." *Science* 127 (1958): 754-5.

Axelrod, Julius, S. Senoh, and B. Witkop. "O-Methylation of Catecholamines *In Vivo*." *Journal of Biological Chemistry* 233 (1958): 697-701.

Axelrod, Julius, Irwin J. Kopin, and J. D. Mann. "3-Methoxy-4hydroxyphenyl Glycol, a New Metabolite of Epinephrine and Norepinephrine." *Biochimica et Biophysica Acta* 36 (1959): 576-7.

Hertting, Georg, Julius Axelrod, Irwin J. Kopin, and L. G. Whitby. "Lack of Uptake of Catecholamines After Chronic Denervation of Sympathetic Nerves." *Nature* 189 (1961): 66.

Kety, Seymour S. "A Biologist Examines the Mind and Behavior." *Science* 132, no. 3443 (23 December 1960): 1861-70.

Kopin, Irwin J., and Julius Axelrod. "Dihydroxyphenylglycol, a Metabolite of Epinephrine." *Archives of Biochemistry and Biophysics* 40 (1960): 377-8.

Sokoloff, Louis. "Local Cerebral Circulation at Rest and During Altered Cerebral Activity Induced by Anesthesia or Visual Stimulation." In *The Regional Chemistry, Physiology, and Pharmacology of the Nervous System*, edited by Seymour S. Kety and Joel Elkes, 107-17. Oxford: Pergamon Press, 1961.

Sokoloff, Louis, and Seymour Kaufman. "Thyroxine stimulation of Amino Acid Incorporation Into Protein." *Journal of Biological Chemistry* 236 (1961): 795-803.

Electroencephalography Branch, NINDB

Abraham, Kristof, and Cosimo Ajmone-Marsan. "Patterns of Cortical Discharges and Their Relation to Routine Scalp Electroencephalography." *Electroencephalography and Clinical Neurophysiology* 10 (1958): 447-61.

Ajmone-Marsan, Cosimo, and Bruce L. Ralston. *The Epileptic Seizure: Its Functional Morphology and Diagnostic Significance.* Springfield, Ill: Charles C. Thomas, 1957.

Ajmone-Marsan, Cosimo, and John Van Buren. "Epileptiform Activity in Cortical and Subcortical Structures in the Temporal Lobe of Man." In *Temporal Lobe Epilepsy, A Colloquium.* Springfield, Ill: Charles C. Thomas, 1958.

Ajmone-Marsan, Cosimo, and Kristof Abraham. "A Seizure Atlas." *Electroencephalography and Clinical Neurophysiology* Suppl. no. 15 (1960): 215.

Enamoto, T. Francis, and Cosimo Ajmone-Marsan. "Epileptic Activity of Single Cortical Neurons and Their Relationship With Electroencephalographic Discharges." *Electroencephalography and Clinical Neurophysiology* 11 (1959): 199-218.

Jasper, Herbert H., and Cosimo Ajmone-Marsan. *A Stereotaxic Atlas of the Diencephalon of the Cat.* Ottawa: National Research Council of Canada, 1954.

Matsumoto, Hideo, and Cosimo Ajmone-Marsan. "Cortical Cellular Phenomena in Experimental Epilepsy: Interictal Manifestations." *Experimental Neurology* 9 (1964): 286-304.

Matsumoto, Hideo, and Cosimo Ajmone-Marsan, "Cortical Cellular Phenomena in Experimental Epilepsy: Ictal Manifestations." *Experimental Neurology* 9 (1964): 305-26.

Pollen, Daniel and Cosimo Ajmone-Marsan. "Cortical Inhibitory Post-Synaptic Potentials and Strychninization." *Journal of Neurophysiology* 28 (1965): 342-58.

Laboratory of Neuroanatomical Sciences, NINDB

Angevine, Jr., J. B., and Richard L. Sidman. "Autoradiographic Study of Cell Migration During Histogenesis of Cerebral Cortex in the Mouse." *Nature* 192 (1961): 766-8.

Clemente, C. D. and William F. Windle. "Regeneration of Severed Nerve Fibers in the Spinal Cord of the Adult Cat." *Journal of Comparative Neurology* 101 (154): 691-731.

Guth, Lloyd. "Regeneration in the Mammalian Peripheral Nervous System." *Physiological Reviews* 36 (1956): 441-78.

Miale, I. L., and Richard L. Sidman. "An Autoradiographic Analysis of Histogenesis in the Mouse Cerebellum." *Experimental Neurology* 4 (1961): 277-96.

Palay, Sanford L. "Synapses in the Central Nervous System." *Journal of Biophysical and Biochemical Cytology* 2 (1956): 193-201.

Palay, Sanford L. "The Morphology of Synapses in the Central Nervous System." *Experimental Cell Research* 5, Suppl. (1958): 275-93.

Palay, Sanford L. "An Electron Microscopic Study of Neuroglia." In *Biology of Neuroglia*, edited by William F. Windle, 24-38. Springfield: Charles C. Thomas, 1958.

Palay, Sanford L., S. M. McGee-Russell, S. Gordon, and M. A. Grillo. "Fixation of Neural Tissues for Electron Microscopy by Perfusion with Solutions of Osmium Tetroxide." *Journal of Cell Biology* 12 (1962): 385-410.

Sidman, Richard. "Histogenesis of Mouse Retina Studied with Thymidine-H³." In *The Structure of the Eye*, edited by G. K. Smelser, 487-506. New York: Academic Press, 1961.

Sidman, Richard, I. L. Miale, and N. Feder. "Cell Proliferation and Migration in the Primitive Ependymal Zone: An Autoradiographic Study of Histogenesis in the Nervous System." *Experimental Neurology* 1 (1959): 322-33.

Windle, William F., ed. *Regeneration in the Central Nervous System.* Springfield, Illinois: Charles C. Thomas, 1955.

Windle, William F. "Regeneration of Axons in the Vertebrate Central Nervous System." *Physiological Reviews* 36 (1956): 427-40.

Laboratory of Neurochemistry, NIMH-NINDB

Brady, Roscoe O., J. Kanfer, and D. Shapiro. "The Metabolism of Glucocerebrosides. I. Purification and Properties of a Glucocerebroside-Cleaving Enzyme From Spleen Tissue." *Journal of Biological Chemistry* 240 (1965): 39-42.

Felsenfeld, Gary, David R. Davies, and Alexander Rich. "Formation of a Three-stranded Polynucleotide Molecule." *Journal of the American Chemical Society* 79 (1957): 2023-4.

Gernandt, Bo E., and Sid Gilman. "Vestibular and Propriospinal Interactions and Protracted Spinal Inhibition by Brain Stem Activation." *Journal of Neurophysiology* 23 (1960): 269-87.

Gernandt, Bo E., and Sid Gilman. "Interactions of Vestibular, Pyramidal, and Cortically Evoked Extrapyramidal Activities." *Journal of Neurophysiology* 23 (1960): 516-33.

Landau, William M., Walter H. Freygang, Jr., Lewis P. Rowland, Louis Sokoloff, and Seymour S. Kety. "The Local Circulation of the Living Brain; Values in the Unanesthetized and Anesthetized Cat." *Transactions of the American Neurological Association* 80 (1955): 125-9.

Trams, Eberhard G., and Roscoe O. Brady. "Cerebroside Synthesis in Gaucher's Disease." *Journal of Clinical Investigations* 39 (1960): 1546-50.

Laboratory of Neurophysiology, NIMH-NINDB

MacLean, Paul D., and Detlev W. Ploog. "Cerebral Representation of Penile Erection." *Neurophysiology* 25 (1962): 29-55.

Ploog, Detlev W., and Paul D. MacLean. "Display of Penile Erection in Squirrel Monkey (Saimiri Sciureus)." *Animal Behaviour* 11 (1963): 32-9.

Ploog, Detlev W., J. Blitz, and F. Ploog. "Studies on Social and Sexual Behavior of the Squirrel Monkey (Saimiri Sciureus)." *Folia Primatologica* 1 (1963): 29-66.

Ploog, Detlev W., and Paul D. MacLean. "On Functions of the Mamillary Bodies in the Squirrel Monkey." *Experimental Neurology* 7 (1963): 76-85.

Tasaki, Ichiji, and Karl Frank. "Measurement of the Action Potential of Myelinated Nerve Fiber." *American Journal of Physiology* 182 (1955): 572-8.

Tasaki, Ichiji, and Walter H. Freygang, Jr. "The Parallelism Between the Action Potential, Action Current, and Membrane Resistance at a Node of Ranvier." *Journal of General Physiology* 39 (1955): 211-23.

Tasaki, Ichiji. "Conduction of the Nerve Impulse, Chapter III." In *Handbook of Physiology, Section 1: Neurophysiology, Vol. 1*, edited by J. Field, H. W. Magoun, and V. E. Hall, 75-121. *American Physiological Society*, 1958.

Laboratory of Psychology, NIMH

Battig, Karl, Haldor E. Rosvold, and Mortimer Mishkin. "Comparison of Effects of Frontal and Caudate Lesions on Delayed Response and Alternation in Monkeys." *Journal of Comparative and Physiological Psychology* 53 (1960): 400-4.

Birren, James E., Robert N. Butler, Samuel W. Greenhouse, Louis Sokoloff, and Marian R. Yarrow, eds. *Human Aging*. Washington, D. C.: Public Health Publication, No. 986, Government Printing Office, 1963.

Birren, James E., H. A. Imus, and William F. Windle, eds. *The Process of Aging in the Nervous System*. Springfield, IL: Charles C. Thomas, 1959.

Blough, Donald S. "Spectral Sensitivity in the Pigeon." *Journal of the Optical Society of America* 47 (1957): 827-33.

Blough, Donald S. "Delayed Matching in the Pigeon." *Journal of the Experimental Analysis of Behavior* 2 (1959): 151-60.

Blough, Donald S. "Animal Psychophysics." *Scientific American* 205 (1961), 113-22.

Botwinick, Jack, J. S. Robbin, and Joseph F. Brinley. "Age Differences in Card-sorting Performance in Relation to Task Difficulty Task Set, and Practice." *Journal of Experimental Psychology* 59 (1960): 10-18.

Handlon, Joseph H. "A Metatheoretical View of Assumptions Regarding the Etiology of Schizophrenia: Implications for Research." *Archives of General Psychiatry* 2 (1960): 43-60.

Jerome, Edward A. "Age and Learning: Experimental Studies." In *Handbook of Aging and the Individual: Psychological and Biological Aspects*, edited by James E. Birren, 655-99. Chicago: University of Chicago Press, 1960.

Lansdell, Herbert, and Allan F. Mirsky. "Attention in Focal and Centrencephalic Epilepsy." *Experimental Neurology* 9 (1964): 463-9.

Mirsky, Allan F. "Studies of the Effects of Brain Lesions on Social Behavior in *Macaca Mulatta*: Methodological and Theoretical Considerations." *Annals of the New York Academy of Sciences* 85 (1960): 785-94.

Mirsky, Allan F., D. W. Primac, Cosimo Ajmone Marsan, Haldor E. Rosvold, and J. A. Stevens. "A Comparison of the Psychological Test Performance of Patients With Focal and Nonfocal Epilepsy." *Experimental Neurology* 2 (1960): 75-89.

Mirsky, Allan F., and John M. Van Buren. "On the Nature of the 'Absence' in Centrencephalic Epilepsy: A Study of Some Behavioral, Electroencephalographic and Autonomic Factors." *Electroencephalography and Clinical Neurophysiology* 19 (1965), 334-48.

Mishkin, Mortimer. "Perseveration of Central Sets After Frontal Lesions In Monkeys." In *The Frontal Granular Cortex and Behavior*, edited by J. M. Warren and K. Akert, 271-94. New York: McGraw-Hill, 1964.

Mishkin, Mortimer, E. S. Prockop, and Haldor E. Rosvold. "One Trial Object Discrimination Learning in Monkeys With Frontal Lesions." *Journal of Comparative and Physiological Psychology* 55 (1962): 178-81.

Parloff, Morris B. "The Family in Psychotherapy." *Archives of General Psychiatry* 4 (1961): 445-51.

Rosenthal, David. "Problems of Sampling and Diagnosis in the Major Twin Studies of Schizophrenia." *Journal of Psychiatric Research* 1 (1962): 116-34.

Rosenthal, David, ed. *The Genain Quadruplets: A Case Study and Theoretical Analysis of Heredity and Environment in Schizophrenia*. New York: Basic Books, 1963.

Rosvold, Haldor E., Mortimer Mishkin, and Maria K. Szwarcbart. "Effects of Subcortical Lesions in Monkeys on Visual Discrimination and Single Alternation Performance." *Journal of Comparative and Physiological Psychology* 51 (1958): 437-44.

Rosvold, Haldor E., and Maria K. Szwarcbart. "Neural Structures Involved in Delayed-Response Performance." In *The Frontal Granular Cortex and Behavior*, edited by J. M. Warren and K. Akert, 1-15. New York: McGraw-Hill, Inc. 1964.

Rosvold, Haldor E., Maria K. Szwarcbart, Allan F. Mirsky, and Mortimer Mishkin. "The Effect of Frontal Lobe Damage on Delayed Response Performance in Chimpanzees." *Journal of Comparative and Physiological Psychology*, 54 (1961): 368-74.

Shakow, David. "Segmental Set: A Theory of the Formal Psychological Deficit in Schizophrenia." *Archives of General Psychiatry* 6 (1962): 1-17.

Zahn, Theodore P., David Rosenthal, and David Shakow. "Reaction Time in Schizophrenic and Normal Subjects in Relation to the Sequence of Series of Regular Preparatory Intervals." *Journal of Abnormal and Social Psychology* 63 (1961): 161-8.

Zahn, Theodore P., David Rosenthal, and David Shakow. "Effects of Irregular Preparatory Intervals on Reaction Time in Schizophrenia." *Journal of Abnormal and Social Psychology* 67 (1963): 44-52.

Laboratory of Socio-Environmental Studies, NIMH

Clausen, John A., and Marian Radke Yarrow, issue eds. "The Impact of Mental Illness on the Family." *Journal of Social Issues* 11, no. 4 (1955): entire issue.

Goffman, Erving. *Asylums: Essays on the Social Situation of Mental Patients and Other Inmates.* Oxford, England: Doubleday (Anchor), 1961.

Goffman, Erving. "The Moral Career of the Mental Patient." *Psychiatry: Journal for the Study of Interpersonal Processes* 22 (1959): 123-42.

Kohn, Melvin L. and John A. Clausen. "Social Isolation and Schizophrenia." *American Sociological Review* 20 (June 1955): 265-73.

Kohn, Melvin L. "Social Class and Parental Values." *American Journal of Sociology* 64 (January 1959): 337-51.

Appendix D

Available Resources

Available Published Sources

Bailey, Pearce. "The Present Outlook for Neurology in the United States: A Factual Evaluation." *Journal of the Association of Medical Colleges* 24 (1949): 214-28.

Bailey, Pearce. "America's First National Neurologic Institute." *Neurology* 3 (1953): 321.

Berry, Frank B. "The Story of 'The Berry Plan.'" *Bulletin of the National Academy of Medicine* 52, no. 3 (1976): 278-82.

Brown, Bertram S. "The Federal Mental Health Program: Past, Present, and Future." *Hospital and Community Psychiatry* 27, no. 7 (1976): 512-4.

DeJong, Russell N. *A History of American Neurology.* New York: Raven Press, 1982.

Denny-Brown D., Adolph L. Sahs, Augustus Steele Rose, eds. *Centennial Anniversary Volume of the American Neurological Association.* New York: Springer, 1975.

Furman, Bess. *A Profile of the United States Public Health Service, 1798-1948.* Washington, D.C.: U.S. Department of Health, Education, and Welfare, 1973.

Grob, Gerald N. *From Asylum to Community: Mental Health Policy in Modern America.* Princeton: Princeton University Press, 1991.

Grob, Gerald N. "Creation of the National Institute of Mental Health." *Public Health Reports* 111 (1996): 378-81.

Judd, Lewis L. "Historical Highlights of the National Institute of Mental Health From 1946 to the Present." *American Journal of Psychiatry* 155 Suppl (1998): 3-8.

Mental Health Challenges: Past and Future. Proceedings of a Conference on the Twenty-Fifth Anniversary of the National Mental Health Act. June 28 and 29, 1971, Washington, D.C., 1971.

Mullan, Fitzhugh. *Plagues and Politics: The Story of the United States Public Health Service*. New York: Basic Books, 1989.

McHenry, Lawrence C. "The Founding of the American Neurological Association and the Origin of American Neurology." *Annals of Neurology* 14, no. 1 (1983): 153-4.

National Institute of Mental Health. *Research in the Service of Mental Health: Summary Report of the Research Task Force of the National Institute of Mental Health*. Publication No. (ADM) 75-237, 1975.

Park, Buhm Soon. "The Development of the Intramural Research Program at the National Institutes of Health After World War II." *Perspectives in Biology and Medicine* 46, no. 3 (2003): 383-402.

Pickren, Wade and Stanley Schneider, eds. *Psychology and the National Institute of Mental Health: A Historical Analysis of Science, Practice, and Policy* (Washington, D.C.: American Psychological Association Press, forthcoming).

Quen, Jacques M. "Asylum Psychiatry, Neurology, Social Work, and Mental Hygiene – An Exploratory Study in Interprofessional History." *Journal of the History of the Behavioral Sciences* 13, no. 1 (1977): 3-11.

Rowland, Lewis P. *NINDS At 50: An Incomplete History Celebrating the Fiftieth Anniversary of the National Institute of Neurological Disorders and Stroke*. NIH Publication No. 01-4161, 2001.

Rubinstein, Eli A., and George V. Coelho. "Mental Health and Behavioral Sciences: One Federal Agency's Role in the Behavioral Sciences." *American Psychologist 25 (1970):* 517-23.

Sapir, Philip, and Jeanne Brand. "The National Institutes of Health Research Grant Program and the History and Sociocultural Aspects of Medicine." *Bulletin of the History of Medicine* 33, no. 1 (1959): 67-74.

Schneider, Stanley F. "National Institute of Mental Health." In the *Encyclopedia of Psychology*, Volume 5, 391-394. Washington, D.C.: American Psychological Association and Oxford University Press, 2000.

Sokoloff, Louis. "Seymour S. Kety, 1915-2000." *Biographical Memoirs* 83 (2003): 1-21.

Stetten, DeWitt, Jr., and W. T. Carrigan, eds. *NIH: An Account of Research in Its Laboratories and Clinics.* New York: Academic Press, 1984.

Tower, Donald B., ed. *The Nervous System: A Three-Volume Work Commemorating the 25th Anniversary of the National Institute of Neurological and Communicative Disorders and Stroke.* 3 vols. New York: Raven Press, 1975.

Williams, Ralph Chester. *The United States Public Health Service, 1798-1950.* Washington, D.C.: Commissioned Officers Association of the United States Public Health Service, 1951.

Windle, William F., ed. "The Beginning of Experimental Neurology," *Experimental Neurology* 51, no. 2 (1976): 277-80.

NIH National Library of Medicine,
History of Medicine Division (Bethesda, MD)
(*http://www.nlm.nih.gov/hmd/index.html*)

Personal Papers: Julius Axelrod, Bertram Brown, Robert Felix, Lawrence Kolb, Paul MacLean, James Shannon.

NIMH Oral History Collection, 1975-1978 (OH 144): John Adams, Robert Atwell, John E. Bell, Frank Braceland, Bertram Brown, Ewald Busse, Dale Cameron, Jerry Carter, John Clausen, Louis Cohen, Robert Cohen, Leonard Duhl, John Eberhart, Will Edgerton, Robert Felix, Esther Garrison, Eli Ginzberg, Robert Hewitt, Nicholas Hobbs, Herbert Kelman, George Kingman, Lawrence Kolb, Gerald Kurtz, Gardner Lindzey, Ivan Mensh, Alan Miller, Quigg Newton, Donald Oken, Eliot Rodnick, John Romano, Philip Sapir, George Saslow, David Shakow, Edwin Shneidman, Alberta Siegel, Joseph Speisman, Robert Stubblefield, George Tarjan, George Van Staden, Louis J. West, Richard Williams, Stanley F. Yolles.

Images from the History of Medicine.

Office of NIH History (Bethesda, MD) (*http://history.nih.gov*)

Klein, Melissa K. "The Legacy of the 'Yellow Berets': The Vietnam War, the Doctor Draft, and the NIH Associate Training Program." Unpublished typescript, 1998.

Parascandola, John. "Background Report on the Organizational History of Mental Health and Substance Abuse Programs in PHS." Unpublished typescript, additional copy in the historical reference files of the Office of the Public Health Service Historian, 1993.

NIH Almanacs (1965-1976, 1978-1981, 1983-2001): provide historical data (events, legislative, and NIMH director chronology), information on offices and divisions, and grant appropriation information by fiscal year. Published annually. Available on-line at *http://www.nih.gov/welcome/ 97_Almanac/main.htm.*

NIH Data Books: Basic Data Relating to the NIH (1954, 1961-1994): provide information on NIH extramural awards and research grants, NIH appropriations and obligations, NIH research training appointments, positions, and personnel, national health expenditures, and national mortality and morbidity data.

NIH Record (1949-present): in-house newspaper. [Issues since July 1996 are available online at *http://www.nih.gov/news/NIH-Record/ archives.htm*].

NIH Scientific Director Meetings' Minutes (1950-1983): minutes of biweekly meetings involving all institute scientific directors.

NIH Telephone Directories (1948-current): provides names, affiliations, and locations of laboratory, branch, and section chiefs.

NIMH and NINDB oral histories and biographical files

NIH Library (Bethesda, MD)
(http://nihlibrary.nih.gov)

NIMH Annual Reports (1950-1952, 1954-1960, 1967-1968, 1971-1989, 1992-current): NIMH Director, NIMH Scientific Director, NIMH Clinical Director, and Laboratory and Branch Chiefs' annual reports; individual study abstracts.

NINDB Annual Reports (1954-1988): NINDB Director, NINDB Scientific Director, NINDB Clinical Director, and Laboratory and Branch Chiefs' annual reports; individual study abstracts.

NIH Reports for the fiscal years, 1950-51, and 1951-52: unpublished internal documents.

NIH Scientific Directories and Annual Bibliographies (1956, 1959-1991): provide names of all laboratory, branch and section chiefs and individual members as well as yearly bibliography of published work.

American Psychological Association Archives (Washington, D.C.)
(http://www.apa.org/archives)

Brand, Jeanne L., and Philip Sapir. "An Historical Perspective on the National Institute of Mental Health (prepared as sec. 1 of the NIMH Report to the Woolridge Committee of the President's Scientific Advisory Committee). Mimeograph." 1964.

U.S. National Archives and Records Administration (College Park, MD)
(*http://www.archives.gov/research_room/federal_records_guide*)

Record Group 90: United States Public Health Service.

Record Group 443: National Institutes of Health.

Record Group 511: Alcohol, Drug Abuse, and Mental Health Administration.

Archives of the History of American Psychology, University of Akron (Akron, OH)
(*http://www3.uakron.edu/ahap*)

David Shakow personal papers.

American Neurological Association Archives (Minneapolis, MN)
(*http://www.aneuroa.org/archives.html*)

Transactions of the American Neurological Association.

Osler Library, McGill University (Montreal, Canada)
(*http://www.health.library.mcgill.ca/osler*)

Wilder Penfield Archive.

American Academy of Neurology Archives and Library Collection
Washington University (St. Louis, MO)
(*http://medicine.wustl.edu/library/aan.htm*)

Neuroscience History Archives-Brain Research Institute,
University of California (Los Angeles, CA)
(*http://www.NeuroscienceArchives.org*)

Columbia University Oral History Research Office (New York, NY)
(*http://www.columbia.edu/cu/lweb/indiv/oral*)

NIH Computer Retrieval of Information on Scientific Projects (CRISP)
(*http://crisp.cit.nih.gov*)

Index

A

Aberle, David F., 312, 321

Abraham, Kristof, 159, 162, 314

Adelman, W. J., Jr., 309

Adland, Marvin, 321

Adrian, R. H., 318

Agranoff, Bernard W., 312, 317, 319

Aichhorn, August, 81

Ajmone-Marsan, Cosimo, xix, 97, 151-168, 224, 296, 314, 324

Albers, R. Wayne, 235, 312, 316

Alexander, Franz, 321

Alexander, Irving, 307

Allen, Gordon, 317, 321, 323

Alphen, Gerard van, 320

Altman, Albert S., 14

Altmann, Stuart A., 316

Altrocchi, Paul H., 314

Alvord, Ellsworth C., Jr., 66, 145, 312, 314, 324

American Academy of Neurology (AAN), 20, 24

American Medical Association (AMA), 6, 47, 65

American Neurological Association (ANA), 19, 20, 21, 22, 24, 30, 272

American Psychiatric Association, 7

Ames, Bruce N., 309

Antosiewicz, H. A., 309, 317

Aronson, Samuel, 320

Arvanitaki-Chalazonitis, A., 319

Ashburner, Roberta, 316

Assembly of Scientists, 42-45, 49-50, 233

Associates Training Program (*See* National Institutes of Health)

Auster, Simon, 307, 323

Axelrod, Julius, 61, 91, 93, 191, 194, 195, 210, 216, 246, 256, 268, 269, 271, 272, 273, 274, 275, 276, 277, 278, 311, 312, 317, 321

B

Bach, Sven A., 324

Bacon, M., 318

Bailey, Clark J., 316

Bailey, Pearce (father), 22

Bailey, Pearce (son), 22-24, 34, 65, 67, 107, 143, 151, 153, 187, 227, 232, 295, 301

Bairati, Angelo, 316

Baird, Robert L., 324

Bak, Anthony, 318, 319

Baker, A., 204

Baker, Abe B., 20, 24

Baldwin, Maitland, 50, 65, 66, 67, 97, 143-144, 152-153, 154, 155, 156, 224, 295-296, 314, 324